Neurology

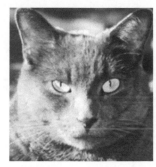

for the Small Animal Practitioner

Cheryl Chrisman, DVM, MS, Ed.S.,
Diplomate ACVIM (Neurology)

Christopher Mariani, DVM,
Diplomate ACVIM (Neurology)

Simon Platt, BVM&S, MRCVS,
Diplomate ACVIM (Neurology),
Diplomate ECVN, RCVS (Neurology)

Roger Clemmons, DVM, Ph.D.

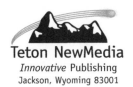

Teton NewMedia
Innovative Publishing
Jackson, Wyoming 83001

Executive Editor: Carroll C. Cann
Development Editor: Susan L. Hunsberger
Editor: Nicole Giandomenico
Art Director & Production Manager: Anita B. Sykes

Design & Layout: 5640 Design, Alpine, WY
Illustrations by Anne Rains

Made Easy Series Editors:
Larry P. Tilley, DVM, Diplomate ACVIM (Internal Medicine)
Francis W. K. Smith Jr., DVM, Diplomate ACVIM (Cardiology and Internal Medicine)

Teton NewMedia
P.O. Box 4833
Jackson, WY 83001
1-888-770-3165

ISBN # 1-893441-82-2

Library of Congress Cataloging-in-Publication Data on file.

Dedication

This is dedicated to the ones we love.... including each other.

Special blessings to Drs. Heidi Barnes, Ron Johnson, John Meeks, Shirley Shelton, Laurie Pearce, Gillian Irving, Julia Blackmore, Linda Shell, and Tom Schubert. Many of the cases illustrated in this book were seen when they were neurology residents at the University of Florida, and we gratefully acknowledge their contributions.

We also dedicate this book to the small animal practitioners who have consulted with us, referred the cases presented in this book, or may have always been a bit uncomfortable dealing with neurology.

This book was written for you.

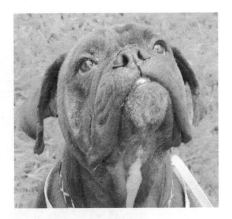

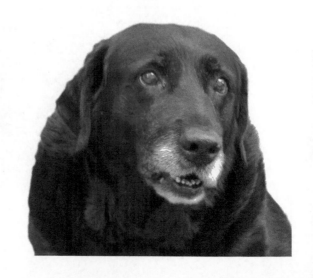

Acknowledgments

The definitions in this book were adapted from Dorland's Medical Dictionary 29th Edition, WB Saunders, Philadelphia, 2000.

Drug dosages in this book are based on recommendations found in: Plumb DC: Veterinary Drug Handbook, 3rd ed., Iowa State University Press, 1999.

Some of the photographs were gifts from other veterinarians and have been used in our teaching over the years. They are acknowledged as best as can be remembered; our apologies to anyone we forgot to acknowledge.

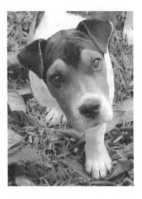

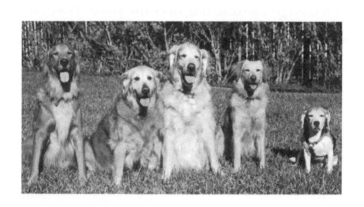

Preface

This book is the culmination of the authors' 65 years of combined experience practicing clinical veterinary neurology and neurosurgery, teaching neurology to veterinary students, and providing general practitioners with hundreds of hours of phone consultations and continuing education in neurology. All the authors have been in general small animal practice at some time in their careers, and this book was designed as a practical, quick reference handbook of common neurologic problems for the busy small animal practitioner.

The first section is a review of the clinical approach to patients, the neurologic examination, and an overview of lesion localization. The following sections begin with a chief complaint, definitions related to the problem, the location of the lesion, and the differential diagnosis. The frequency of occurrence of each disorder is indicated, and the focus of the text is on common and occasional disorders. Rare disorders are usually listed in a table or presented in a brief paragraph at the end of the section for completeness. For each problem, important historical questions, abnormal physical and neurologic examination findings and applicable diagnostic tests are initially reviewed. Finally, the important diagnostic, therapeutic, and prognostic features of each disorder are presented.

Many sections have quick–reference, emergency treatment tables with specific drugs and doses. Charts of lesion localization, common treatment approaches, and nursing care and physical therapy are also included. Other treatments are bolded in the discussion for repeated quick reference. Warning boxes are placed throughout the text, emphasizing problems in specific situations that occur in practice. Advice to owners for special situations can be found in other tables. A companion CD is available. Please see "Some Helpful Hints" on page 3.

As in other specialties, all neurologists may not agree on diagnostic criteria, treatments, and prognoses for various disorders, and the information in this book is based on the scientific literature as well as our combined clinical experience. It was our intent to have this book live up to its name "Neurology Made Easy" for the small animal practitioner. It is our wish that this handbook will be a useful practical guide to help veterinarians deal more effectively with small animal neurologic patients and clients and be an educated part of the team when assistance from a specialist is required.

Table of Contents

Section 1 Introduction

Section 2 Dementia, Stupor, and Coma

Section 3 Seizures

Section 4 Tremors

Section 5 Head Tilt, Dysequilibrium and Nystagmus

Section 6   Cranial Neuropathies and Myopathies

Section 7 Neck or Back Pain

Section 8 Ataxia

Section 9 Acute Quadriparesis, Quadriplegia, Hemiparesis, or Hemiplegia

Section 10 Chronic Quadriparesis

Section 11 Episodic and Exercise-induced Weakness

Section 12 Acute Paraparesis or Paraplegia

Section 13 Chronic Paraparesis

Spinal Cord Disorders 305

Neuromuscular Disorders. 316

Section 14 Monoparesis and Monoplegia

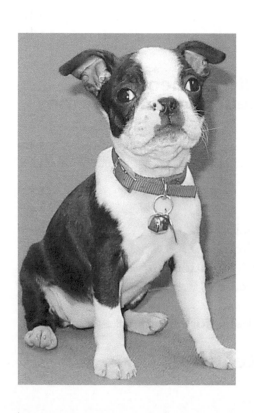

Section 1
Introduction

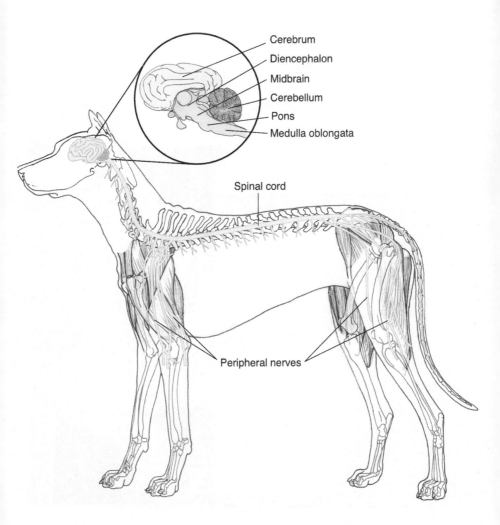

Cerebrum
Diencephalon
Midbrain
Cerebellum
Pons
Medulla oblongata

Spinal cord

Peripheral nerves

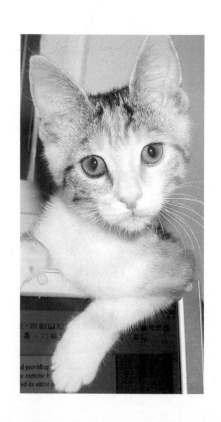

Introduction

The goals of this book are to be a quick reference easy to use text for the general practitioner.

Some Helpful Hints

The following icons are used in this book to indicate important concepts:

✓ Routine. This feature is routine, something you should know.

♥ Important. This concept strikes at the heart of the matter.

⚷ Key. This concept is a key one and is necessary for full understanding.

💣 Something serious will happen if you don't remember this, possibly resulting in the loss of both patient and client.

✋ Stop. This doesn't look important but it can really make a difference when trying to sort out unusual situations.

⊙ A companion CD is available for purchase by calling 877-306-9793. The CD contains the full text, figures, and tables of this book formatted for easy search and retrieval. In addition, the CD contains Section Specific case studies and teaching videos.

Neuroanatomy

🔑— The **nervous system** (Figure 1-1) is composed of billions of **neurons**. Each **neuron** consists of a **cell body** with one or more processes known as **dendrites** and **axons. Dendrites** bring information to the cell body, and another process, known as an **axon**, transmits information to other neurons or muscles. Neurons connect and form electrochemical circuits that receive and transmit electrical signals and ensure proper function of all body systems.

✓ **Glial cells** outnumber neurons in the nervous system and consist of three main types: **oligodendrocytes, astrocytes,** and **microglia.** The glial cells surround the neurons and perform many important functions, such as structural support, myelination, formation of the blood-brain barrier, regulation of metabolic function, and immunologic defense.

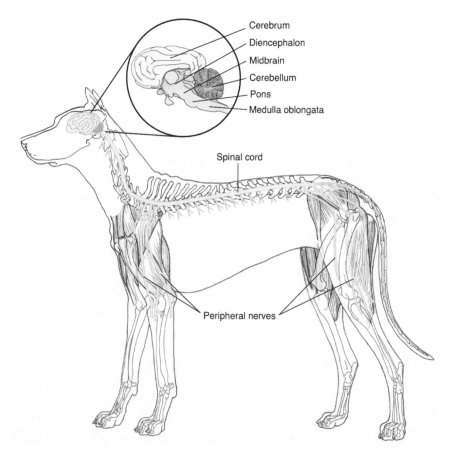

Cerebrum
Diencephalon
Midbrain
Cerebellum
Pons
Medulla oblongata

Spinal cord

Peripheral nerves

Figure 1-1 The major divisions of the nervous system.

❧ The **central nervous system** (CNS) consists of the brain and spinal cord. The protective covering of the CNS, called the **meninges,** consists of three layers: the **dura mater, arachnoid membrane,** and **pia mater**. The area between the arachnoid membrane and pia mater is the subarachnoid space.

❧ **Cerebrospinal fluid** (CSF) surrounds the CNS in the subarachnoid space. CSF is also found inside the CNS in a series of four connecting cavities within the brain, known as ventricles, and a central canal in the spinal cord. CSF is produced inside the ventricles by structures known as the **choroid plexuses** and flows caudally into the subarachnoid space where it is absorbed. CSF provides structural and metabolic support and environmental protection for the CNS.

❧ The **peripheral nervous system** (PNS) connects the CNS to the rest of the body and is formed by neurons entering and leaving the brainstem (cranial nerves) and spinal cord (spinal nerves).

❧ The **brain** resides within the protective covering of the skull and consists of the **cerebrum, cerebellum,** and **brainstem.** The **brainstem** is subdivided from rostral to caudal into the **diencephalon** (includes the thalamus, epithalamus, subthalamus, and hypothalamus), **midbrain, pons,** and **medulla oblongata** (Figure 1-1). **Cranial nerves** are associated with specific brain or brainstem regions and form the PNS of the head. There are 12 pairs of cranial nerves.

❧ The **spinal cord** resides within the protective covering of the bony vertebral column. **Spinal nerves** enter and exit between the vertebrae to form the PNS of the trunk and limbs. The spinal cord and corresponding **nerve roots** (the most proximal part of each spinal nerve) are divided into 8 cervical (C), 13 thoracic (T), 7 lumbar (L), 3 sacral (S), and usually 5 or more caudal (Cd) segments. Each vertebra, spinal cord segment, and group of nerve roots is numbered as follows: C1-8, T1-13, L1-7, S1-3, and Cd1-5. Thus, C2 means the second cervical vertebra, spinal cord segment, or nerve root and L5 means the fifth lumbar vertebra, spinal cord segment, or nerve root.

❧ The **spinal cord segments** and **nerve roots** do not directly align with the **vertebrae** of the same number. There are eight cervical spinal cord segments and nerve roots and only seven cervical vertebrae. The nerve roots C1-C7 enter and exit the spinal canal along the cranial edge of the vertebrae of the same number, and nerve roots caudal to C8 enter and exit along the caudal edge of the vertebrae of the same number. The spinal cord segments generally lie slightly cranial to the vertebrae of the same number except from T11-L3 (Figure 1-2). Caudal to L3, the spinal cord segments shorten and end at approximately the L6 vertebra in dogs and the L7 vertebra in cats. The collection of nerve roots from L7-Cd5 continues in the vertebral canal and forms the **cauda equina.** The neurologic examination localizes the lesion to certain spinal cord segments and nerve roots, but the corresponding vertebral localization must be considered in order to radiograph the correct area.

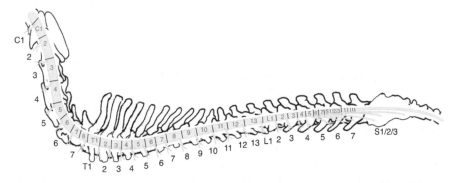

Figure 1-2 The correlation of the spinal cord segments and vertebrae in the dog.

✓ The **foramen magnum** is the caudal opening in the skull at the junction of the brain and spinal cord. Lesions may be localized above the foramen magnum (brain) or below the foramen magnum (spinal cord, nerve roots, peripheral nerves, and muscles).

☞ **Sensory, or afferent, nerves** of the PNS and CNS transmit special senses such as olfaction, vision, equilibrium, hearing, and taste as well as the somatic senses of touch, pain, temperature, and proprioception (Figure 1-3). The PNS sensory nerves receive stimulation either directly or from special receptor cells. The stimulus is then transmitted to their cell bodies located in PNS **ganglia.** Sensory nerve axons enter the CNS and connect with **nuclei** (groups of neuronal cell bodies in the CNS) in the brainstem or spinal cord. CNS sensory neurons leave the nuclei and ascend to the brain in organized **sensory tracts** often named by where they begin and end. Examples include the spinocerebellar tract (beginning in the spinal cord and ending in the cerebellum) or the spinothalamic tract (beginning in the spinal cord and ending in the thalamic portion of the diencephalon). The main sensory tracts of the spinal cord are shown in Figure 1-4.

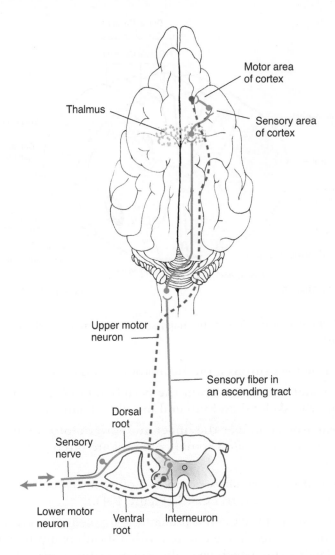

Figure 1-3 Color Illustration of the relationship of the sensory nerves and pathways and upper motor neurons and lower motor neurons as well as the reflex arc (sensory nerve, dorsal root, interneuron, ventral root and lower motor neuron).

Motor or efferent nerves are responsible for the **movements** of all skeletal and smooth muscles. Motor nerves originate in the nuclei of the cerebrum and brainstem and descend through organized tracts. These tracts are often named by where they begin and end, such as the vestibulospinal tract (beginning in the vestibular nuclei of the medulla oblongata and ending in the spinal cord). The main motor tracts of the spinal cord are shown in Figure 1-4.

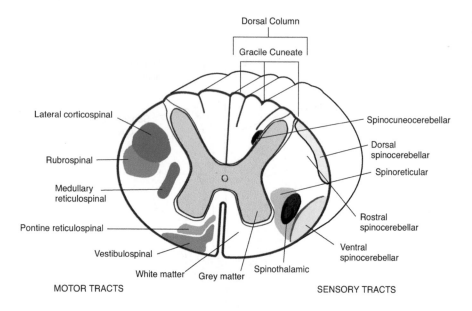

Figure 1-4 Color illustration of the major sensory and motor pathways in the spinal cord.

✓ **Upper motor neurons** form the motor tracts (Figures 1-3 and 1-4).

✓ **Lower motor neurons** form the peripheral nerves that innervate the skeletal and visceral muscles (Figure 1-3).

✓ **Interneurons** connect the upper and lower motor neurons within the brainstem and spinal cord and are often part of the reflex arc.

✓ **Gray matter** is primarily composed of neuronal cell bodies and their dendrites within the CNS (Figure 1-4).

✓ **White matter** of the CNS is primarily composed of axons (Figure 1-4). Many of the axons are covered with a sheath of myelin formed by oligodendrocytes, which gives the region a white color.

✓ A **reflex arc** is composed of a peripheral sensory nerve and a lower motor neuron and their connection within a specific brainstem or spinal cord segment. Most spinal reflexes are multi-synaptic and include an interneuron (Figure 1-3). The patellar reflex discussed below is monosynaptic and has no interneuron. If all the components of the reflex arc are functional, then the reflex will be present even if the upper motor neurons are severely damaged.

Overview of the Patient Evaluation

✓ The **signalment** is the species, age, breed, gender, and coat and eye color, which are considered when determining potential causes of impairment (Table 1-1).

Table 1-1
Mechanisms of Disease by the DAMNNIITTV Scheme with Typical Signalment, History, and Symmetry of the Neurologic Deficits

MECHANISM	SIGNALMENT	ONSET AND PROGRESSION	NEUROLOGIC DEFICITS
Degenerative (acquired not congenital or familial)	Often adult	Usually chronic progressive	Symmetric or asymmetric
Anomalous (Congenital or Familial)	Often purebred, young	Neonatal nonprogressive or chronic progressive	Symmetric or asymmetric
Metabolic	Any age, breed, gender	Acute or chronic progressive	Usually symmetric
Nutritional	Any age, breed, gender	Acute or chronic progressive	Usually symmetric
Neoplastic	Often adult	Usually chronic progressive	Often asymmetric Occasionally symmetric
Inflammatory or Infectious	Any age, breed, gender	Acute or chronic progressive	Often asymmetric Occasionally symmetric
Idiopathic	Varies with the syndrome	Acute or episodic	Symmetric or asymmetric
Toxic	Any age, breed, gender	Acute progressive	Usually symmetric
Traumatic	Any age, breed, gender	Acute nonprogressive	Symmetric or asymmetric
Vascular	Any age, breed, gender	Acute nonprogressive	Usually asymmetric

✓ The **primary complaint** is the reason for seeking medical assistance, such as seizures, dysequilibrium, and paraplegia. The most common primary complaints are listed in the Table of Contents as the title for each section of this book.

♥ The **history** is a series of questions to determine the most likely cause of the primary complaint and to assist in making a definitive diagnosis, a treatment plan, and an accurate prognosis. Onset and progression of the primary complaint may be neonatal nonprogressive, acute nonprogressive, acute progressive, chronic progressive, or episodic (Table 1-1). Neonatal nonprogressive disorders become apparent shortly after birth and remain unchanged. Animals with acute nonprogressive disorders develop signs immediately or within 72 hours of the eliciting cause and then remain unchanged. Animals with acute progressive disorders develop signs that progressively worsen immediately or within 72 hours of the event. Animals with chronic progressive disorders develop signs that continue to worsen over several days, weeks, or months. Animals with episodic disorders are normal between signs. Duration of the signs may affect treatment options. A thorough investigation of other neurologic signs, concurrent or previous illness, vaccination status, the possibility of trauma or exposure to toxins, similar familial problems, travel history, current medications and supplements, and lifestyle are essential to accurately determine the cause of the primary complaint. Important historical questions are outlined for each primary complaint in the following chapters.

♥ A complete **physical examination** is essential to detect abnormalities in other body systems that might cause a disorder that also affects the nervous system. Diseases that may mimic primary neurologic diseases, such as arrhythmias and orthopedic disease, can also be identified. Since some diagnostic tests are performed under anesthesia, the physical examination is important to assess anesthetic risks.

♥ The **neurologic examination** is a special series of observations and tests to determine if there is a neurologic problem, its location in the nervous system, its severity, and whether the deficit is symmetric or asymmetric. Some mechanisms of disease produce primarily symmetric or asymmetric signs (Table 1-1).

♥ The **differential diagnosis** is a list of possible mechanisms of disease and the specific diseases for each mechanism that are most compatible with the information obtained in the history and physical and neurologic examinations (Table 1-1).

♥ The **diagnostic plan** may initially include a complete blood count (CBC), serum chemistry profile, and urinalysis to detect systemic disease and to further evaluate the animal for potential anesthesia and additional diagnostic tests. It is assumed that routine parasite monitoring and prevention are ongoing. Evaluation of the thoracic and abdominal cavities by radiography and ultrasonography is often performed if neoplasia is on the differential diagnosis list or if historical or physical examination abnormalities warrant further investigation. Further diagnostic tests can be performed to determine the most likely diagnosis (Table 1-2). Suggested diagnostic tests for specific problems are listed in each chapter of this book.

✓ Once the **differential diagnosis, diagnostic plan,** and likely **prognoses** are established, they are presented to the pet owner, and the potential benefits and risks and estimate of the charges are discussed.

💣 Anesthesia carries some risk in any animal and varies with age, body condition, and concurrent illness. Anesthesia is required for most advanced neurologic tests.

💣 CSF collection is avoided in animals suspected to have increased intracranial pressure, as the cerebellum may herniate through the foramen magnum, compress the caudal brainstem, and cause death. Caution is also exerted in animals with increased bleeding tendencies. Significant hemorrhage and worsening of neurologic deficits are very rare complications of CSF collection.

💣 Myelography may transiently worsen neurologic deficits but improvement is often seen within 24 to 72 hours.

💣 Surgical biopsy carries the usual risks of hemorrhage or infection.

♥ **Final diagnosis:** The results of all diagnostic tests are evaluated, and the most likely diagnosis is established.

♥ **Therapeutic plan:** A therapeutic plan is developed on the basis of the diagnosis and therapeutic history. For the welfare of the animal, some therapeutic interventions may be necessary before the results of all the diagnostic tests have been obtained and a final diagnosis is secured. Therapy may be medical, surgical, or a combination of both.

♥ **Commmunication plan:** Once established, the diagnosis, therapeutic plan, and prognosis are presented to the pet owner. The communication plan involves a clear explanation of the risks, benefits, and costs of all treatments.

Table 1-2 Further Diagnostic Tests

Test	Description (Diseases Evaluated)
Tests on blood and serum	Serum bile acids (hepatic encephalopathy), serum cholinesterase (organophosphate intoxication), serum thyroxine and thyroid-stimulating hormone levels (hypothyroidism), immunoassays for specific organisms (meningoen cephalomyelitis), and assays for toxicity (e.g., lead, phenobarbital, bromide)
Cerebrospinal fluid analysis (CSF)	Evaluate cell number, cell type, total protein, presence of organisms, bacterial and fungal cultures, organism immunoassays, immunoglobulins, immunoglobulin G index, and albumin quota (neoplasia, meningoen-cephalomyelitis, other encephalopathies, and spinal cord compression)
Electroencephalography (EEG)	Evaluation of the electrical activity of the brain (hydrocephalus, encephalitis, head injury, other encephalopathies, neoplasia, and epilepsy)
Electromyography (EMG) Includes nerve conduction velocity, repetitive nerve stimulation and F wave evaluation	Evaluation of the electrical activity of peripheral nerves and muscles (locate and indicate severity of nerve injuries, nerve root compression, and diffuse disorders of the peripheral nerves, neuromuscular junctions, and muscles)
Brainstem auditory evoked response (BAER)	Evaluation of the electrical activity of the auditory nerve and pathway through the brainstem (hearing testing and brainstem diseases)
Spinal cord-evoked responses	Stimulation of peripheral nerves and recording of dorsal spinal cord potentials (nerve root and spinal cord lesions)
Radiography (routine)	Skull and vertebral column (malformation, infection, fracture, and neoplasia of bones; degenerated and infected intervertebral disks)
Myelography	Injection of iohexol (Omnipaque) 240 mg of iodine/ml into subarachnoid space (spinal cord compression, swelling, or other abnormalities, vertebral or spinal cord malformations, intervertebral disk degeneration, trauma, and neoplasia)
Computed tomography (CT)	Cross-sectional radiographic imaging with computerized reconstruction; intravenous diatrizoate meglumine and diatrizoate sodium (Hypaque-76) is administered to enhance inflammatory or neoplastic diseases; can be used in conjunction with myelography; superior to magnetic resonance imaging for bone detail and acute hemorrhage (trauma; vascular disease; and spinal cord and vertebral column lesions, including intervertebral disk degeneration)
Magnetic resonance imaging (MRI)	Multiple plane images based on electromagnetic technology and the water content of various tissues; better soft tissue detail than computed tomography; intravenous gadolinium is given to accentuate areas in which the blood-brain barrier is disrupted (most brain and spinal cord neoplasia and inflammation and nerve tumors)
Surgical biopsy	Diagnostic excision of lesions and subsequent cytologic and histopathologic evaluation, immunocytochemistry, or culture and sensitivity; useful for lesions of the brain, peripheral nerves, muscles and those around the spinal cord (neoplasia, meningoencephalitis, peripheral neuropathies, and myopathies)

The Neurologic Examination Overview and Form

✓ The **neurologic examination** is performed to determine **if** a neurologic problem is present, **where** it is located in the nervous system, **how** severe it is, and **what** might be causing it.

♥ The **neurologic examination**, starting from the front to back of the animal, may be divided into the evaluation of the **head, gait, neck and thoracic limbs, back, pelvic limbs, anus, and tail.** A chart to assist with the examination and to record the results is useful (Table 1-3).

Table 1-3
The Neurologic Examination

L=left, R=right: Y=yes, N=no; N/D/A or N/D/A/I:
N=normal, D=delayed, depressed, or reduced, A=absent, and I=increased.

EVALUATION OF THE HEAD						
Seizures (Y/N)			Mentation (describe)			
Head pressing (Y/N)			Head turn (Y/N and direction)			
Head incoordination or tremors (Y/N)			Head tilt (Y/N and direction)			

EVALUATION OF THE CRANIAL NERVES (1-12)						
	LEFT	**RIGHT**			**LEFT**	**RIGHT**
Olfaction (Y/N)			Menace (Y/N)			
Vision (Y/N)			Midrange pupil size (Y/N)			
Mydriasis (Y/N)			Miosis (Y/N)			
Direct pupillary light reflex (Y/N)			Consensual pupillary light reflex (Y/N)			
Strabismus and direction (Y/N)			Positional strabismus (Y/N)			
Ptosis (Y/N)			Enophthalmos (Y/N)			
Globe retraction (Y/N)			Intranasal sensation (Y/N)			
Temporal/masseter atrophy (Y/N)			Jaw tone (N/D/A/I)			
Jaw range of motion (N/D/A/I)			Palpebral, aural, and buccal reflexes (N/D/A/I)			
Normal nystagmus (Y/N)			Spontaneous nystagmus (Y/N)			
Positional nystagmus (Y/N)			Hearing (Y/N)			
Swallow (Y/N)			Regurgitation (Y/N)			
Voice change (Y/N)			Stridor (Y/N)			
Trapezius atrophy (Y/N)			Tongue atrophy (Y/N)			

13

Table 1-3 Continued

EVALUATION OF THE GAIT
(WALK, TROT, GALLOP, TURN, STEP, HEMIWALK, WHEELBARROW)

Indicate if pacing or circling (note direction), lame, ataxic, paretic—mild, moderate, severe, or paralyzed (no voluntary movement). Ambulatory or nonambulatory. Note asymmetry.

_____

_____

_____

_____

_____

_____

_____

EVALUATION OF THE NECK AND THORACIC LIMBS	LEFT	RIGHT	EVALUATION OF THE BACK, PELVIC LIMBS, ANUS, AND TAIL	LEFT	RIGHT
Postural Reactions			**Postural Reactions**		
Hopping (N/D/A)			Hopping (N/D/A)		
Conscious proprioception (N/D/A)			Conscious proprioception (N/D/A)		
Spinal reflexes			**Spinal reflexes**		
			Patellar (N/D/A/I)		
Biceps (N/D/A/I)			Gastrocnemius (N/D/A/I)		
Triceps (N/D/A/I)			Cranial tibial (N/D/A/I)		
Extensor carpi radialis (N/D/A/I)			Sciatic (N/D/A/I)		
Flexor (N/D/A)			Flexor (N/D/A)		
Crossed extensor (Y/N)			Crossed extensor (Y/N)		
			Anal reflex (N/D/A)		
			Tail reflex (N/D/A)		
Miscellaneous			**Miscellaneous**		
Babinski's sign (Y/N)			Babinski's sign (Y/N)		
Muscle atrophy (Y/N, location)			Muscle atrophy (Y/N, location)		
			Voluntary urinations (Y/N)		
			Voluntary tail wag (Y/N)		
Pain perception			**Pain perception**		
Neck pain (Y/N)			Back pain (Y/N)		
Superficial Sensation (Y/N)			Superficial sensation (Y/N, location)		
Deep pain (Y/N)			Cutaneous trunci (Y/N, location)		
			Deep pain (Y/N)		

LOCATION OF LESION(S):

SEVERITY OF LESION(S): (mild, moderate, severe)

Neurologic Examination Techniques and Lesion Localization

Evaluation of the Head

✓ **Head evaluation** is performed by questioning the owner about seizures and changes in mentation, observation of the animal, palpation of the head, and examination of cranial nerve reflexes.

✓ **Seizures** may be witnessed but are often an historical finding and indicate dysfunction of the **cerebrum** or **diencephalon.**

✓ **Mentation** is a term that describes the animal's state of awareness and ability to respond appropriately to the environment. Mentation can first be observed while collecting the initial history. The owner's opinion of any behavior changes is important to note. A depressed animal is quiet but responds appropriately. A demented animal is awake but dull and responds inappropriately. Pet owners may complain that the personality has changed or that the animal does not recognize them. Delirium is hysterical behavior. Rage or aggression is commonly a behavioral or neuropsychiatric problem but occasionally can result from primary brain disease. Stupor is a somnolent state with reduced responses to most environmental stimuli except pain. Coma is a state of unconsciousness with a lack of response to any environmental stimuli. Lesions of the **cerebrum** and **diencephalon** produce dementia, delirium, rage, stupor, and coma. Lesions of the **midbrain, pons,** and **medulla oblongata** produce stupor and coma.

✓ **Head pressing** occurs when the animal pushes the top of its head against a wall and indicates a lesion of the cerebrum or diencephalon.

✓ **Head turning** occurs toward the side of the lesion and is caused by lesions of the cerebrum and diencephalon. Animals with neck pain may carry the head low and more to one side. In a head turn, both ears are level, which allows this condition to be differentiated from a head tilt. A head turn is often accompanied by circling.

✓ **Head incoordination** and **tremors** may be observed with movement of the head or during attempts to eat and drink. This usually indicates a lesion of the **cerebellum.**

✓ A **head tilt** is when the head is cocked to one side and one ear is closer to the ground. A head tilt indicates a lesion of the vestibular system (the **vestibular nerve [cranial nerve 8]**, the **vestibular nuclei** in the **rostral medulla oblongata,** or the **flocculonodular lobe** of the **cerebellum**). The head tilts toward the lesion in vestibular nerve disease, toward or away from the lesion in medulla oblongata disease, and away from the lesion in cerebellar disease.

✓ Twelve pairs of **cranial nerves (CN)** line the left and right sides of the brain and brainstem. The CN are numbered 1 to 12 as follows: **CN 1 = olfactory, CN 2 = optic, CN 3 = oculomotor, CN 4 = trochlear, CN 5 = trigeminal, CN 6 = abducens, CN 7= facial, CN 8 = vestibular, CN 9 = glossopharyngeal, CN 10 = vagus, CN 11= spinal accessory,** and **CN 12 = hypoglossal.** Signs of dysfunction indicate a disease of the cranial nerve or its nuclei in the brainstem on the same side (ipsilateral), except for olfactory, optic, and the trochlear nerves. Vision and olfaction have some bilateral input; the trochlear nerve crosses to the opposite side within the brainstem. Some reduction of cranial nerve function may be observed in cerebral and diencephalic lesions.

✓ **Olfaction** is the function of the **olfactory nerves (CN 1)** and can be tested by offering food and observing whether the animal can locate the food with its sense of smell (Figure 1-5). Most animals that cannot smell will not eat, so questioning the owner about the appetite is important. Noxious substances should not be used for testing because they evaluate the sensory portion of the trigeminal nerves (CN 5) and not CN 1.

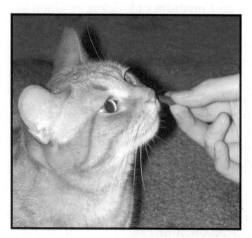

Figure 1-5 Testing smell with food (can blindfold the animal if concerned that it is seeing the food instead of smelling it).

✓ The **menace response** evaluates the **optic nerves (CN 2), facial nerves (CN 7),** and a complex set of pathways through the brainstem, brain, and cerebellum. Advancing a hand or fingers toward the eye and observing an eyelid blink tests the menace response (Figure 1-6). One eye is covered to test each eye separately. Care is taken not to touch the eyelid or whiskers or to make air currents that might stimulate the sensory portion of the **trigeminal nerves (CN 5).**

✓ **Vision** is the function of the **optic nerves (CN 2),** the **diencephalon,** and the occipital lobe of the **cerebrum.** In addition to the menace response, vision is tested by observing the animal in an unfamiliar environment to see if it bumps into objects or by throwing cotton balls (which do not produce a localizing sound) and watching for signs of recognition as they pass through the animal's visual field. Vision may also be tested by observing the animal focus on an object (Figure 1-7).

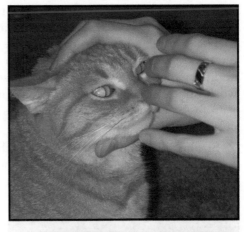

Figure 1-6 Testing the menace response.

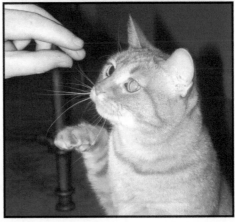

Figure 1-7 Observing the response to a visual stimulus.

✓ The **pupil size** is observed in normal room light. Pupils are usually midrange in normal room light unless the animal is fearful or excited. In normal animals, fear, excitement, and reduction of ambient light cause the pupils to become larger **(mydriasis).** A reduction in pupil diameter **(miosis)** occurs with increases in ambient light if the animal is not fearful or excited or has intraocular disease. Mydriasis may occur with lesions of the **retina, optic nerves (CN 2), oculomotor nerves (CN 3),** or the **midbrain.** Midrange size pupils that do not respond to light may be associated with **midbrain** lesions. **Miotic** pupils may be associated with lesions of the cerebrum, diencephalon, and the CNS and PNS **sympathetic nerves** that innervate the pupil (Section 6).

✓ The **pupillary light reflex** evaluates the **optic nerves (CN 2)** and the **oculomotor nerves (CN 3)** and can be tested by shining a light into one pupil and observing pupillary constriction in the eye tested (the **direct response**) and in the opposite eye (the **consensual response**) (Figure 1-8). If either the direct or consensual responses are absent, then a lesion is affecting **CN 2 or CN 3** and their associated pathways through the **diencephalon** and **midbrain.** Excited or fearful animals may have a reduced direct and consensual pupillary light reflex. A strong light source should be used because a weak light source may not induce pupil constriction. Lesions of CN 2 and CN 3 usually produce mydriasis as well as a reduced or absent pupillary light reflex.

✓ **Strabismus** occurs when one or both eyes deviate into an abnormal position due to paralysis of one or more extraocular muscles.

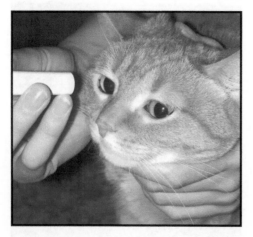

Figure 1-8 Testing the pupillary light reflex.

Ventrolateral strabismus (down and outward position) occurs with lesions of the **oculomotor nerves (CN 3)** or their nuclei in the **midbrain.** A lateral rotation of the eyeball occurs with lesions of the **trochlear nerve (CN 4)** or their nuclei in the **midbrain** but is only obvious in cats because of their vertical pupils. Medial strabismus (inward position) occurs with lesions of the **abducens nerves (CN 6).**

✔ **Positional strabismus** is an abnormal eye position due to a lesion of the **vestibular system (CN 8, medulla oblongata,** and **cerebellum).** If head tilt is also present, when the head is straightened and the nose is elevated, ventral strabismus (eye drop) is observed on the side of the lesion.

✔ **Ptosis** is a weakness of the levator muscles that open the eyelid and results in reduction of the diameter of the palpebral fissure. Ptosis is most commonly associated with lesions of the **oculomotor nerves (CN 3)** or their nuclei in the **midbrain** or the **sympathetic nerves** to the eyelid. Ptosis may be secondary to enophthalmos.

✔ **Enophthalmos** is a backward displacement of the eyeball into the orbit that induces a passive elevation of the third eyelid and a slight reduction in the diameter of the palpebral fissure. Enophthalmos is most commonly associated with lesions of the **sympathetic nerves** to the periorbital muscles but can occur with stimulation of the **abducens nerves (CN 6),** as seen in tetanus.

✔ **Globe retraction** (corneal reflex) occurs when the eyelids are held open and the cornea is gently touched. Loss of this reflex occurs in lesions of the sensory portion of the **trigeminal nerves (CN 5)** and their connections in the **pons** and **medulla oblongata** and lesions of the **abducens nerves (CN 6)** or their nuclei in the rostral **medulla oblongata.**

✔ **Intranasal sensation** is tested by inserting a hemostat into the nostril, which induces the animal to move the head away to avoid the stimulus. Loss of intranasal sensation occurs with lesions of the **trigeminal nerves (CN 5)** as well as of the complex set of pathways through the brainstem, diencephalon, and cerebrum.

✔ **Temporal** and **masseter muscle atrophy** is evaluated by visual observation and palpation and is associated with cachexia as well as with lesions of the **trigeminal nerves (CN 5),** their nuclei in the **pons,** and with primary muscle diseases.

✔ **Jaw tone** and **range of motion** are observed by opening and closing the mouth. Loss of jaw tone is usually associated with bilateral lesions of the **trigeminal nerves (CN 5).** Restricted range of motion is often caused by a primary myopathy.

✓ The **palpebral reflex** is elicited by touching the medial or lateral canthus of the eye, which causes closure of the eyelids (Figure 1-9). The **aural reflexes** are elicited by touching or pinching the ear and the **buccal reflexes** by touching the lip and observing their movement. Facial sensation arises from the **trigeminal nerves (CN 5),** and movement of the facial muscles (the eyelids, ears, and lips) is controlled by the **facial nerves (CN 7).** Loss of the palpebral, aural or buccal reflex indicates a lesion of CN 5, CN 7 or their connections in the **pons** and **rostral medulla oblongata.**

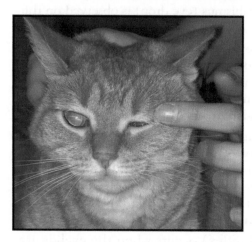

Figure 1-9 Testing the palpebral reflex.

✓ **Normal** or **physiologic nystagmus** is induced when the head is moved. As the head is moving, the eyes move slowly (slow phase) away from the direction of head movement then rapidly snap back (fast phase) toward that side. As the head is moved to the left, the fast phase is to the left; when moved to the right, the fast phase is to the right. As the head is moved up, the fast phase is up; when moved down, the fast phase is down. These eye movements are repeated several times when the head is moved from side to side or up and down. Normal nystagmus requires the integrity of the **vestibular nerves (CN 8), oculomotor nerves (CN 3), trochlear nerves (CN 4), abducens nerves (CN 6)**, and their connections through the brainstem.

✓ **Spontaneous** or **pathologic nystagmus** occurs without head movement with lesions of the **vestibular system** (vestibular nerves [CN 8], rostral medulla oblongata, or cerebellum). **Positional nystagmus** is induced when the animal is placed in lateral or dorsal recumbency and indicates a vestibular system lesion. As with physiologic nystagmus, spontaneous and positional nystagmus have a fast and slow phase. The fast phase often occurs away from the side of the lesion. With **horizontal nystagmus,** the eyes go from side to side in a straight, horizontal plane. With **rotatory nystagmus,** the eyes go side to side in a horizontal plane but form an arc. With **vertical nystagmus,** the eyes go up and down in a vertical direction.

✓ **Hearing** is crudely tested by observing a response to such noises as whistling, yelling, hand clapping, or clanging metal against metal. Care should be taken not to create vibrations or visual cues that would induce a false-positive response. Loss of hearing is usually associated with lesions of the middle ear, inner ear, or **cochlear nerves (CN 8).**

✓ **Swallowing** is evaluated by applying external pressure to the hyoid bones to stimulate swallowing or stimulating the pharynx with a finger to elicit a gag response (Figure 1-10). Swallowing dysfunction is associated with lesions of the pharyngeal muscles, **glossopharyngeal nerves (CN 9), vagus nerves (CN 10),** or caudal **medulla oblongata.**

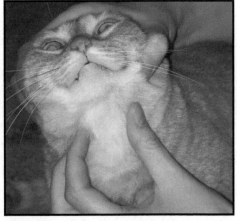

Figure 1-10 Testing the swallowing reflex.

✓ **Regurgitation** may be observed or noted in the history and is often caused by megaesophagus. Megaesophagus can result from lesions of the **vagus nerves (CN 10)** or the **caudal medulla oblongata** but is usually secondary to diseases of the esophageal muscles or neuromuscular junction.

✓ **A voice change (dysphonia)** may be observed or noted in the history and can be due to lesions of the laryngeal muscles, **vagus nerves (CN 10),** or the **caudal medulla oblongata.**

✓ **Stridor**—a harsh, high-pitched respiratory sound often associated with inspiration—can be heard with the bare ear or a stethoscope. This sign is associated with unilateral or bilateral laryngeal paresis or paralysis associated with lesions of the laryngeal muscles, **vagus nerves (CN 10),** or the caudal **medulla oblongata.** Dyspnea with cyanosis can also occur and constitutes an emergency situation.

✓ **Trapezius and brachiocephalicus muscle atrophy** may be palpated in rare instances of lesions affecting the **spinal accessory nerves (CN 11).**

✓ **Tongue atrophy or weakness** may be evaluated when the animal is drinking or by direct visual inspection, manipulation, and palpation. Unilateral lesions of the **hypoglossal nerves (CN 12)** produce these signs. In chronic lesions, the tongue contracts and becomes fibrotic on the affected side.

Evaluation of the Gait

🖐 A **normal gait** requires proper function of sensory and motor **peripheral nerves** and connected pathways through the **spinal cord, brainstem,** and **cerebellum.** The cerebrum is less important for a normal gait in animals, and cerebral lesions usually cause only subtle or temporary gait deficits. It is usually best to have an assistant walk, trot, and turn the animal to maximize the clinician's ability to observe. Watching the animal roam freely is also helpful. If only the pelvic limbs are abnormal, then a lesion below T2 is suspected. If all four limbs are affected, then a lesion above T2 is suspected. If the animal is nonambulatory, it should be supported and an attempt made to assist it in walking so any voluntary movement can be assessed.

✓ **Hemiwalking** involves supporting the animal by picking up the limbs on one side and pushing it forward and sideways so that it is forced to walk on the limbs of one side only (Figure 1-11). By comparing sides, it can be determined if one side is more affected than the other.

✓ **Wheelbarrowing** involves supporting the pelvic limbs and observing the animal's ability to walk on the thoracic limbs alone. This technique can detect thoracic limb deficits not appreciated during the gait evaluation (Figure 1-12). In quadriparetic animals, this test may be used to determine if the thoracic limbs are more or less involved than the pelvic limbs, but supporting the chest is essential to preclude falling and neck injury. Extension of the neck during wheelbarrowing may accentuate thoracic limb deficits. Supporting the thoracic limbs and forcing the animal to walk on the hind limbs alone can be useful to evaluate the hind limbs.

✓ **Lameness** is most often seen with orthopedic disease but may occasionally be caused by lesions that irritate the nerve roots, which innervate the limb.

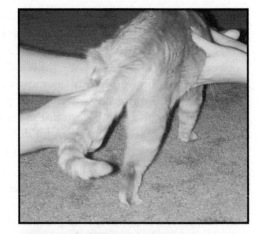

Figure 1-11 Evaluating the ability to hemiwalk.

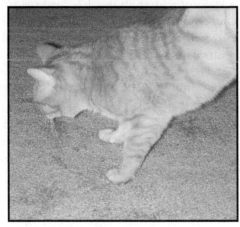

Figure 1-12 Evaluation of wheelbarrowing on thoracic limbs.

✓ **Ataxia** is an uncoordinated gait and is caused by lesions of the sensory peripheral nerves, spinal cord, brainstem, vestibular system, or cerebellum. Hypermetria and hypometria are types of ataxia. **Hypermetria** refers to exaggerated motion and is associated with excessive flexion and over-reaching of the limbs. **Hypometria** is reduced flexion and under-reaching of the limbs during movement.

✓ **Ataxia with limb paresis (weakness)** may be due to peripheral nerve, spinal cord, or brainstem lesions. Paresis is not seen in cerebellar lesions.

🖑 **Paresis** is weakness or impaired motor function due to a neurologic or myopathic cause. The severity may vary from mild weakness to an inability to stand and walk, but paresis implies that some **voluntary** movement is present. Care must be taken not to confuse reflex activity with voluntary movement. The spinal reflexes are preserved and often become exaggerated if the components of the reflex arc are still intact (Figure 1-3). In severe spinal cord lesions between T3 and L3, the pelvic limb reflexes become so exaggerated that reflex flexion and extension can occur with the slightest stimulus and mimic voluntary movement. This phenomenon is known as **spinal walking** and can be present even if the spinal cord is functionally severed. Spinal walking can be difficult to differentiate from voluntary movements unless deep pain is present.

✓ **Paraparesis** is paresis of the pelvic limbs resulting from a lesion located behind T2. **Quadriparesis (tetraparesis)** is paresis of all four limbs caused by a lesion located above T2 or diffuse neuromuscular disease. **Hemiparesis** is paresis of the limbs on one side due to a lesion located above T2. Lesions from the caudal midbrain to T2 cause ipsilateral hemiparesis (the lesion is on the same side as the paresis). Lesions from the rostral midbrain to the cerebrum cause contralateral hemiparesis (the lesion is on the opposite side of the paresis). Paresis of the thoracic limbs is usually more subtle than the pelvic limbs and is often manifested as a choppy, short-strided gait.

✓ **Paralysis** is total loss of all voluntary movement (reflex movements may still be intact but do not indicate spinal cord integrity above the reflex level). **Paraplegia** is paralysis of the pelvic limbs only. **Quadriplegia (tetraplegia)** is paralysis of all four limbs. **Hemiplegia** is paralysis of the limbs on one side.

✓ **Circling** or **pacing** usually indicates a lesion of the **cerebrum** or **diencephalon.** Animals usually circle toward the side of the lesion. In animals with a **head tilt, circling** is usually caused by a lesion of the **vestibular system.**

Evaluation of the Neck, Thoracic Limbs, Back, Pelvic Limbs, Anus, and Tail

🖐 Evaluation of these parts of the patient's anatomy can detect subtle abnormalities that can help determine whether the lesion is located above T2 or below T2. The function of each individual limb can be compared, and asymmetry that can localize the lesion to one side may be noted.

Postural Reactions

✓ **Hopping** is evaluated by lifting three limbs and pushing the animal laterally to observe their ability to walk or hop on each thoracic or pelvic limb independently (Figure 1-13). In large dogs, lifting only the opposite thoracic or pelvic limb is adequate for evaluation, but support is necessary to prevent falling. Most animals do not hop well in a medial direction. Equal responses should be seen on both sides. Minor ataxia or weakness of a thoracic or pelvic limb may be detected.

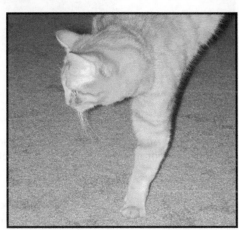

Figure 1-13 Evaluation of the hopping response on one thoracic limb.

✓ **Conscious proprioception (CP)** can be a very important tool to detect subtle dysfunction and confirm that a neurologic disease is present when other signs are minimal. The animal is supported under the chest or between the pelvic limbs, and the paw is turned so that the dorsal surface contacts the ground (Figure 1-14). The animal should return the paw to the correct position within a few seconds. The animal should not lean against the examiner, nor should the examiner support all of the animal's weight. Consistent CP deficits indicate a nervous system lesion and are not caused by an orthopedic disease (Figure 1-15).

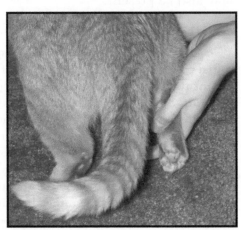

Figure 1-14 Evaluation of conscious proprioception in a pelvic limb.

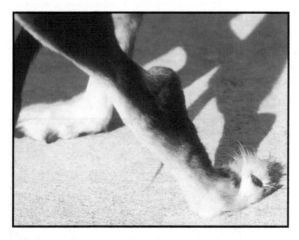

Figure 1-15 Absent conscious proprioception; the dog stays standing on the dorsal surface of the paw indicating a neurologic lesion.

✓ Appropriate CP responses require the integrity of sensory systems (peripheral nerve, spinal cord, brainstem, and cerebral cortex) to perceive the paw position and motor systems (cerebral cortex, brainstem, spinal cord, peripheral nerve, and muscle) to correct the paw position. Therefore, although it is a good test to document neurologic dysfunction, it does not localize a lesion to any specific site. CP deficits found in animals with a cranial nerve problem indicate that the lesion could be in the brainstem segment rather than in the peripheral nerve, which changes the differential diagnosis, diagnostic plan, and prognosis. Deficits of CP found in animals that are having difficulty rising indicate a neurologic disorder and not just an orthopedic disorder, which may also be present.

Spinal Cord Reflexes

🖐 **Spinal cord reflexes** pass through specific peripheral nerves and spinal cord segments (Figure 1-3), so if a **spinal reflex is depressed or absent the lesion is localized to that specific nerve or spinal cord segment.** Spinal reflexes are best tested in a relaxed animal held in lateral recumbency by an assistant. The limb to be tested may be gently flexed and extended to ensure a normal range of motion and relaxation. A percussion hammer (pleximeter) is used to briskly tap tendons and muscles to elicit the appropriate response. If the animal is too tense or the limb has tendon contraction, then spinal reflexes will not be evaluated accurately. It is most important to determine if the spinal reflexes are depressed or absent. Although hyperreflexia may be associated with a lesion of the upper motor neurons, in the absence of other neurologic deficits it means little. Nervous dogs may exhibit hyperactive spinal reflexes.

✓ **Thoracic limb spinal reflexes** and their spinal cord segments, nerve roots, and peripheral nerves include the following:

♥ **Biceps tendon reflex (C6-8 and the musculocutaneous nerves):** Put the thumb on the biceps tendon and tap with a percussion hammer. Feel or observe biceps tendon contraction and elbow flexion (Figure 1-16).

♥ **Triceps tendon reflex (C7-T2 and the radial nerves):** Put the forefinger on the triceps tendon and tap with a percussion hammer, and feel or observe triceps tendon contraction and elbow extension (Figure 1-17).

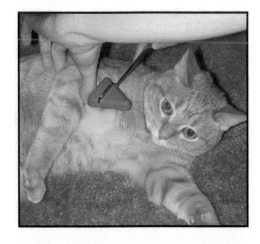

Figure 1-16 Testing the biceps reflex.

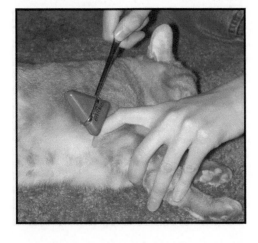

Figure 1-17 Testing the triceps reflex.

♥ **Extensor carpi radialis reflex (C7-T2 and the radial nerves):** Tap the extensor carpi radialis muscle with a percussion hammer, and observe extension of the carpus (Figure 1-18).

♥ **Flexor reflex (C7-T2 and the radial, axillary, musculocutaneous, median, and ulnar nerves):** The flexor reflex is also known as the withdrawal or toe-pinch reflex. Sensory input is through the radial, median, and ulnar nerves, and motor output is through C7-T2 spinal cord segments and nerve roots and the axillary, musculocutaneous, median, and ulnar nerves. The toe is pinched by the examiner's fingers or with a hemostat to elicit flexion of the shoulder, elbow, carpus, and sometimes digits (Figure 1-19). If this reflex is absent, each toe can be tested individually to determine if specific deficits of the radial, median, or ulnar nerves are present (see Section 14).

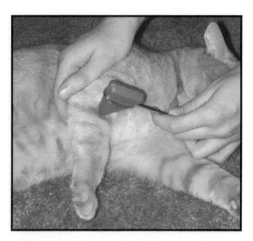

Figure 1-18 Testing the ext carpi radialis reflex.

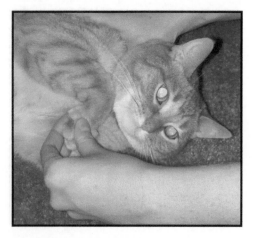

Figure 1-19 Testing the flexor reflex of thoracic limb.

♥ **Crossed extensor reflex:** When the animal is relaxed in lateral recumbency and inducing the flexor reflex results in extension of the limb on the opposite side, a lesion above C7 is suspected. Care should be taken to ensure the animal was not trying to rise during the testing, as this will cause extension of the opposite limb as well.

✓ **Pelvic limb, anal, and tail spinal reflexes** and their spinal cord segments, nerve roots, and nerves include the following:

♥ **Patellar reflex (L4-5** and the **femoral nerves):** Tap the patellar tendon briskly with the percussion hammer to elicit extension of the stifle (Figure 1-20).

♥ **Gastocnemius reflex (L6-S2** and **tibial nerves):** Hold the gastocnemius muscle between the thumb and forefinger, and tap the thumb briskly with the percussion hammer to elicit extension of the hock (Figure 1-21).

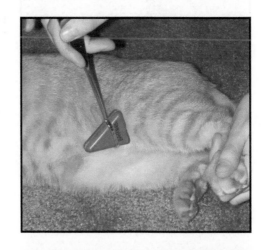

Figure 1-20 Testing the patellar reflex.

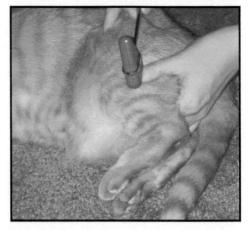

Figure 1-21 Testing the gastroc-nemius reflex.

♥ **Cranial tibial reflex (L6-S2** and the **sciatic and peroneal nerves):** Tap the cranial tibial muscle briskly with the percussion hammer to elicit flexion of the hock (Figure 1-22).

♥ **Sciatic reflex (L6-S2** and the **sciatic and peroneal nerves):** Place a finger on the sciatic nerve in the notch formed by the greater trochanter and the ischiatic tuberosity, and tap the finger to elicit brief extension of the hock (Figure 1-23).

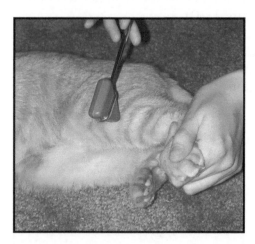

Figure 1-22 Testing the cranial tibial muscle reflex.

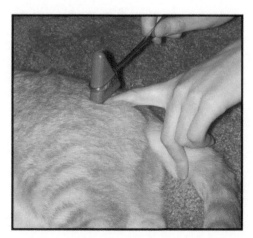

Figure 1-23 Testing the sciatic nerve reflex.

♥ **Flexor reflex (L6-S2** and the **sciatic and peroneal nerves):** On a pelvic limb, the examiner pinches the toe with fingers or a hemostat, and flexion of the hip, stifle, hock, and sometimes the digits is elicited (Figure 1-24).

♥ **Crossed extensor reflex:** If the opposite limb extends when the flexor reflex is elicited (Figure 1-25), then a crossed extensor reflex is observed. When the animal is in lateral recumbency and not trying to rise, a crossed extensor reflex of the pelvic limb usually indicates a lesion above spinal cord segment L6.

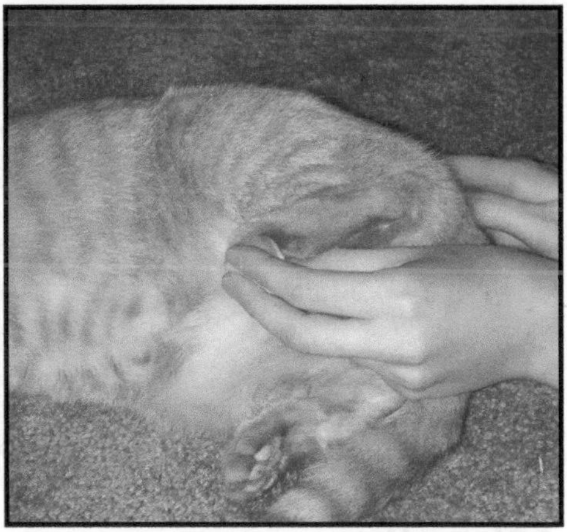

Figure 1-24 Testing the flexor reflex of the pelvic limb.

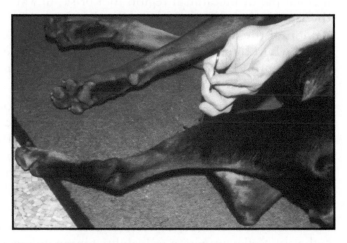

Figure 1-25 A crossed extensor reflex.

♥ **Anal reflex (S1-3 and pudendal nerves):** The perineal area on each side is pinched with a hemostat, and the anal sphincter will constrict (Figure 1-26). If a reduced reflex is suspected, a gloved finger is inserted into the anus. If the reflex is normal, a strong contraction of the anal sphincter will occur.

♥ **Tail reflex (S1-Cd5 and the caudal nerves of the tail):** As the perineal area is stimulated with a hemostat or finger, flexion of the tail toward the anus will occur.

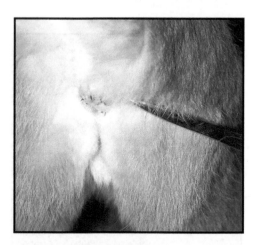

Figure 1-26
Testing the anal reflex.

Miscellaneous

♥ The **Babinski's sign** can be tested in the thoracic and pelvic limbs by stroking the plantar and palmar surface of the metacarpal or metatarsal region in a brisk, upward motion with the tip of a percussion hammer handle (Figure 1-27). A slight flexion of the digits is normally seen. A positive Babinski's sign is noted when the digits extend and flare out, indicating an upper motor neuron lesion above C6 for the thoracic limb and above L6 for the pelvic limb.

♥ **Muscle atrophy** may be associated with disuse or from lower motor neuron or muscle disease. Disuse of a limb causes a symmetric reduction in muscle size diffusely over the limb. Muscle atrophy associated with specific nerve or muscle disease is usually focal and more severe than disuse atrophy. Generalized muscle atrophy occurs in polyneuropathies and polymyopathies (see Sections 10 and 11).

♥ **Urination** is observed to detect involvement of the micturition pathways. Reflex urination or inability to urinate is common in animals with spinal cord lesions and must be properly managed.

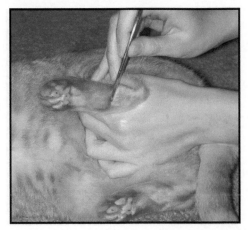

Figure 1-27 Testing for Babinski's sign.

♥ **Tail wagging** when the dog is spoken to or offered food is usually voluntary and indicates integrity of the nervous system from head to tail. Reflex tail wagging may occur with lesions above the caudal segments when the limb spinal reflexes are tested.

Pain Perception

🖐 Palpation and manipulation to detect painful areas and testing pain perception are usually performed last so that the animal will remain cooperative during the rest of the neurologic examination. If the animal exhibits severe neck or back pain, the neurologic examination may be modified so that undue stress to the pet or owner is avoided.

♥ **Neck pain** may be observed as a reluctance to move the head or to look upward. In severe cases, the animal may hold the head down with the neck extended. Spontaneous muscle spasms of the neck may cause jerky neck movements and vocalization. Deep palpation of the cervical musculature or movement of the neck in dorsal, ventral, and side-to-side directions may also elicit tensing, muscle spasms, and vocalization (Figure 1-28). Neck pain is most often associated with cervical lesions but occasionally may be associated with intracranial disease (see Section 7). Diseases affecting the cervical vertebrae, sensory nerve roots, or meninges usually cause some degree of discomfort.

♥ **Back pain** may be expressed by arching the back, muscle tension or spasms, and vocalizing when the paravertebral musculature is palpated. Careful palpation can usually narrow the area of discomfort to within two to three spinal segments. Disorders affecting thoracolumbar vertebrae, sensory nerve roots, or meninges are the most common causes of back pain.

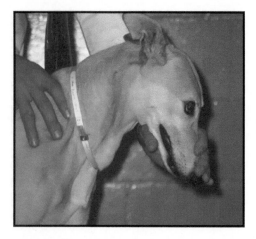

Figure 1-28 Evaluating range of motion of the neck to evaluate for pain.

♥ **Superficial sensation** is evaluated by pinching the skin with a hemostat or pricking the skin with a needle to elicit a behavioral response indicating the sensation was perceived. Vocalizing, trying to bite, or avoiding the stimulus is an appropriate response to a painful stimulus. Each spinal nerve carries superficial pain sensations from a discrete region of skin known as a dermatome. **Hyperesthesia** is an increased sensitivity to stimulation resulting in a negative behavioral reaction from the animal and is usually located at the site of a lesion. **Hypesthesia** or **anesthesia** are reduced or absent sensation, which may be located within three spinal segments from the lesion. Superficial sensation is a localizing sharp pain carried by large fibers from the skin and is often lost prior to deep pain in spinal cord lesions.

♥ A **cutaneous trunci response** or **panniculus response** is elicited when the dorsal skin of the trunk between T2-L4 is pinched and a twitch of the cutaneous muscles is observed (Figure 1-29). From the site tested, sensory nerves travel to the spinal cord and ascend to C8-T1 where they synapse on cell bodies of the lateral thoracic nerve. The lateral thoracic nerve exits the spinal cord and stimulates the cutaneous trunci muscles to contract (Figure 1-30). A lesion anywhere along this pathway may cause a reduction or loss of the cutaneous trunci response. This response is used mainly to further localize lesions between T3-L3 but can be absent on the side of a brachial plexus avulsion (see Section 14). In normal animals, it can easily be elicited just caudal to the shoulders and just cranial to the pelvic limb. The cutaneous trunci response is lost only at one site in nerve root lesions but may be completely absent caudal to the lesion with some spinal cord lesions. The presence of this response caudal to a lesion indicates that some spinal cord integrity remains even when superficial sensation and deep pain are lost. The cutaneous trunci response may be completely absent in polyneuropathies.

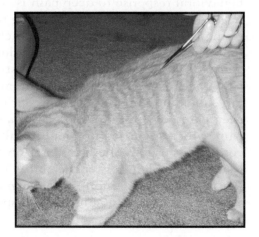

Figure 1-29 Testing the cutaneous trunci response.

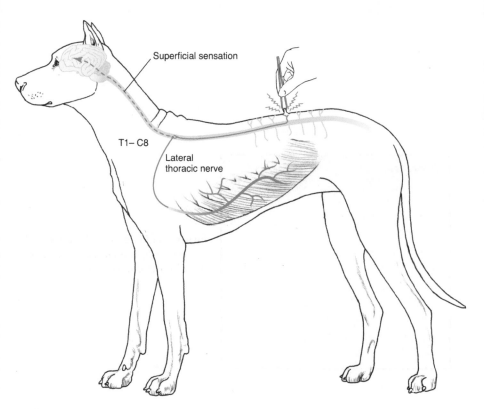

Figure 1-30 The cutaneous trunci response pathway.

♥ **Deep pain** is tested by applying firm pressure to the **bones of the digits** of a thoracic or pelvic limb with the fingers or a hemostat to elicit a behavioral response (Figure 1-31). A positive behavioral response to deep pain is consistent turning of the head and looking, vocalizing, trying to bite the examiner, or trying to escape when the toe is pinched. **Withdrawal of the limb is only the flexor reflex and does not mean the animal consciously perceives the painful stimulus.** If response to deep pain appears absent from one digit, all remaining digits and the tail should be tested to determine if there is a complete loss of deep pain perception. Deep pain is a small-fiber, nonlocalizing pain, which is carried in a multifocal network within the spinal cord and is usually the last sensation that remains in spinal cord lesions. Complete loss of the ability to feel deep pain signifies a severe spinal cord lesion. If the deep pain sensation is absent for a month or longer in animals with spinal cord lesions, recovery of function is unlikely.

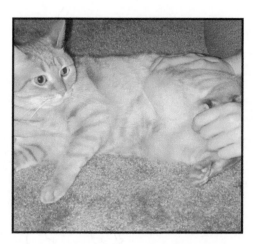

Figure 1-31 Testing deep pain of a hind limb; the cat reacts to the pain by turning or complaining.

Lesion Localization

♥ When the neurologic examination is complete, an attempt should be made to explain all abnormal findings by a lesion at one anatomic site. If this cannot be done, then the animal may have a multifocal or diffuse disease process and the differential diagnosis should reflect this. Two separate and distinct lesion sites from two different diseases is an unlikely scenario in clinical neurology unless one can be explained by a history of a long-standing problem unrelated to the current primary complaint. Each anatomic region has specific signs, which localize lesions to that region.

✔ **Polyneuropathies** are disorders that affect multiple peripheral nerves, and **polymyopathies** are disorders that affect multiple muscles. An overview of these localizing signs and consequent alterations of gait, conscious proprioception and hopping, and spinal cord reflexes is outlined in Table 1-4.

Table 1-4 Localization of Neurologic and Neuromuscular Lesions

Anatomic Location of the Lesion	Signs That Localize the Lesion Above the Foramen Magnum (One or More)	Alterations of the Gait: Strength and Coordination	Conscious Proprioception and Hopping	Spinal Cord Reflexes
Cerebrum and diencephalon	Seizures; behavior change, dementia, delirium, depression, stupor or coma with normal or miotic pupils; head press; pacing; circling; loss of smell (CN 1); blind with dilated pupils (CN 2) or normal pupils.	Acute lesions-(transient) contralateral hemiparesis or quadriparesis; Chronic lesions-normal	Normal or Contralateral ↓↓ in one or both limbs of one side, ↓↓ in both pelvic limbs or in all four limbs	Normal or ↑↑ in all four limbs
Midbrain (mesencephalon)	Stupor, coma, dilated (CN 3) or midrange fixed pupils; ventrolateral strabismus (CN 3); absent pupillary light reflex (CN 3)	Rostral midbrain lesions-contralateral hemiparesis; Caudal midbrain lesions-ipsilateral hemiparesis; Quadriparesis with bilateral lesions	Contralateral or ipsilateral ↓↓ in one or both limbs, ↓↓ in the pelvic limbs or in all four limbs	Normal or ↑↑ in all four limbs
Pons (metencephalon)	Depression, stupor, coma or normal mentation; atrophy of temporal and masseter muscles or ↓↓ or ↑↑ facial sensation (CN 5)	Ipsilateral hemiparesis, quadriparesis or normal depending on the size of the lesion	Ipsilateral ↓↓ in one or both limbs, ↓↓ in only the pelvic limbs or in all four limbs	Normal or ↑↑ in all four limbs
Rostral medulla oblongata (myelencephalon)	Depressed or normal mentation; medial strabismus (CN 6); reduced blink, lip and ear reflex (CN 7); head tilt	Ipsilateral hemiparesis, quadriparesis or normal depending on the size of lesion, Ipsilateral hypermetria or hypometria	Ipsilateral ↓↓ in one or both limbs, ↓↓ in the pelvic limbs or in all four limbs	Normal or ↑↑ in all four limbs

Location	Cranial nerve / mentation signs	Gait / posture	Postural reactions	Spinal reflexes
Caudal medulla oblongata (myelencephalon)	(CN 8), nystagmus and dysequilibrium (CN 8) Depressed or normal mentation; dysphagia (CN 9 or 10); megaesophagus (CN 10); laryngeal paresis (CN 10); tongue atrophy or paralysis (CN 12)	Ipsilateral hemiparesis, quadriparesis or normal depending on the size of lesion; Ipsilateral or bilateral hypermetria or hypometria	Ipsilateral ↓↓ in one or both limbs; ↓↓ in only the pelvic limbs or in all four limbs	Normal or ↑↑ in all four limbs
Cerebellum	Intention tremors and ataxia of the head; head tilt away from lesion; nystagmus; loss of menace response	Ipsilateral or bilateral ataxia (hypermetria and hypometria); Normal limb strength	Normal	Normal
Spinal cord C1-C5 (vertebrae C1- C4 dog)	No "head signs" except perhaps ptosis, miosis, enophthalmos (Horner's syndrome); crossed extensor reflex thoracic and pelvic limbs; neck pain	Ataxia ipsilateral or all four limbs; Ipsilateral hemiparesis; Quadriparesis with or without respiratory depression	Normal, Ipsilateral ↓↓ in one or both limbs; ↓↓ in only the pelvic limbs or in all four limbs	Normal or ↑↑ in all four limbs
Spinal cord C6-T2 (vertebrae C5-T2 dog)	No "head signs" except perhaps ptosis, miosis, enophthalmos (Horner's syndrome); neck pain; ↓↓ thoracic limb spinal reflexes; atrophy of supra and infraspinatus muscles.	Dysmetria (incoordination); Ataxia ipsilateral or all four limbs; Ipsilateral hemiparesis; Quadriparesis; respiratory depression; thoracic limbs may be worse than the pelvic limbs	Normal; Ipsilateral ↓↓ in one or both limbs; ↓↓ in only the thoracic or pelvic limbs or in all four	Normal or ↓↓ in thoracic limbs; Normal or ↑↑ in pelvic limbs
Spinal cord T3-L3 (vertebrae T3-L2 dog)	No "head signs"; no thoracic limb signs; back pain; paraplegia with normal or ↑↑ spinal reflexes; loss of cutaneous trunci response at the cranial aspect of the lesion	Ataxia of pelvic limbs; Paraparesis (can be asymmetric—worse on the side of the lesion); Paraplegia	Normal; Ipsilateral or bilateral ↓↓ in one or both pelvic limbs	Normal in thoracic limbs; Normal or ↑↑ in pelvic limbs

Table 1-4 Continued

Anatomic Location of the Lesion	Signs That Localize the Lesion below the Foramen Magnum (one or more)	Alterations of the Gait: Strength and Coordination	Conscious Proprioception and Hopping	Spinal Cord Reflexes
Spinal cord and nerve roots L4-S2 (vertebrae L3- L7 dog)	No "head signs"; no thoracic limb signs; paraplegia with ↓↓ of one or more spinal reflexes of the pelvic limbs; loss of cutaneous trunci response at cranial aspect of lesion	Ataxia of pelvic limbs; Paraparesis (can be asymmetrical-worse on side of lesion): Paraplegia	Normal; Ipsilateral or bilateral ↓↓ in one or both pelvic limbs	Normal in thoracic limbs; ↓↓ patellar reflex – L4-5 (vertebrae L3-5) lesion); ↓↓ flexor, gastrocnemius, cranial tibial reflexes – L6-S2 (vertebrae L5-7) lesion; ↓↓ anal reflex – S1-3 (vertebrae L5-S3) lesion
Nerve roots S1-Cd5 (vertebrae L7-S3 dog)	No "head signs"; no thoracic limb signs; lumbosacral pain; pelvic limbs normal or slight paresis; ↓↓ anal and tail tone	Normal; May be mild pelvic limb ataxia or paresis	Normal; May be pelvic limb conscious proprioceptive deficits unilateral or bilateral	Normal in thoracic and pelvic limbs; ↓↓ Anal reflex – S1-3 (vertebrae L5-S3); ↓↓ Tail reflex Cd 1-5 (vertebrae L6-Cd)
Polyneuropathy	Normal "head signs" or one or more CN deficits; Quadriparesis or quadriplegia with depressed or absent spinal reflexes	Paraparesis (mild cases); Quadriparesis Quadriplegia	May be reduced in all four limbs	Patellar reflex may be the only reflex ↓↓; ↓↓ of spinal reflexes in all four limbs
Polymyopathy	Normal "head signs" or may have temporalis and masseter muscle atrophy; Quadriparesis or quadriplegia with generalized muscle atrophy	Paraparesis (mild cases); Quadriparesis Quadriplegia	Conscious proprioception is usually normal; Hopping may be reduced or absent	Spinal reflexes are usually normal; In severe cases spinal reflexes may be depressed

CN = cranial nerves (CN signs are ipsilateral); contralateral = signs on side opposite lesion; ipsilateral = signs on the same side as lesion; ↓↓ = reduced or absent responses or reflexes; ↑↑ = hyperactive reflexes, which includes the crossed extensor reflex and a positive Babinski's sign; "Head signs" = abnormalities related to the brain.

Section 2
Dementia, Stupor, and Coma

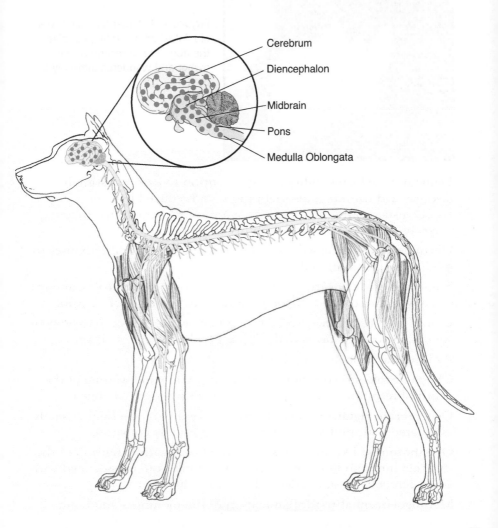

Cerebrum

Diencephalon

Midbrain

Pons

Medulla Oblongata

Definitions

Depression: Lethargy with reduced activity but no reduction in mental ability.

Dementia: Loss of mental and intellectual abilities, memory, and usual personality; often manifests as inability to perform trained activities and inability to recognize the owner or other familiar objects (Figure 2-1).

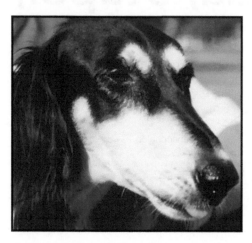

Figure 2-1 Dementia in an 8-year-old Saluki with cerebral neoplasia; the dog did not recognize the owner and wandered aimlessly to the left.

Delirium: Reduced ability to pay attention to external stimuli, disorganized thinking, disorientation, and reduced level of consciousness; often manifests as agitation, hyperactivity, hysteria, excessive vocalization, and inability to be calmed.

Obtundation: Decreased consciousness and behavioral responses to mild sensory stimuli; dull, sleepy.

Stupor: Partial or nearly complete unconsciousness; animal maintains a behavioral response to vigorous or noxious stimuli, such as pain.

Coma: Unconsciousness and an absent behavioral response to noxious stimuli, including pain; spinal reflexes may be present or absent.

Anisocoria: Unequal pupil size.

Cheyne-Stokes respiration: Rhythmic waxing and waning of the depth of respiration with regularly recurring periods of apnea.

Decerebrate rigidity: Marked extensor rigidity of the limbs, usually associated with midbrain lesions; animal usually comatose.

Opisthotonus: Dorsal extension of the head, with extension of the thoracic limbs and flexion of the pelvic limbs; often associated with acute cerebellar lesions (decerebellate rigidity).

Meningoencephalitis: Inflammation of the meninges and brain.

Encephalitis: Inflammation of the brain.

Meningoencephalomyelitis: Inflammation of the brain, meninges, and spinal cord.

Meningomyelitis: Inflammation of the meninges and spinal cord.

Meningitis: Inflammation of the meninges.

Myelitis: Inflammation of the spinal cord.

Lesion Localization

✓ Location of lesions that cause stupor or coma is shown in Figure 2-2.

✓ Dementia and delirium result from lesions of the:

    Cerebrum

    Diencephalon

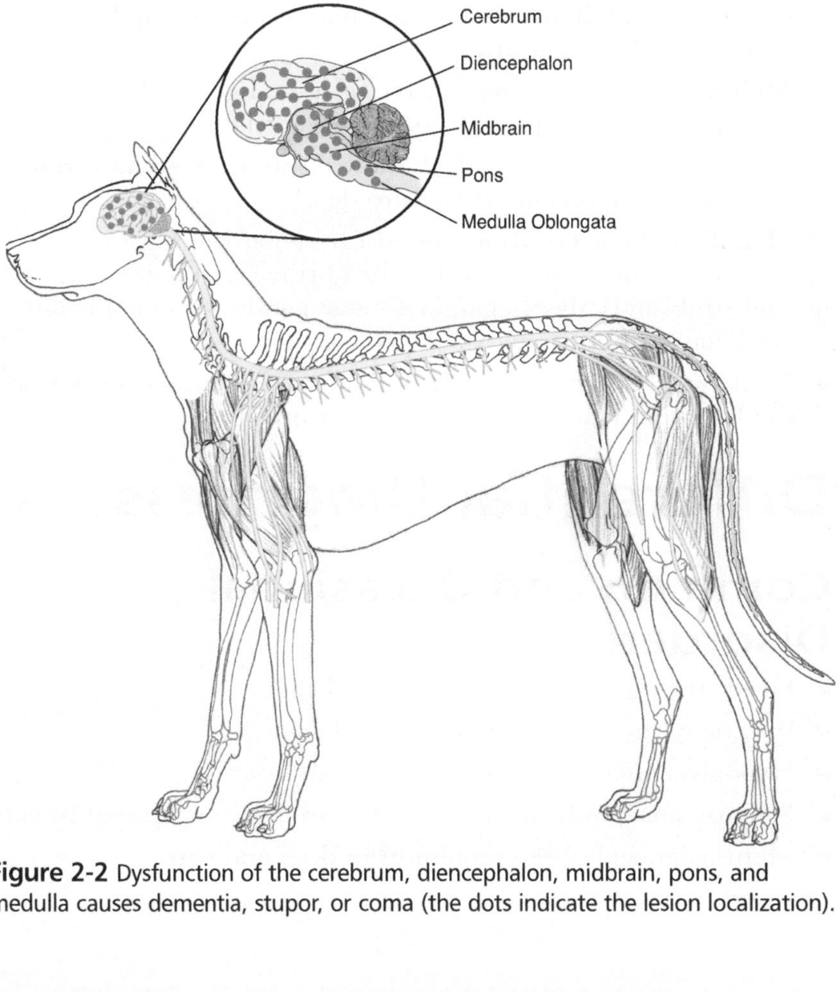

Figure 2-2 Dysfunction of the cerebrum, diencephalon, midbrain, pons, and medulla causes dementia, stupor, or coma (the dots indicate the lesion localization).

✓ Stupor or coma is caused by lesions of the:

Cerebrum

Diencephalon

Midbrain

Pons

Medulla oblongata (stupor)

Differentiation of Lesions Causing Stupor or Coma

✓ Figure 2-3 is an algorithm using changes in pupils and respiration to assist in localizing lesions that cause stupor or coma on the basis of clinical signs.

✓ **Cerebrum and diencephalon:** Normal or miotic pupils; normal or Cheyne-Stokes respiration

✓ **Midbrain:** Dilated, unresponsive or midrange fixed, unresponsive pupils; normal respiration or hyperventilation

✓ **Pons:** Miotic pupils; rapid, shallow respiration; coma is rare, as vital center involvement leads to death

✓ **Medulla oblongata:** Miotic pupils; irregular respiration or apnea; cranial nerve deficits (i.e., head tilt, facial paralysis, medial strabismus, dysphagia, or tongue paralysis); coma is rare, as vital center involvement leads to death

✓ Unilateral lesions at all sites will affect one pupil on the side of the lesion and cause anisocoria (Section 6)

Differential Diagnosis

Common and Occasional Disorders

✓ Head trauma—common in dogs and cats

✓ Intoxication—common in dogs and cats

✓ Hypoglycemia—common in dogs and cats

✓ Hepatic encephalopathy—common in dogs, occasional in cats

✓ Meningoencephalitis—common in dogs and cats

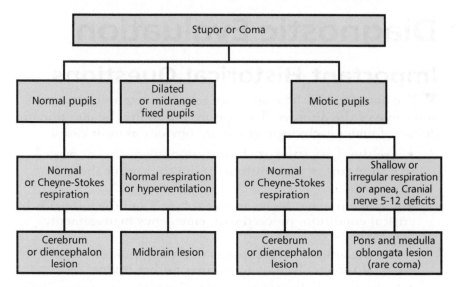

Figure 2-3 Algorithm outlining lesion localization of stupor or coma

✓ Hydrocephalus—common in toy-breed dogs, occasional in other dogs and cats

✓ Neoplasia—common in dogs and cats

✓ Cerebrovascular disorders—occasional in dogs and cats

✓ Hypoxia and anoxia—occasional in dogs and cats

✓ Cognitive dysfunction syndrome—common in dogs

Rare Causes of Stupor and Coma

✓ Diabetes mellitus

✓ Hypothyroidism

✓ Hyponatremia

✓ Hypernatremia

✓ Uremic encephalopathy

✓ Thiamine deficiency

✓ Lysosomal storage disease

✓ Epidermoid, dermoid, and arachnoid cysts

✓ Lissencephaly

Diagnostic Evaluation

Important Historical Questions

♥ The questions in the history are asked to determine the type and cause of the disorder. The reasons for asking the question are discussed under each disorder but are obvious in most cases.

- Are the signs acute or chronic, nonprogressive or progressive, constant or intermittent, or did they occur shortly after birth?

- Possible trauma? If the answer is "yes," and the animal is in critical condition, proceed with emergency management. See Table 2-1.

- Has the animal been exposed to prescription or illegal drugs, antifreeze, lead, ivermectin, or other toxins?

- Is the animal allowed to wander outside?

- Does the animal recognize and respond to the owner?

- Is the animal head pressing, circling, pacing compulsively, or showing increased or reduced activity?

- Does the animal have seizures or other neurologic abnormalities?

- Are there signs of disease in other systems, such as anorexia, polyphagia, polyuria/polydipsia, coughing, sneezing, vomiting, or diarrhea?

- Is there any current or past illness or neoplasia?

- Does the animal receive an all-fish, cooked-meat, or other type of diet deficient in thiamine?

- What is the boarding or travel history (exposure to infectious agents)?

- What recent or current medications, nutriceuticals, herbal supplements or vaccinations has the animal been given?

Physical Examination

♥ Evidence of multisystemic disease, such as fever, icterus, pallor, cyanosis, petechiae or ecchymoses, chorioretinitis, increased lung sounds, heart murmur, abdominal or other masses, renomegaly, alopecia, enlarged lymph nodes, or trauma, should be thoroughly investigated.

✓ Bacterial meningitis can result from hematogenous spread of infections of the endocardium, uterus, bladder, prostate, or elsewhere in the body or directly from sinus or ear infections and animal bites.

Table 2-1
Emergency Management And Monitoring Of Acute Head Injury

1. Ensure animal is breathing and the airway is patent; Intubate and ventilate with oxygen if animal is comatose and in respiratory arrest

2. Evaluate heart rate and rhythm, mucous membrane color, capillary refill time, and pulse strength; attempt resuscitation if in cardiac arrest

3. Administer oxygen by mask or flow-by nose (avoid nasal catheters as sneezing increases intracranial pressure [ICP]); an oxygen cage may be useful for longer term administration

4. Evaluate and monitor blood pressure, and try to keep within normal limits

5. Place an intravenous catheter (avoid jugular vein compression, as this increases ICP)

6. Begin low-volume fluid resuscitation if needed with colloids or hypertonic saline and crystalloids intravenously to maintain normal blood pressure and cerebral blood flow (avoid excessive fluid volume as this may increase ICP)

7. Triage for other life-threatening situations, such as internal hemorrhage or other thoracic or abdominal injuries

8. **Consider therapy to reduce ICP: mannitol as a bolus dose 0.25–2.0 g/kg IV over 10-15 minutes followed in 15 minutes with furosemide, 0.7 mg/kg IV.**

9. Monitor arterial blood gases for ventilation and oxygenation; pulse oximetry may also be useful

10. Keep the head elevated 30 degrees above the heart to ensure venous return from the brain

11. Monitor electrocardiogram (ECG), and treat life-threatening cardiac arrhythmias

12. Monitor body temperature (avoid overheating)

13. Initiate IV antibiotic therapy if a penetrating injury is present

14. Monitor level of consciousness, pupil size and response to light, and respiratory pattern

Neurologic Examination

✓ Animals with cerebral or diencephalic lesions often pace or circle toward the side of the lesion, stand in a corner, or press their head against the wall (Figure 2-4).

✓ Demented animals may appear blind, have no menace response, and do not follow cotton balls but often avoid table legs or walls. Demented, blind animals bump into walls and table legs. If the pupillary light reflex is reduced or absent, an optic nerve lesion is likely. If the pupils are normal, then the lesion is located in the optic radiations or occipital cortex.

✓ Unilateral conscious proprioceptive and other postural reaction deficits are contralateral (on the side opposite the lesion) in cerebral, diencephalic, and rostral midbrain lesions and ipsilateral (on the same side as the lesion) in caudal midbrain, pons, and medulla oblongata lesions.

✓ A deficit of CN 5 localizes the lesion to the pons, and deficits of CN 6-12 localize the lesion to the medulla oblongata (Sections 1 and 6).

✓ Evidence of neck pain may suggest meningoencephalitis or increased intracranial pressure (ICP) secondary to trauma, neoplasia, or other mass lesions.

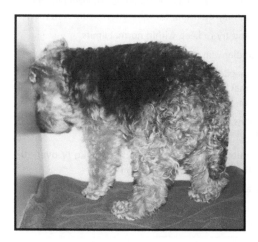

Figure 2-4
A dog that is head pressing.

Applicable Diagnostic Tests

✓ A complete blood count (CBC); serum chemistry profile that includes glucose, blood urea nitrogen (BUN), creatinine, sodium, potassium, calcium, chloride, liver enzymes (such as alanine aminotransferase, aspartate aminotransferase, α-glutamyl transferase, and alkaline phosphatase) and cholesterol and urinalysis can be useful to detect hypoglycemia, renal dysfunction, hepatic dysfunction, and electrolyte abnormalities that may secondarily affect the brain.

✓ Fungal hyphae associated with systemic aspergillosis may be found on cytologic examination of the urine. Ammonium biurate crystals may be found in the urine of animals with hepatic encephalopathy secondary to portosystemic shunts (PSS), and calcium oxalate monohydrate crystals may be found with ethylene glycol intoxication.

✓ A fasting and 2-hour postprandial serum bile acids and blood ammonia level are useful to evaluate liver function and are elevated in hepatic encephalopathy.

✓ An adrenocorticotropic hormone (ACTH) stimulation test may demonstrate hypoadrenocorticism.

✓ Blood gas analysis is useful to detect hypoxemia, acidosis or alkalosis.

✓ Coagulation and platelet function tests, including prothrombin time, partial thromboplastin time, activated clotting time, fibrin split products, mucosal bleeding time, and platelet counts, may be indicated if a cerebrovascular disorder is suspected.

✓ Thoracic radiography and abdominal radiography and ultrasonography may be used to evaluate liver size, examine for portosystemic shunts, or detect neoplasia.

✓ Transcolonic scintigraphy or a venous portogram can be useful to demonstrate portosystemic shunting associated with hepatic encephalopathy.

✓ Histologic examination of a liver biopsy may be necessary to diagnose hepatic microvascular dysplasia or specific causes of liver failure.

✓ Ultrasonography of the brain through a persistent fontanelle can demonstrate hydrocephalus.

✓ Serum total thyroxine (T4) and free T4 levels are usually low and thyroid-stimulating hormone (TSH) levels are often elevated in hypothyroidism.

✓ When overmedication or intoxication is suspected, assays for specific drugs and intoxicants (e.g., phenobarbital, bromide, ethylene glycol, lead) may be performed.

✓ An electroencephalogram (EEG) is usually abnormal in trauma, meningoencephalitis, hydrocephalus, cerebral neoplasia, and severe metabolic disorders.

✓ In comatose animals with respiratory arrest but preserved cardiac function, brain death is indicated by the absence of electrical activity on the EEG or the brainstem auditory-evoked response (BAER) test.

✓ The following are tests that are performed under general anesthesia (unless the animal is comatose), as well as their findings:

• Computed tomography (CT) or magnetic resonance imaging (MRI) can demonstrate hydrocephalus, lissencephaly, focal or multifocal mass lesions, inflammatory or degenerative lesions, edema, and hemorrhage.

• Cerebrospinal fluid (CSF) analysis is performed following CT or MRI if the animal does not have head trauma and other causes of increased ICP are not suspected. The CSF often has increased leukocytes and protein levels in menin-goencephalitis and increased protein levels in neoplasia.

- Brain biopsy with histologic examination of tissue collected may provide a definitive diagnosis and characterize the disease process.

✓ Serum and CSF assays for specific organisms are obtained if meningoencephalitis is documented or an infection is suspected.

✓ Bacterial or fungal cultures of CSF and blood are obtained if an infection is suspected.

Common and Occasional Disorders

Head Trauma

🦴➤ Head trauma from motor vehicle accidents, animal bites, gunshot wounds, or malicious attacks commonly causes dementia, stupor, or coma (Figure 2-5). Concussion is a transient loss of consciousness without structural brain lesions. Structural lesions occurring at the time of trauma may include tearing of brain tissue by bony edges or penetrating injuries or hemorrhage into or around brain parenchyma. Contusion is brain hemorrhage and edema with disruption of nerve fibers. Stupor and coma that persists is most likely caused by contusion. Contusion of the brain tissue can stimulate excessive release of excitatory amino acids, which begin a cascade of events involving intracellular calcium influx, free radical production, cerebral edema, increased intracranial pressure (ICP),

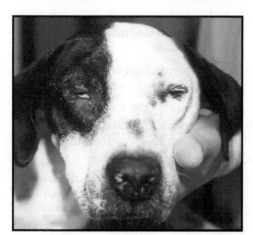

Figure 2-5 A dog with stupor from a head injury.

and cell death. Increased ICP leads to impaired cerebral blood flow and can cause portions of the cerebral cortex to herniate under the tentorium cerebelli and compress the midbrain, producing coma (Figures 2-6 and 2-7). If left untreated, the cerebellum may herniate through the foramen magnum and compress the caudal medulla, causing death (Figures 2-6 and 2-7).

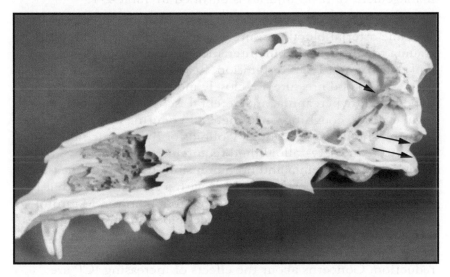

Figure 2-6 A sagittal section of the dog's skull showing the bony tentorium cerebelli (single arrow) and foramen magnum (double arrows).

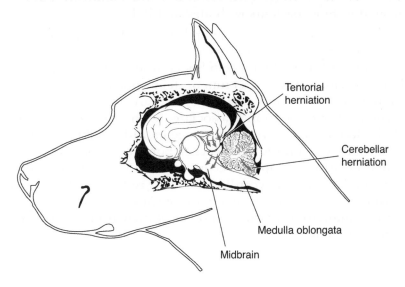

Tentorial herniation

Cerebellar herniation

Medulla oblongata

Midbrain

Figure 2-7 An illustration of tentorial and cerebellar herniation from increased intracranial pressure.

💣 As head injuries are often accompanied by trauma to other body systems, shock, hemorrhage, and other life-threatening problems must be rapidly identified and managed appropriately. Movement of the neck is avoided in comatose animals as combined head and neck injuries can occur. The emergency management of head injuries is outlined in Table 2-1.

🔑 Cerebral blood flow depends upon a balance between systemic arterial blood pressure and ICP, and therapy for head trauma revolves around maintenance of normal blood pressure and reduction of ICP. Respiration, heart rate and rhythm, blood gases, and blood pressure are closely monitored to avoid hypoxemia, hypercapnia, and cerebral ischemia. Pressure on the jugular veins, coughing, sneezing, and vomiting can all elevate ICP and should be prevented. Colloids or hypertonic saline are given to reduce crystalloid fluid requirements and achieve the goals of normovolemia and normotension. ICP can be measured directly in some specialty hospitals with a special probe that is inserted into the brain and connected to a monitor. Mannitol has an osmotic diuretic effect, reduces blood viscosity, improves oxygen delivery to the brain, and is effective for lowering ICP. Furosemide can increase the magnitude and duration of the ICP reduction. Concerns about the effects of increasing ICP are greater than those regarding the theoretic exacerbation of intracranial hemorrhage with mannitol, and administration is indicated in most patients with elevated ICP.

✋ The level of consciousness, pupil size, cardiac rate and rhythm, and respiratory patterns are ideally monitored every 15 to 30 minutes for the first 4 to 6 hours in severely affected patients. Lesions of the cerebrum or diencephalon are better tolerated than those affecting the other parts of the brainstem. Cheyne-Stokes respiration is associated with cerebral and dien-cephalic lesions. Hyperventilation occurs with midbrain lesions. Rapid, shallow respiration indicates a pontine lesion and irregular breathing or apnea occurs with lesions of the medulla oblongata. Marked bradycardia may occur reflexively because of hypertension, which is secondary to increased ICP (Cushing's reflex). Examination findings in order of increasing severity are outlined in Table 2-2.

Table 2-2
Examination Findings in Order of Increasing Severity

MENTATION	PUPILS	CARDIAC RATE	CARDIAC RHYTHM	RESPIRATION
Normal	Normal	Normal	Normal	Normal
Dementia	Miotic	Tachycardia	Ventricular	Cheyne-Stokes
Delirium	Mydriatic	Bradycardia	premature	Hyperventilation
Obtundation	Midrange	Arrest	contractions	Shallow, erratic
Stupor	and fixed		Loss of normal	Apnea
Coma			sinus rhythm	
			Arrest	

🖐 If the pupils are normal or miotic, cardiac rate and rhythm are stable, and respiration is normal or Cheyne-Stokes respiration is present, even severely stuporous or comatose animals may eventually recover if their signs do not worsen within the first 24 hours. If the animal is presented in an acute coma with unresponsive pupils of midrange size and decerebrate rigidity, then a midbrain contusion is likely and the prognosis for recovery is grave. Opisthotonus with preserved consciousness occurs with cerebellar lesions (decerebellate rigidity). Loss of spinal reflexes can occur in a comatose animal with severe brain injury due to release of descending inhibitory pathways that suppress such reflexes. This should be differentiated from reflex loss secondary to concurrent spinal cord or peripheral nerve injuries. Neck or back pain may be associated with a concurrent vertebral fracture; when such pain is noted, vertebral radiographs should be obtained as soon as the patient is stable (see Sections 7, 9, and 12). If the animal is conscious, the cranial nerves can be evaluated and voluntary movement of the limbs should be noted. If the animal is ambulatory and there is no evidence of concurrent spinal trauma, a more complete neurologic examination can be performed (see Section 1).

🖐 Although plain radiographs may detect skull fractures, CT is preferred to demonstrate fractures, acute hemorrhage or edema and to determine the prognosis in patients with deteriorating signs. MRI may be helpful at a later time to delineate the extent of injury. CSF collection is avoided because of the increased risk of brain herniation.

✓ In the absence of an objective measure of ICP, therapeutic decisions must be made on the basis of serial neurologic examination, which is an insensitive evaluation of increasing ICP. If serial neurologic evaluations reveal a decreasing level of consciousness and dilatation of the pupils, herniation of the cerebral cortex under the tentorium cerebelli due to increasing ICP is suspected (Figure 2-7), and aggressive treatment to rapidly reduce ICP is needed

(Table 2-1). Surgery to explore the area and decompress the brain should be considered with penetrating injuries and compressive skull fractures and in animals with intractable elevations of ICP. Corticosteroid administration for head trauma remains a controversial topic. No clinical benefit has been proven following their administration, and in some cases, administration has been associated with a worsened outcome.

✓ The caloric test of brainstem integrity may be performed in comatose animals by warm-water lavage into the external ear canal. If nystagmus is induced, the medulla oblongata, pons, and midbrain are intact. BAER testing can evaluate brainstem integrity and EEG can evaluate cerebral cortex integrity (Section 1). These tests are useful in animals with respiratory arrest but preserved cardiac function. The absence of electrical activity on these tests indicates brain death and a hopeless prognosis.

✓ With adequate nursing care and support, animals with severe cerebral and diencephalic lesions and less severe lesions of the midbrain, pons, and medulla oblongata can recover completely or become acceptable pets. Improvement may continue over 9 to 12 months. Epilepsy may appear as long as 2 years after the head injury but can usually be controlled with anticonvulsant drug therapy (Section 3).

Intoxication

✓ Many substances can cause dementia, delirium, stupor, or coma, and a thorough history of current and recent medications and exposure to prescription, over-the-counter, and illegal drugs and other intoxicants should be obtained. The adverse side effects of all current medications, nutriceuticals, and herbal supplements should be reviewed. The ASPCA National Animal Poison Control Center (888-426-4435) or other poison control centers can provide additional information on potential toxicity and treatment. An overview of some common causes of intoxication is found in Table 2-3 and Section 3, Table 3-3. The emergency treatment of recent oral intoxication is outlined in Table 2-4.

✓ If topical pesticide intoxication is suspected, the animal should be bathed to remove any residual toxin. Assays for anticonvulsants and certain other drugs may be performed to determine if the serum levels are excessive so that the doses may be adjusted (Section 3). Animals that are delirious or seizing from stimulants may have to be sedated (Section 3). A discussion of some common neurologic toxins follows.

Table 2-3
Common Causes of Intoxication

Dementia, stupor, or coma

• Adverse drug reaction from a current medication, nutraceutical, or herbal supplement

• Overdose of prescribed anticonvulsants

• Overdose of other prescription drugs

• Overdose of ivermectin

• Overdose or adverse reaction to pesticides

• Accidental ingestion of owner's alcohol, sedatives, or over-the-counter drugs (e.g., sleep aids, antihistamines)

• Accidental ingestion of marijuana or other illegal drugs

• Accidental ingestion of antifreeze, methanol, cleaning supplies, or industrial solvents

Hyperactivity and delirium

• Adverse reaction from a current medication, nutraceutical, or herbal supplement

• Overdose of prescribed stimulants

• Overdose of ivermectin

• Other pesticide overdose or adverse reaction

• Accidental ingestion of owner's stimulants or over-the-counter drugs (e.g., chocolate, caffeine, antihistamines, tobacco, nicotine gum, etc.)

• Accidental ingestion of amphetamines, cocaine, or other illegal stimulants

• Lead intoxication

Phone number of the ASPCA National Animal Poison Control Center: 888-426-4435

Table 2-4
Emergency Treatment of Recent Oral Intoxication

• Stop seizures if present (Section 3)

• If the animal is conscious, induce vomiting with 1 ml/kg (not to excede 30 ml) of 3% hydrogen peroxide PO or 2 ml/kg (do not exceed 15 ml) syrup of ipecac PO; do not induce vomiting for caustic substances)

• If comatose, perform gastric lavage; intubate trachea to avoid aspiration

• Administer activated charcoal (ToxiBan; Vet-a-Mix) 2–8 g/kg PO or through tube into stomach to reduce further absorption of toxin

• Consider IV fluid therapy to promote renal excretion of the toxin

• Monitor respiration and heart rate; give ventilatory assistance, and treat cardiac arrhythmias as needed

• Give specific antidotes and treatment when indicated

♥ **Ivermectin intoxication** commonly occurs due to dosing errors when owners treat their dogs and cats with a concentrated preparation marketed for use in sheep and cattle (Ivomec, Merial). Although single doses of 2 mg/kg or less may be safe in most dogs, death often occurs with doses over 80 mg/kg. The blood-brain barrier of collies, Shetland sheepdogs, Old English sheepdogs, Australian shepherds, and potentially other breeds appears to be more permeable to ivermectin, and intoxication can be manifested at off-label doses recommended for heartworm microfilaria or other parasites. Signs of intoxication begin within 10 hours and include dilated pupils, agitation, tremors, vocalization, delirium, blindness, head pressing, stupor, and coma. Recent ingestion is treated as outlined in Table 2-4. **There is no specific antidote, and therapy is mainly supportive in nature.** Fluid therapy, nutritional support, and general nursing care should all be provided. Ventilatory support may be required in some cases. Diazepam may act synergistically with ivermectin and should probably be avoided in these animals. Recovery can be prolonged and may take up to several weeks in some cases, but with adequate supportive care, most animals can make a full recovery.

♥ **Pyrethrin and pyrethroid insecticides** may cause depression, hypersalivation, tremors, ataxia, and rarely seizures. Atropine sulfate is not recommended as an antidote for pyrethrin or pyrethroid intoxication. Organophosphate and carbamate intoxication may cause depression, but muscle tremors and seizures are more common. This is discussed in Sections 3 and 4.

♥ **Ethylene glycol intoxication** commonly occurs from ingestion of antifreeze preparations and several other industrial solvents, particularly in the fall and spring when car fluids are replaced to prepare for a change in seasons. One tablespoon of antifreeze can be lethal for a cat. The brain can be directly affected by the toxin or secondarily affected as a result of hypocalcemia, acidosis, and acute renal failure. Vomiting frequently occurs. Neurologic signs begin with ataxia and rapidly progress to tremors, seizures, stupor, and coma. Renal failure follows the onset of neurologic signs and is detectable from 24 to 96 hours after toxin ingestion.

🖐 Hypocalcemia, azotemia, and a large anion gap are found on the serum chemistry profile, and severe metabolic acidosis is found on blood gas analysis. **Numerous calcium oxalate monohydrate crystals, which are characteristic of ethylene glycol intoxication, are often found in the urine, and should not be confused with triple phosphate crystals** (Figure 2-8). If no urine is available, the crystals may be demonstrated in fluid collected from the bladder after catheterization and instillation of a small amount of saline. A colorimetric test for ethylene glycol is available for testing blood or urine samples but is most accurate if used within 24 hours of ingestion. False-positive results may result from ingestion of propylene glycol, which is an additive in some semimoist pet foods. Companies manufacturing antifreeze add a substance that causes it to fluoresce under ultraviolet light, and a Wood's lamp can be used to detect staining around an animals paws or muzzle or fluorescence in a urine sample.

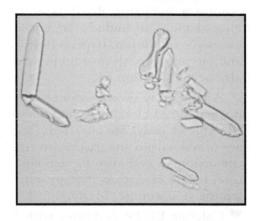

Figure 2-8 Calcium oxalate monohydrate crystals in the urine of a dog with ethylene glycol intoxication. Note the characteristic spindle and dumbell shapes (Courtesy of Drs Rick Alleman, Rose Raskin, and Perry Bain)

🖐 If animals have been observed ingesting the toxin or ingestion is suspected and a positive colorimetric or Wood's lamp test is obtained before clinical signs are evident, early initiation of treatment can be curative. In alert animals that are able to swallow, the standard therapy for intoxication outlined in Table 2-4 can be instituted. Fluid therapy is essential to eliminate toxins and correct dehydration or acidosis. Sodium bicarbonate therapy may be considered in some cases to treat severe acidosis. **The treatment of choice for dogs diagnosed within 24 hours of ingestion is IV fomepizole (Antizol-Vet, Orphan Medical) or 4-methylpyrazole in a 20 mg/kg loading dose, then 15 mg/kg at 12 and 24 hours and 5 mg/kg at 36 hours. For cats treated within 3 hours of toxin ingestion, fomepizole 125 mg/kg IV initially followed by 30 mg/kg at 12, 24 and 36 hours may be effective. Ethanol is recommended for cats (20% at 5 ml/kg IV every 6 hours for five treatments, then every 8 hours for four treatments) or dogs (5.5 ml/kg every 4 hours for five treatments, then every 6 hours for four treatments) when 4-methylpyrazole is not available.** Animals receiving ethanol must be monitored very closely and the dose adjusted if necessary to avoid ethanol toxicosis.

✓ If the animal is in renal failure, blood dialysis is the best option but is available at only a few select referral centers. Peritoneal dialysis is a second option, although it is typically very labor intensive. The prognosis is fair in animals diagnosed and treated early in the course of the illness, but is poor if renal failure is present unless dialysis is available.

♥ **Lead intoxication** can occur from ingestion of lead-based paints, putty, linoleum, roofing material, fishing weights, old batteries, and improperly glazed ceramic dishes. Young dogs are most commonly affected, and intoxication is rare in cats. Anorexia, vomiting, diarrhea, and abdominal pain often occur. Neurologic signs include dementia, blindness, chewing motions, excessive salivation, hyperactivity, and seizures. Megaesophagus and laryngeal paralysis from peripheral nerve involvement may also occur (Section 6).

✓ A CBC may show evidence of mild regenerative anemia with nucleated red blood cells and basophilic stippling of erythrocytes. Blood lead assays are elevated. Occasionally, metallic substances are noted within the gastrointestinal tract with radiography of the abdomen and must be removed from the gastrointestinal tract before chelation therapy with calcium EDTA or D-penicillamine (Cuprimine, Merck).

♥ **Calcium EDTA is diluted with 5% dextrose to a 1% solution (10 mg/ml), and 25 mg/kg SQ is given every 6 hours for 5 days then discontinued for 5 days. The process is repeated if blood lead levels are still elevated. Oral D-penicillamine may be given after or instead of EDTA at 10 to 30 mg/kg every 8 hours on an empty stomach for 1 to 2 weeks.** Gastrointestinal upset can occur and may necessitate use of lower doses. Excessive use of calcium EDTA can result in renal tubular necrosis, and adequate hydration during therapy is essential. A newer therapy, succimer (Chemet, Sanofi), at 10 mg/kg PO every 8 hours for 5 days then every 12 hours for 2 weeks has shown promise as a superior treatment for lead intoxication. The prognosis is fair to good with proper therapy in most animals.

Hypoglycemia

⚕ As glucose is the main energy supply for the proper function of nerve cells, hypoglycemia results in weakness, ataxia, muscle tremors, seizures, dementia, stupor, or coma. Prolonged hypoglycemia leads to neuronal death and permanent brain damage. Clinical signs may be episodic in nature. The causes of hypoglycemia in dogs and cats are listed in Table 2-5.

Table 2-5
Causes of Hypoglycemia

- Inadequate glycogen storage in toy-breed dogs (juvenile hypoglycemia)
- Insulin overdose
- Insulinoma
- Excessive exercise in fasted hunting dogs
- Hepatic failure
- Sepsis
- Hypoadrenocorticism
- Paraneoplastic syndrome (hepatic tumors, leiomyosarcoma)
- Excessive parasitism
- Starvation (rare)

👋 A serum glucose level below 50 mg/dl indicates hypoglycemia, but levels can become normal between hypoglycemic episodes. A sample taken after a 24 to 48-hour fast may be necessary to document hypoglycemia. Other biochemical or CBC abnormalities are usually present in hepatic failure, hypoadrenocorticism, or sepsis. Elevated pre- and 2-hour postprandial bile acids support a diagnosis of hepatic failure. An ACTH-stimulation test may be useful to document hypoadrenocorticism. If an insulin-secreting tumor is suspected, the animal is fasted under supervision until blood glucose falls below 60 mg/dl, and blood is collected in a sodium fluoride tube for a paired plasma insulin and glucose determination. A high-normal or elevated insulin level (greater than 10 µU/ml) in the presence of hypoglycemia is suggestive of an insulin-secreting tumor. An amended insulin-glucose ratio can also be calculated (Table 2-6).

✔ Abdominal ultrasonography is superior to plain radiography to visualize insulinomas or other masses, but because of the small size of these tumors, surgical exploration with gross examination and palpation of the pancreas may be necessary for diagnosis.

Table 2-6
Amended Insulin-Glucose Ratio

$$\frac{\text{Plasma insulin } (\mu U/ml) \times 100}{\text{Plasma glucose } (mg/dl) - 30mg} = X\mu U/mg$$

Note: A ratio of greater than 30 µU/mg is suggestive of an insulin-secreting tumor

♥ Fifty percent dextrose 1–2 ml/kg IV diluted 1:1 in saline and administered slowly is indicated to correct hypoglycemia in animals with stupor or coma. Fifty percent dextrose 1–2 ml/kg PO may be used in animals able to swallow. Owners may apply a sugar solution (corn syrup) directly to the oral mucous membranes if signs occur at home. In cases of juvenile hypoglycemia, exercise-induced hypoglycemia, or insulin overdoses, dextrose therapy alone may be adequate. Obviously, the reasons for the decompensation or overdose should be investigated, and the need for continued insulin therapy fully evaluated, especially in cats, where transient insulin resistance is a possibility. Animals with hepatic failure, hypoadrenocorticism, sepsis, or a paraneoplastic syndrome will require additional specific therapy for these underlying conditions.

♥ Administration of dextrose to dogs with insulinomas may temporarily alleviate clinical signs but can stimulate the tumor to secrete more insulin, resulting in severe hypoglycemia within a few hours. The goal in such cases should be to alleviate clinical signs rather than attempt to normalize blood glucose. If the response to dextrose administration is adequate, the animal should be fed a small, high-protein meal every 4 to 6 hours. Some animals may require a constant-rate infusion of 2.5% to 5% dextrose at 3–4 ml/kg/hr IV to control clinical signs. In refractory cases, it may be necessary to add dexamethasone 0.5–1.0 mg/kg in the IV fluids over 6 hours or octreotide 20–40 µg SQ every 8 to 12 hours may be necessary.

♥ Surgical removal of the primary tumor and all visible metastases is the treatment of choice and offers the best long-term prognosis. When the tumor has been removed, hypoglycemia is often at least temporarily resolved. However, many insulinomas have metastasized at the time of diagnosis and the long-term diagnosis may be guarded to poor. Metastatic foci may not secrete insulin for several months.

✓ Long-term medical therapy consists of feeding three to six small meals daily, limiting exercise, and administering prednisone 0.25 mg/kg/day PO. Animals refractory to prednisone and dietary therapy may be given diazoxide (Proglycem, Baker Norton) 5–13 mg/kg PO every 12 hours. Serum glucose levels are monitored closely until stable. With early diagnosis, surgical therapy, and medical management, even dogs with metastatic insulinomas may retain a reasonable quality of life for a year or more. The prognosis may be better for paraneoplastic processes associated with other tumors, as hypoglycemia often resolves with complete surgical excision.

Hepatic Encephalopathy

⚡ The pathophysiology of hepatic encephalopathy is complex and multifactorial and remains the subject of considerable debate. The disorder results from failure of the liver to filter portal blood from the intestinal tract before it enters systemic circulation. Ammonia and other toxic products from the intestines enter the circulation and reach the brain, where they alter cerebral function. Other factors, such as the formation of false neurotransmitters and cerebral edema, may also play a role. The causes of hepatic encephalopathy are outlined in Table 2-7.

Table 2-7
Causes of Hepatic Encephalopathy

Congenital

- Extrahepatic or intrahepatic portosystemic shunts
- Hepatic microvascular dysplasia

Acquired

- Acute hepatitis
- Chronic active hepatitis
- Hepatic lipidosis
- Toxic hepatic necrosis
- Cirrhosis
- Liver neoplasia

🖐 Congenital PSS occurs most commonly in small- and toy-breed dogs and occasionally in cats. Larger dogs tend to have intrahepatic PSS. Hepatic microvascular dysplasia (MVD) occurs most commonly in Yorkshire and Cairn terriers and other small-breed dogs. Clinical signs of PSS usually occur within the first year of life, but can be delayed until middle age. MVD often occurs later than PSS, and many dogs remain asymptomatic for life. Acquired liver failure may occur at any age.

✓ The history may reveal episodes of dementia after feeding or signs compatible with chronic hepatic dysfunction. Acute stupor or coma can occur. Intermittent seizure activity alone is very unusual with hepatic encephalopathy. Many animals do not have seizures, and if present, alterations in mentation are usually obvious. The physical examination often shows poor growth with PSS or may reveal abnormalities related to liver disease. Ptyalism is common in cats, and the iris is frequently a striking copper color (Figure 2-9). The neurologic examination may be normal or may show dementia, stupor, coma, apparent blindness, pacing, circling, head pressing, and ataxia.

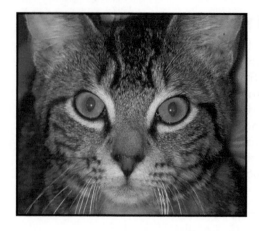

Figure 2-9 A cat with copper colored irises associated with hepatic encephalopathy.

✔ The CBC typically shows microcytosis with PSS or may be inflammatory in cases of hepatitis. Serum biochemical evaluation may show increases in liver enzymes and decreases in BUN, cholesterol, albumin, and glucose. Ammonium biurate crystals are often found in the urine of animals with PSS. Pre- and postprandial serum bile acid assays are usually markedly elevated in all cases with signs of hepatic encephalopathy. Blood ammonia testing can also be useful, but sample handling is critical—the sample should be placed into a chilled tube and separated immediately after collection. Animals with MVD may not have elevated blood ammonia.

✋ Abdominal radiographs typically show a small liver with PSS, while cases with hepatitis or hepatic neoplasia may show hepatomegaly. In hepatic MVD and other hepatopathies, liver size can be normal. Abdominal ultrasonography can further delineate these abnormalities, and visualization of a shunting vessel is often possible. Transcolonic scintigraphy is useful to document shunting of blood around the liver. CT or MRI of the brain may show evidence of cerebral edema but are most useful to rule-out other disease processes. The definitive diagnosis is often made with surgery through gross visualization of abnormal vasculature or with the aid of a portogram. Histologic examination of a liver biopsy may be necessary to make a diagnosis of hepatic MVD or acquired acute or chronic liver failure.

♥ Medical therapy consists of correction of fluid and electrolyte disturbances and reduction of absorption of toxic substances from the intestinal tract. Hypokalemia, metabolic alkalosis, and hypoglycemia can all exacerbate hepatic encephalopathy and must be corrected if present. A well-balanced, low-protein, high-complex carbohydrate diet is provided. **Lactulose 0.25–0.5 ml/kg PO**

every 8 to 12 hours can be given to dogs and cats and the dose
adjusted so that the stool is slightly soft. Lactulose is a semisyn-
thetic disaccharide that acidifies intestinal contents, alters
bacterial flora, shortens intestinal transit time, and reduces
ammonia absorption within the colon. **Lactulose may be used
alone or in conjunction with oral neomycin 20 mg/kg every 8 to
12 hours, ampicillin 22 mg/kg every 8 hours, or metronidazole 7
mg/kg every 12 hours to reduce the anaerobic and urea-splitting
bacterial flora in the gastrointestinal tract.**

✔ In comatose animals that are unable to swallow, lactulose may
be given as a retention enema. After a cleansing enema is given,
an inflated Foley catheter is inserted into the rectum and 20
ml/kg of a mixture of three parts lactulose with seven parts water
is instilled into the lower colon and left in place for 15 to 20
minutes. If lactulose is unavailable, a 10% povodone-iodine
solution may be substituted. **If cerebral edema is suspected,
administration of mannitol as a bolus dose 0.25–2.0 g/kg IV over
10 to 15 minutes followed in 15 minutes by furosemide 0.7
mg/kg IV can be considered.**

♥ **The surgical treatment of choice for animals with congenital
PSS is partial ligation or attenuation of the anomalous vessel.
Extrahepatic PSS are easier to repair than are intrahepatic
shunts.** Severe seizures and status epilepticus are uncommon
complications after partial ligation of a PSS and may require
aggressive therapy with potassium bromide or propofol or isoflurane
anesthesia (Section 3). If episodic seizures continue after surgery,
potassium bromide at 22 to 44 mg/kg PO every 12 hours is the
preferred anticonvulsant, as it is excreted by the kidneys and not
metabolized by the liver (Section 3). Specific therapy for hepatitis,
hepatic neoplasia, or intoxication should be given as needed. The
prognosis for hepatic encephalopathy varies greatly and depends on
the underlying cause and severity of the clinical signs.

Meningoencephalitis

🤚 Meningoencephalitis or encephalitis is on the differential
diagnosis list for any dog or cat presented with dementia, compulsive circling or pacing, stupor, or coma as well as seizures, head tilt,
or other signs of cranial neuropathy, generalized incoordination,
and head tremors (Sections 3 through 6 and 8). Meningitis,
meningomyelitis, or myelitis can cause neck or back pain, paresis,
or paralysis (Sections 7 through 13). The organisms that most
commonly cause meningoencephalitis, encephalitis, meningoencephalomyelitis, meningitis, meningomyelitis, and myelitis in dogs
and cats are listed in Table 2-8.

Table 2-8

Specific Organisms, Diagnosis, and Prognosis of Central Nervous System Infections of Dogs and Cats

INFECTIOUS AGENTS	MOST COMMON ORGANISMS	CYTOLOGIC RESULTS OF CEREBROSPINAL FLUID (CSF)	OTHER TESTS	PROGNOSIS
Viruses-Dogs	Distemper (canine distemper virus- CDV) Rabies Pseudorabies	Lymphocytic pleocytosis or normal	Specific serum and CSF assays, CT, and MRI; Conjunctival cytologic studies for CDV; None-Rabies and Pseudorabies	Distemper: fair to poor; Rabies: dead in 10 days; Pseudorabies: dead in 3 days
Viruses-Cats	Feline infectious peritonitis (FIP), Feline immunodeficiency virus (FIV), Rabies, Undetermined ("viral non-FIP")	FIP: neutrophilic leukocytosis; FIV: normal or mild pleocytosis; Rabies: lymphocytic pleocytosis; Undetermined: neutrophilic or lymphocytic pleocytosis	Specific serum and CSF assays (unreliable for FIP but reliable for FIV); None-Rabies	FIP: poor; FIV: guarded; Rabies: dead in10 days; Undetermined: good
Protozoa	*Toxoplasma gondii* *Neospora caninum* (dogs)	Mixed cell, neutrophilic, or eosinophilic pleocytosis	Specific serum and CSF assays; CT and MRI	Guarded
Fungi	*Crytococcus neoformans* *Aspergillus spp.* (dogs) *Blastomyces dermatidis* *Coccidiodes inmitis* *Cladosporium spp.*	Mixed cell, neutrophilic, or rarely eosinophilic pleocytosis may be visible organisms (Cryptococcus)	Specific serum and CSF special stains for organisms; CSF culture; Urinalysis (may see hyphae); CT and MRI	Guarded
Bacteria	*Streptococcus spp.* *Staphylococcus spp.* *Pasteurella spp.* Anaerobes	Neutrophilic pleocytosis; may be mixed-cell population if animal on antibiotics	Gram stain CSF; CSF and blood cultures	Guarded-poor
Rickettsia and spirochetes of Dogs	*Erhlichia canis, Rickettsia rickettsia* (Rocky mountain spotted fever), *Borrelia burgdorferi* (Lyme disease)	Neutrophilic, mixed, or monocytic pleocytosis	Specific serum and CSF assays	Fair-guarded
Parasites	*Cuterebra spp.* *Dirofilaria immitis*	Neutrophilic or eosinophilic pleocytosis	CT and MRI	Guarded

✔ Although there are many infectious causes of meningoencephalitis in dogs, most cases are not associated with a known organism (Table 2-9).

♥ Steroid-responsive meningoencephalitis (SRME) can occur in dogs of any breed or age and probably represents atypical or mild cases of steroid-responsive meningitis/arteritis (SRMA), granulomatous meningoencephalitis (GME), necrotizing meningoencephalitis (NME), an immune-mediated disorder, or an unclassified viral infection. Beagles, Boxers, Bernese mountain dogs, and German shorthaired pointers younger than 2 years of age are most commonly infected with SRMA, but it does affect other dogs as well. Many cases of SRMA have severe neck pain without other neurologic signs. The diagnosis, prognosis and treatment are discussed in Section 7. NME, also known as pug encephalitis, affects Pugs, and Maltese and Yorkshire terriers from 2 months to 10 years of age. Neurologic signs in Pugs and Maltese terriers are similar and primarily reflect involvement of the cerebrum (seizures, circling, head pressing, stupor, coma), whereas Yorkshire terriers typically have brainstem involvement. A steroid-responsive eosinophilic meningoencephalomyelitis (EME) occurs in Golden retrievers.

Table 2-9
Noninfectious Causes of Inflammation of the Central Nervous System in Dogs

DISEASE	MOST COMMON CYTOLOGIC RESULTS OF CEREBROSPINAL FLUID	OTHER TESTS	PROGNOSIS
Steroid-responsive meningoencephalitis	Mixed, lymphocytic, or monocytic pleocytosis	CT or MRI	Excellent
Steroid responsive meningitis/arteritis	Neutrophilic pleocytosis	CT or MRI	Excellent
Granulomatous meningoencephalitis	Mononuclear, mixed-cell, or neutrophilic pleocytosis	CT or MRI; Histologic examination of brain biopsy	Poor
Necrotizing meningoencephalitis	Lymphocytic pleocytosis	CT or MRI; Histologic examination of brain biopsy	Poor
Eosinophilic meningoencephalomyelitis	Eosinophilic pleocytosis	CT or MRI	Excellent

🖑 Body temperature is often normal in animals with meningoencephalitis except in cases with systemic infections. A cardiac murmur may be found in cases of bacterial endocarditis that have showered bacterial emboli to the brain. Bacterial meningitis can also result from hematogenous spread of infection from the uterus, bladder, prostate, or elsewhere in the body or from direct extension of bacteria from sinus or ear infections, animal bites, and neurosurgical procedures. Chorioretinitis can be found with many infectious agents and GME (Figure 2-10).

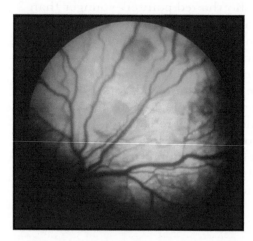

Figure 2-10
Chorioretinitis in a dog with distemper meningoencephalitis.

🖑 Neurologic signs are usually multifocal in nature, and seizures, cranial nerve deficits, postural-reaction deficits, and spinal hyperpathia frequently accompany changes in mentation. The CBC is usually normal, although leukocytosis may be seen with bacterial or fungal infections and thrombocytopenia is often noted with rickettsial disease. An elevated fibrinogen level is often seen regardless of cause. Diagnosis rests upon the demonstration of inflammatory CSF, which usually consists of elevations in both the white blood cell count and protein. In cases of severe stupor or coma, CT or MRI is performed prior to CSF collection, if possible, to note cerebral edema, mass lesions, or shifts in brain tissue associated with increased ICP.

🖑 Many cases of meningoencephalitis show patchy, diffuse, or multifocal lesions on CT or MRI, helping to distinguish them from primary neoplasia (Figure 2-11). Occasionally, a protozoal or fungal granuloma, GME, or abcess may appear as a mass indistinguishable from neoplasia on CT and MRI (Figure 2-12). Histologic examination of a biopsy specimen may be necessary for a definitive diagnosis.

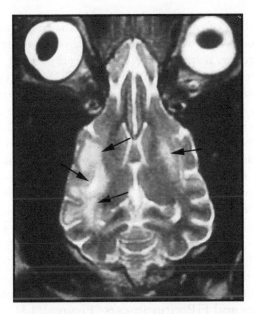

Figure 2-11 Dorsal T2–weighted MRI of the brain showing multifocal lesions (arrows) in the cerebral white matter associated with granulomatous meningoencephalitis. Fluid is white on T2–weighted images; note the white aqueous and vitreous humor of the left and right eyes at the top of the picture (the left cerebrum is on the viewer's right, and the right cerebrum is on the viewer's left).

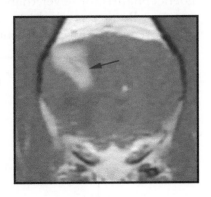

Figure 2-12
Transverse post-contrast T1–weighted MRI of focal granulomatous meningoencephalitis in the right cerebrum (arrow) that might be mistaken for neoplasia.

💣☀ Collection of CSF from the cerebellomedullary cistern in animals with increased ICP can lead to brain herniation (Figure 2-7) into the low-pressure area created by CSF removal, resulting in coma, apnea, or death. Collection of CSF from the lumbar region may be safer in these animals, although herniation can still occur. **If increased ICP is suspected, IV mannitol as a bolus dose 0.25–2.0 g/kg is administered over 10 to 15 minutes followed in 15 minutes with furosemide 0.7 mg/kg prior to CSF collection.**

The diagnosis of meningoencephalitis is suspected when leukocytic pleocytosis (more than 6 cells/µl) is found on CSF analysis. However, normal CSF or elevated protein alone may be seen in cases of canine distemper virus (CDV) encephalitis, other focal parenchymal infections, or GME that does not communicate with the CSF. Leukocytic pleocytosis can also be associated with trauma, intervertebral disk herniation, and neoplasia, although meningoencephalitis is strongly suspected when cell counts exceed 50 cells/µl. Cytologic results of CSF can be similar for many different causes of meningoencephalitis (Tables 2-8 and 2-9). When neutrophilic pleocytosis is present, blood and CSF culture for aerobic and anaerobic bacteria or fungi can be considered. This can be unrewarding, however, even in cases of bacterial meningoencephalitis. As much CSF fluid as possible should be submitted for culture, although the total amount of CSF removed should not exceed 1 ml/5 kg of body weight. The most common causes of neutrophilic pleocytosis are SRMA in dogs and FIP virus in cats (Figure 2-13).

Meningoencephalitis caused by the rabies virus is often clinically indistinguishable from other viral encephalitides. The potential for transmission to humans and invariably fatal course dictate that unvaccinated animals with clinical signs of meningoencephalitis for fewer than 10 days should be handled with caution. Protective clothing and gloves should be worn and appropriate quarantine measures taken. Serum antibody titers are

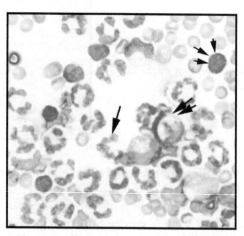

Figure 2-13 Pleocytosis consisting of neutrophils (single arrow), macrophages (double arrow), and lymphocytes (triple arrows) with red blood cells in the background in a cat with meningoencephalitis associated with the feline infectious peritonitis virus.

usually not elevated in unvaccinated dogs as the rapid disease progression does not allow time to mount an antibody response. Although no reliable premortem diagnostic test for rabies is available, infected animals deteriorate and die within 3 to 10 days. If death occurs in a suspect animal, the brain should be examined by the necessary public health officials. Diagnosis is made with a fluorescent antibody test and by demonstrating typical negri bodies on histologic examination of brain tissue.

✓ Serum and CSF assays are available for many infectious organisms (Table 2-8). If antibody titers are used, immunoglobulin (Ig) G and IgM determinations are obtained if available. Elevated IgG levels indicate previous exposure, vaccination, or chronic infection. An elevated IgM level suggests recent exposure or vaccination (within 3 weeks) or an active disease process. Polymerase chain reaction tests for specific organisms may be more accurate, if available. Antibody titers are usually higher in the serum than in the CSF, although some organisms, notably CDV, may cause intrathecal production of immunoglobulins, leading to higher CSF titers. In animals with elevated CSF protein, the presence of CSF IgG may represent compromise of the blood-brain barrier, especially when serum IgG levels are elevated.

✓ Corticosteroid therapy is the usual treatment for SRME, SRMA, GME, NME, and EME. Since many dogs have some type of steroid-responsive meninogoencephalitis and it may take several days to obtain the results of infectious organism assays, corticosteroid therapy as outlined in Table 2-10 is initiated if there is no evidence of a bacterial, fungal or protozoal infection. Several doses of corticosteroids may even be beneficial to reduce inflammation in patients with infectious encephalitis. Oral trimethoprim-sulfadiazine and occasionally doxycycline may be given for 5 to 7 days while assay results are pending. If the assays indicate an infectious process, corticosteroid therapy is discontinued and the appropriate antimicrobial therapy listed in Table 2-11 administered.

✓ **If GME is suspected or confirmed through histologic examination of a brain biopsy, the antineoplastic drug procarbazine (Matulene, Sigma Tau) may be given PO at 2–4 mg/kg/day for 1 week then increased to 4–6 mg/kg/day.** The CBC and platelet numbers should initially be monitored every week. If the leukocyte count falls below 4000 cells/µl or platelets are less than 100,000 /µl, the drug is discontinued until the leukocyte count returns to normal. Therapy may be needed for 6 to 12 months to control clinical signs. Periodically withdrawing the drug may be tried to test for relapse. Radiation therapy is useful for focal lesions and can prolong survival time for more than a year in some cases. Dogs with focal signs have significantly longer survival times than those with multifocal signs. GME may not be a single disease process, and some lesions have histopathologic features suggestive of neoplasia.

✓ Parasite migration may be treated with prednisone 0.25–0.5 mg/kg PO every 12 hours to reduce inflammation related to movement of the organism through the tissues.

✓ The prognosis for meningoencephalitis varies with the cause and is outlined in Tables 2-8 and 2-9. Since many dogs have SRME, the prognosis for eventual recovery is often excellent.

Table 2-10
Treatment of Meningoencephalitis in Dogs When No Organism Can Be Identified

- Intravenous **methylprednisolone sodium succinate** (Solu Medrol, Pharmacia & Upjohn) 10-15 mg/kg every 6-8 hours is given for 24 hours if the dog is severely stuporous, comatose, or has severe seizures or other life-threatening neurologic dysfunction

- Oral **prednisone** 1-2 mg/kg every 12 hours is given in milder cases or following intravenous therapy (signs often improve in 3-5 days)

- Oral or intravenous **famotidine** (Pepcid AC, Merck) 0.5-1 mg/kg every 12-24 hours, or **cimetidine** (Tagamet, SmithKline Beecham) 5-10 mg/kg every 8 hours is given to protect the gastrointestinal tract from the deleterious effects of the prednisone; oral **sucralfate** (Carafate, Hoechst Marion Roussel) 0.25 g for cats or 0.5-1.0 g for dogs every 8-12 hours can also be used, but it must be separated from other oral medications by several hours, as it may bind them and reduce efficacy

- Oral or intravenous **trimethoprim-sulfadiazine** 15 mg/kg every 12 hours is often given while the results of infectious organism assays are awaited and is discontinued if assay results are normal

- Oral or intravenous **doxycycline** (Vibramycin, Pfizer) 5 mg/kg every 12 hours may be given while rickettsial assay results are awaited if infection with these organisms is suspected

- Oral **prednisone** is continued for 3-4 weeks or until signs resolve and then reduced by 25%-50% every 2-4 weeks until alternate-day therapy is feasible; if signs return as the dose is reduced, the drug is increased to the original amount for a few days and then reduced to the last effective dose; many dogs are tapered from prednisone therapy after 3-6 months and remain free of clinical signs

- In refractory cases consider the addition of procarbazine (see text for details)

Table 2-11
Antimicrobial Therapy for Infectious Meningoencephalitis

Bacterial infections (provide oral therapy for 4-6 weeks with one or more of the following):
- **Trimethoprim-sulfadiazine** 15-30 mg/kg every 12 hours or **ormetoprim-sulfadimethoxine** (Primor, Pfizer) 15 mg/kg every 12 hours

- **Chloramphenicol** (Chloromycetin, Monarch) 45-60 mg/kg every 8 hours for dogs and 25-50 mg/kg every 12 hours in cats (chloramphenicol should not be used in conjunction with pentobarbital, phenobarbital, primidone, or diphenylhydantoin)

- **Metronidazole** (Flagyl, SCS) 10-15 mg/kg every 8 hours in dogs and 10 mg/kg every 12 hours in cats (monitor for additional CNS signs, which may be caused by neurotoxicity – Section 5)

- **Enrofloxacin** (Baytril, Bayer) or **ciprofloxacin** (Cipro, Bayer) 2.5-5 mg/kg every 12 hours in dogs or cats (monitor visual impairment from retinal degeneration in cats [Section 6])

Protozoal infections (provide oral therapy for 2-4 weeks with one or more of the following):
- **Trimethoprim-sulfadiazine** 15-30 mg/kg every 12 hours or **ormetoprim-sulfadimethoxine** (Primor) 15 mg/kg every 12 hours

- **Clindamycin** (Antirobe, Pfizer) 5-10 mg/kg every 12 hours in dogs and cats (may add to trimethoprim-sulfadiazine therapy)

- **Pyrimethamine** (Daraprim, Glaxo Wellcome) 0.5-1.0 mg/kg once daily for 3 days then reduced to 0.25 mg/kg once daily for 14 days in dogs and cats (may add to trimethoprim-sulfadiazine therapy). Some immunosuppression may be seen; animals should be closely monitored.

Rickettsial and spirochete infections (provide oral therapy for 10-14 days)
- **Doxycycline** (Vibramycin, Pfizer) 5 mg/kg every 12 hours for dogs or cats

Fungal infections (provide oral therapy for 3-6 months with one of the following):
- **Fluconazole** (Diflucan, Pfizer) 2.5–5.0 mg/kg once daily in dogs or 2.5–10 mg/kg every 12 hours in cats (best CNS penetration)

- **Itraconazole** (Sporanox, Janssen) 5 mg/kg once daily in dogs and 10 mg/kg once daily in cats

- *Ketoconazole is not recommended*

FIV infections (oral therapy)
- AZT or zidovudine 15-20 mg/kg every 12 hours indefinitely.

Hydrocephalus

☙ Hydrocephalus is dilatation of the ventricular system of the brain and is most commonly observed as a congenital disorder in toy breed or brachycephalic dogs younger than 1 year of age. Hydrocephalus can also occur secondary to an acquired obstruction of CSF flow by cerebral neoplasia or meningoencephalitis, decreased CSF absorption by meningoencephalitis or trauma, and overproduction of CSF associated with a choroid plexus tumor. Loss of brain tissue from inflammation or degeneration adjacent to the ventricular system results in passively enlarged ventricles.

✓ Clinical signs are often chronic and progressive but may be episodic or acute in nature. Such behavioral abnormalities as dementia, aggression, compulsive circling or pacing, and difficulty in training are common (Figure 2-14). Seizures may also occur (Section 3). In cases of congenital hydrocephalus, a persistent fontanelle, due to failure of the sutures of the skull to close completely, and bilateral ventrolateral strabismus are often noted. Some hydrocephalic dogs have a normally formed skull, and some dogs with a persistent fontanelle do not have congenital hydrocephalus. The gait may be normal, ataxic, or paretic, and some animals have visual deficits. Hippus (rhythmic dilation and constriction of the pupils) may be noted.

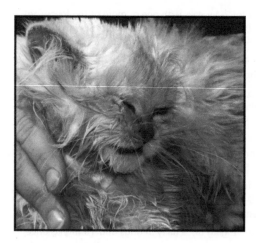

Figure 2-14
A kitten with dementia associated with hydrocephalus.

✓ Lack of the normal gyral pattern caused by smoothing of the inner calvarium in congenital hydrocephalus may be visible on plain skull radiographs. Enlarged ventricles may be detected with ultrasonography through a persistent fontanelle. Ventricular dilatation is obvious on CT and MRI (Figure 2-15). Increased amplitude and decreased frequency of waveforms seen on EEG are characteristic of but not pathognomonic for hydrocephalus. Leukocytic pleocytosis or elevations of protein may be found on CSF evaluation if hydrocephalus is secondary to meningoencephalitis or neoplasia.

✋ In animals with acquired hydrocephalus, the underlying cause should be addressed accordingly. **Medical therapy of congenital hydrocephalus consists of prednisone 0.25–0.5 mg/kg PO every 12 hours for 1 week. Therapy should be tapered to the lowest alternate-day dose able to control the neurologic signs.** Response

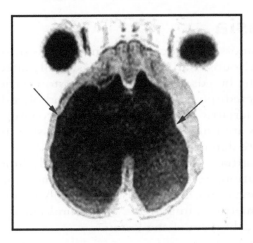

Figure 2-15 Dorsal T1–weighted MRI of the kitten in Figure 2-14 showing massive ventricular enlargement (arrows) (fluid is dark on T1–weighted images; see the two eyeballs at the top of the picture).

to medical therapy is often good, and prednisone may eventually be discontinued after several months. Anticonvulsant therapy with oral phenobarbital 2–4 mg/kg every 12 hours or potassium bromide 22 to 44 mg/kg every 12 hours should be provided if the animal has seizures (Section 3). This therapy may have to be continued indefinitely.

💣☀ Dogs with a persistent fontanelle and thin calvarium are more susceptible to hemorrhage from head injuries, and mild trauma can exacerbate the clinical signs. Exacerbation of the signs can also occur spontaneously and may require the prednisone therapy to be repeated. **If severe stupor, coma, or cluster seizures occur, the animal may be treated with IV mannitol 0.25–1.0 g/kg over 10-15 minutes and methylprednisolone sodium succinate 10 to 15 mg/kg every 8 hours for 24 hours followed by oral prednisone.**

✓ Surgical placement of a ventriculoperitoneal shunt, which drains excess CSF from a lateral ventricle into the peritoneal cavity, may provide long-term control of hydrocephalus. Occlusion of the shunt tubing and infection are potential complications of this procedure. The prognosis depends mainly on the degree of neurologic impairment, and varies widely. Some dogs with severe ventricular dilatation only have mild behavioral abnormalities while others can decompensate and progress to a comatose state that is unresponsive to therapy.

Neoplasia

Brain tumors are typically seen in animals over 5 years of age, although younger animals are occasionally affected. Brachycephalic breeds, such as Boxers, Boston terriers, and Bulldogs are predisposed to astrocytomas and oligodendrogliomas. Geriatric cats often have slow-growing meningiomas. Clinical signs are usually chronic and progressive in nature, although acute deteriorations—sometimes associated with spontaneous hemorrhage—can be seen. Cerebral dysfunction and altered mentation are related both to the tumor and to the secondary edema. Seizures are also commonly observed (Section 3), and asymmetric cranial nerve or postural-reaction deficits may aid in localization of the lesion.

✓ CT or MRI usually demonstrates a mass lesion (Figure 2-16). However, although certain tumors have characteristic imaging appearances, it should be remembered that other causes, including infectious disease and hemorrhage, can produce mass lesions in the brain. Thus, definitive diagnosis may require biopsy and histologic analysis. Ultrasonography or CT-guided biopsies of lesions may allow definitive diagnosis so that an optimal therapeutic plan can be made.

As discussed with meningoencephalitis, collection of CSF is risky in patients with increased ICP, as brain herniation is possible (Figure 2-7). **If increased ICP is suspected, IV mannitol as a bolus dose 0.25 to 2.0 g/kg is administered over 10 to 15 minutes followed in 15 minutes with furosemide 0.7 mg/kg prior to CSF collection.** Elevation of CSF protein without concurrent pleocytosis is typical with neoplasia, although occasionally mild-to-marked elevations of leukocytes in the CSF confuse the diagnosis. Several different tumors found in dogs and cats are listed in Table 2-12.

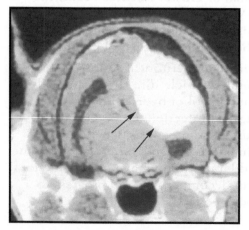

Figure 2-16 Transverse post contrast T1–weighted MRI showing a mass that is compressing the left cerebrum (arrows) of a cat with progressive dementia.

Table 2-12
Types of Cerebral Neoplasia

- Meningioma
- Astrocytoma
- Oligodendroglioma
- Choroid plexus papilloma/carcinoma
- Ependymoma
- Pituitary adenoma
- Lymphoma
- Primitive neuroectodermal tumor
- Metastatic neoplasia

✓ Treatment of cerebral neoplasia involves combinations of surgery, radiation therapy, and chemotherapy. Although craniotomy for the removal of meningioma is often very effective in cats (Figure 2-17), this group of tumors tends to be aggressive in dogs, and adjunctive radiation therapy is usually indicated. Radiation therapy without excisional surgery can be considered for some tumors. Oral lomustine is believed to slow tumor growth and may be an option for some animals. **Lomustine 60 mg/m^2 PO is given, and a CBC and platelet count is performed every week for 5 weeks. If the leukocyte count is 5000 cells/µl or above and platelets are in the normal range, then the lomustine dose is increased to 80 mg/m^2.** Monitoring the CBC and platelets continues, and treatments are repeated every 5 to 8 weeks. If the CBC and platelet counts remain stable, they are then monitored every 1 to 3 months. **Prednisone 0.25–0.5 mg/kg PO every 12 hours can reduce secondary cerebral edema and relieve clinical signs for several months in some cases.** New advances in surgery, radiation therapy, and chemotherapy are improving the prognosis for cerebral neoplasia.

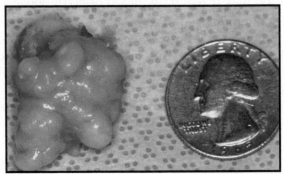

Figure 2-17 The mass shown in Figure 2-16 removed; histopathologic examination showed it to be a meningioma, and the cat recovered completely.

Cerebrovascular Disorders

🔒 Cerebrovascular disorders (strokes) include brain infarction or ischemia, and spontaneous hemorrhage. Although common in humans, these disorders occur only occasionally in dogs and cats. Thrombus formation secondary to coagulopathies, sepsis, neoplasia, localized vasospasm, or heartworm infection can obstruct the flow of blood to specific brain regions. Atherosclerosis associated with hypothyroidism, idiopathic hyperlipidemia, polycythemia, and angiocentric lymphoma are rare causes of cerebral infarction or ischemia in small animals. Feline ischemic encephalopathy appears to be related to migration of the parasite *Cuterebra spp.* through the cerebrum in cats. Spontaneous hemorrhage may occur secondary to hypertension, arteriovenous malformations or similar congenital anomalies, cerebral neoplasia, vasculitis, or coagulopathies.

✓ Acute onset of dementia, stupor, or coma is typically noted. Seizures and other neurologic signs are often seen depending on the brain region affected. Examination may reveal evidence of an underlying systemic disease or asymmetric neurologic deficits.

✓ Acute hemorrhage is best visualized on a CT scan, although MRI is more sensitive in detecting edema related to infarctions and in the visualization of brainstem lesions (Figure 2-18). Blood pressure should be evaluated to rule out hypertension. Bleeding times and platelet counts and function tests should be evaluated for possible coagulopathies prior to CSF collection. The underlying etiology of a cerebrovascular accident often cannot be found. **If increased ICP is suspected, intravenous mannitol as a bolus dose 0.25–2.0 g/kg is administered over 10 to 15 minutes followed in 15 minutes with furosemide 0.7 mg/kg prior to CSF collection.** CSF evaluation may reveal frank blood or erythrophagocytosis.

✓ Treatment should be tailored to address the underlying disease, if one exists. **Prednisone 0.25–0.5 mg/kg PO every 12 hours for 3 to 5 days with subsequent tapering may be considered in such cases as animals with aberrant parasite migration.** The prognosis for cerebrovascular disorders depends on the severity of the neurologic signs, location of the lesion, and ability to correct underlying disease.

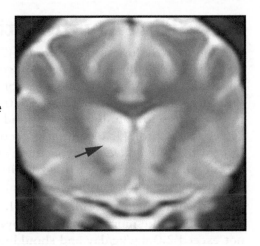

Figure 2-18
Transverse flair MRI of a transverse section of the brain showing infarction in the right caudate nucleus in a dog (arrow).

Hypoxia and Anoxia

Hypoxic and anoxic brain insults can occur secondary to anesthetic accidents, respiratory depression from drugs or head trauma, smoke inhalation, severe pulmonary disease, and suffocation from aspiration of vomitus or foreign bodies. Since oxygen is necessary for proper energy metabolism of the brain, hypoxia or anoxia leads to neuronal death and cerebrocortical necrosis. Reperfusion and reoxygenation during resuscitation or recovery can lead to the excessive release of excitatory amino acids and production of free radicals, which cause further injury to the brain. Dementia, stupor, coma, seizures, and blindness may occur. The diagnosis is usually obvious, but tests such as pulse oximetry, arterial blood gas analysis, and measurement of blood carboxyhemoglobin levels, can help to characterize the problem. Pulmonary disease or aspiration pneumonia may be assessed with thoracic radiographs. MRI of the brain may be useful in determining the extent of cerebral edema initially and cerebrocortical necrosis later.

✓ Oxygen therapy should be administered as soon as possible after the injury. Systemic hypotension, acidosis, and dysfunction of other body systems are treated accordingly. The use of corticosteroids in this setting is controversial and has not shown clear benefits. Newer treatments for reperfusion injury are currently being investigated. As with head-injured animals, some animals suffering severe brain damage can recover with time and adequate nursing care. Recovery may continue for 9 to 12 months. In other cases, neurologic deficits, such as blindness and changes in mentation or behavior, may persist.

Cognitive Dysfunction Syndrome

✓ Cognitive dysfunction syndrome (CDS) may be suspected when no cause can be found for progressive dementia in elderly dogs. Clinical signs of CDS include a loss of training, inappropriate urination or defecation, decreased activity and attention, altered interactions with family members, and changes in the sleep-wake cycle. The neurologic examination is otherwise normal. Blood tests, urinalysis, and CSF analysis are also normal, and there are no specific diagnostic tests for this condition. Brain atrophy with ventricular enlargement may be found on CT or MRI.

✦※ **Selegiline hydrochloride (Anipryl, Pfizer) 0.5–1.0 mg/kg PO once daily in the morning may improve mentation. The dose should not exceed 2.0 mg/kg/day and should not be used concurrently with tricyclic antidepressants, such as clomipramine, amitriptyline, and imipramine, or serotonin reuptake blockers, such as fluoxetine (Prozac, Dista), as toxicosis and death can occur. Improvement is typically noted within 1 month of the initiation of therapy. Vitamin E 30 IU/kg/day not to exceed 400 IU every 12 hours is a potent and readily available antioxidant with neuroprotective effects and may be beneficial in CDS. Gingko biloba standardized extract 2–4 mg/kg every 8 to 12 hours is an herbal preparation that increases cerebral blood flow, and may also be useful for CDS.** Prescription diets are available to support brain function.

Rare Causes of Stupor and Coma

Diabetes Mellitus

✓ Some dogs and cats with diabetes mellitus may develop dementia, stupor, or coma due to a hyperosmolar syndrome with or without ketoacidosis. Concurrent clinical signs often include severe dehydration, weakness, tachypnea, and vomiting, and an acetone odor may be detected on the breath. Serum glucose is often profoundly elevated (greater than 600 mg/dl). Other laboratory abnormalities include increased serum osmolality (greater than 350 mOsm/kg), hypernatremia, prerenal azotemia, metabolic acidosis, and glucosuria. The therapy, which consists of rehydration and **gradual** reduction of blood glucose, is complex and beyond the scope of this text. Serum electrolytes, particularly potassium and phosphorus, must be monitored closely to avoid additional complications. The prognosis for most animals is fair to good with aggressive medical therapy.

Hypothyroidism

✓ Myxedema coma associated with hypothyroidism occurs rarely in dogs. Stupor or coma is accompanied by bradycardia, hypothermia, and occasionally seizures. If pitting edema is present, and microcytic anemia and elevated cholesterol are found on the CBC and chemistry profile, respectively, the diagnosis may be suspected but serum total T4, free T4, and TSH levels should be evaluated on all dogs with stupor or coma of unknown cause. Other complications, such as hyponatremia and hypoventilation, can be seen. The serum total T4 or free T4 levels are very low or undetectable, and serum TSH levels are elevated. The EEG appears flat. Ventilatory support may be needed, and the animal may appear to be near death. Levothyroxine sodium (Synthroid, Knoll Pharmaceutical) 5 mg/kg IV every 12 hours is given for 1 to 2 days as soon as the diagnosis has been established. **Levothyroxine sodium is then given 0.02 mg/kg PO every 12 hours, and serum levels are monitored every 2 weeks until the patient is stable.** Additional treatment consists of correcting hypothermia and electrolyte imbalances and general nursing care. The prognosis is good if therapy is initiated early, and marked improvement is usually seen within 24 hours. Thyroid replacement therapy is often needed indefinitely.

Hyponatremia

✓ Low serum sodium, or hyponatremia, affects the osmotic balance of the brain and vascular system and causes cerebral edema. Ataxia, dementia, stupor, coma, and seizures may result. Hyponatremia can be associated with hypoadrenocorticism, chronic diarrhea secondary to endoparasitism, or loss of sodium-rich fluids from severe burns or chronic effusions. A syndrome of inappropriate secretion of antidiuretic hormone is also recognized after head trauma and cerebrovascular accidents.

✓ The diagnosis is usually straightforward after examination of a serum biochemical profile, and levels less than 130 mEq/l are considered dangerous. An ACTH-stimulation test may be useful to document hypoadrenocorticism. Fecal flotation facilitates the diagnosis of endoparasitism. CT or MRI can be considered if a cerebrovascular accident is a possibility or to investigate the extent of known head trauma.

🖐 It is useful to consider hyponatremia in light of serum osmolarity. Hyponatremia with a normal or increased serum osmolality suggests that other substances, such as lipids, glucose, protein, urea, or toxins, are attracting water into the vascular space and diluting the sodium. Hyponatremia with hypoosmolarity (<280 mOsm/kg) suggests increased total body water relative to sodium from the mechanisms listed above.

✓ Treatment consists of correcting the sodium deficit and treating any underlying disease. Rapid correction of chronic hyponatremia can lead to damage of the myelin sheaths of neurons (myelinolysis) and further neurologic deterioration. Some guidelines for correction of hyponatremia are outlined in Table 2-13.

✓ The prognosis for hyponatremia is good with appropriate therapy if the underlying condition can be successfully treated.

Table 2-13
Guidelines for the Correction of Hyponatremia

- If hypovolemia is present, correct with intravenous 0.9% saline
- If hypervolemia is present, give intravenous furosemide 2-4 mg/kg

Calculate the sodium deficit as follows:
$$Na^+ \text{ deficit (mEq/l)} = (140 - \text{serum } Na^+) \times \text{(body weight in kilograms)} \times 0.3$$

- Replace the sodium deficit over 12-24 hours using 0.9% saline or hypertonic saline (3%-5%), if necessary (avoid rapid correction as myelinolysis and further deterioration is possible)
- Mild cases with excessive intravascular volume may respond to cautious water restriction

Hypernatremia

✓ Elevated serum sodium, or hypernatremia, adversely affects the osmotic balance between the brain and vascular system and causes cerebral dehydration. Cerebral hemorrhage may also occur from damaged blood vessels due to shifts in brain tissue. Ataxia, dementia, stupor, coma, and seizures are the most common signs, but cranial nerve deficits may be seen secondary to hemorrhage. Hypernatremia can be associated with decreased water intake, diabetes insipidus, diabetes mellitus, heat stroke, renal failure, or rarely from the ingestion of toxic quantities of salt.

🖐 Sodium values greater than 180 mEq/L can cause severe brain dehydration. Elevated BUN, creatinine, or glucose on the serum chemistry profile with isosthenuria or glucosuria supports a diagnosis of renal failure or diabetes mellitus. Examination of urine specific gravity in association with water deprivation and possibly antidiuretic hormone administration can aid in a diagnosis of diabetes insipidus if the animal is alert enough for this procedure.

✓ If hypernatremia is chronic, correction of the sodium imbalance is cautiously performed to avoid iatrogenic cerebral edema. The plan for fluid replacement therapy should be considered in light of the body systems, as multiple systems are often involved. Some guidelines for fluid replacement therapy for hypernatremia are outlined in Table 2-14.

✓ If the underlying disease can be treated, appropriate correction of the hypernatremia usually results in a functional recovery.

Table 2-14
Guidelines for Fluid Replacement Therapy for Hypernatremia

- If perfusion is poor, correct volume deficits rapidly with sodium-containing crystalloids or colloids:

- *Correct dehydration over 12-24 hours with lactated Ringer's solution, 0.9% saline, or 0.45% saline*

- Re-measure sodium and correct remaining extracellular water deficit with the following formula:

Water deficit (liters) = [(New Na$^+$ - 140)/140] x (body weight in kg) x 0.6

Uremic Encephalopathy

✓ Uremic encephalopathy can be associated with severe acute or chronic renal failure and azotemia. The pathogenesis is not entirely clear, but as with hepatic encephalopathy, it may be associated with failure to clear toxic metabolites and development of cerebral edema. Clinical signs include depression, stupor, coma, weakness, and seizures. The diagnosis is presumptive, and is based on biochemical evidence of renal failure. Systemic hypertension leading to cerebral hemorrhage may contribute to clinical signs in some animals with chronic renal failure. Treatment is focused on the correction of azotemia and other concurrent problems, such as hypertension and electrolyte abnormalities. The prognosis is usually poor.

Thiamine Deficiency

✓ Routine feeding of well-balanced pet foods has made deficiency of thiamine (vitamin B1) a rare condition. However, this disorder can still occur in animals fed all fish or cooked-meat diets. Thiamine, like glucose and oxygen, is necessary for normal energy metabolism in the brain, and deficiency leads to neuronal necrosis and brainstem hemorrhage. Dementia, stupor, seizures, blindness, mydriasis, dysequilibrium, and ventroflexion of the neck may be seen. **IV thiamine 10–20 mg in cats and 25–50 mg in dogs is given and then repeated SQ daily until signs resolve. Thiamine 2 mg/kg PO once daily may be given to supplement the diet.** If therapy is initiated early, complete recovery is usually seen.

Lysosomal Storage Disorders

✓ Lysosomal storage disorders result from the congenital absence or inactivity of a specific lysosomal enzyme. The substrate normally metabolized by that enzyme accumulates within the cells leading to cellular death or dysfunction. Although the cells of many body systems can be affected, neuronal cell death causes progressive and permanent neurologic deficits. Animals are typically younger than 1 year of age, although clinical signs may not manifest until middle age or later in some diseases.

🖐 Many breeds of dogs and cats are affected, and the clinical signs vary with the specific enzyme deficit (Table 2-15). Initial signs of dementia or aggression are most commonly associated with GM2 gangliosidosis, fucosidosis, and ceroid lipofuscinosis. With some disorders, connective tissue or skeletal involvement or hepatosplenomegaly may be evident. Diagnosis of these diseases has traditionally been difficult without necropsy and histologic examination of the brain. However, CT and MRI studies may show characteristic changes with some diseases, making a presumptive diagnosis possible in an appropriate breed. Other potential diagnostic tests are also listed in Table 2-15.

✓ Finding a laboratory that assays leukocytes for a specific enzyme can be difficult, and obtaining results can be slow. Lymph node, liver, muscle, peripheral nerve, or brain biopsy may show accumulation of storage material within various cells, and special histologic stains may help differentiate the type of substrate stored. No effective therapy is currently available. The prognosis for these diseases, because of their progressive nature, is poor.

Table 2-15 Lysosomal Storage Disorders

DISEASE/DEFICIENT ENZYME	STORAGE MATERIAL	SPECIES	CLINICAL SIGNS	POTENTIAL DIAGNOSTIC TESTS
GM1 gangliosidosis (type 1 and 2)/ β-galactosidase	Ganglioside	Dogs and cats	Tremor, incoordination, spastic paraparesis, ataxia, nystagmus	Assay enzyme in leukocytes; Biopsy lymph node or cerebellum
GM2 Gangliosidosis (type 1-3)/ hexosaminidase A, B or both	Ganglioside	Dogs and cats	Ataxia, incoordination, dementia, blindness, tremors, nystagmus	Assay enzyme in leukocytes; Biopsy lymph node, liver or cerebellum
Glucocerebrosidosis/ β-glucocerebrosidase (Gaucher's Disease)	Glucocerebroside	Dogs	Ataxia, incoordination, tremors	Assay enzyme in leukocytes; Biopsy lymph node or cerebellum
Sphingomyelinosis/ Sphingomyelinase (Niemann Pick Disease)	Sphingomyelin	Dogs and cats	Ataxia, incoordiation, tremors; Paraparesis	Assay enzyme in leukocytes; Biopsy lymph node, liver or cerebellum
Globoid cell leukodystrophy/ galactosylceramidase (Krabbe's Disease)	Galactocerebroside	Dogs and cats	Ataxia, incoordination, progressive paraparesis	Assay enzyme in leukocytes; Biopsy lymph node or peripheral nerve; CSF analysis; MRI
Metachromatic leukodystrophy/ arylsulfatase	Sulfatide	Cats	Seizures, opisthotonus	None
Mucopolysaccharidosis/ arylsulfatase B or α-L--iduronidase and others	Mucopolysaccharide	Dogs and cats	Progressive paraparesis	Assay enzymes in leukocytes; Assay substrate in urine
Mannosidosis/ α-mannosidase	Mannoside	Cats	Ataxia, incoordination, and tremors	Assay urine oligosaccharide
Glycogenosis/α-glucosidase (Pompe's Disease)	Type II glycogen	Dogs and cats	Incoordination, paraparesis, tetraplegia	Assay enzymes in leukocytes
Fucosidosis/ α-L-fucosidase	Fucoglycoproteins	Dogs	Behavior changes, dementia, seizures, ataxia, hearing and vision loss, dysphagia	Assay enzyme in leukocytes and CSF
Ceroid lipofuscinosis	Ceroid and lipofuscin	Dogs and cats	Behavior changes, blindness, ataxia, tremors dementia, seizures	Biopsy lymph node, liver or cerebellum

Epidermoid, Dermoid, and Arachnoid Cysts

✓ Epidermoid, dermoid, and arachnoid cysts may rarely occur in the brain and cause neurologic signs. They are sometimes found incidentally at necropsy. Increased availability of CT and MRI has led to increased recognition of these structures in small animals. Surgical removal may be successful in some cases. Arachnoid cysts can cause progressive compression of the spinal cord and are discussed in Section 13.

Lissencephaly

✓ Lissencephaly is a congenital absence of the normal gyri and sulci of the brain (Figure 2-19). The cerebral cortex is also missing certain cell layers and is thinner than normal. Lhasa Apsos are most frequently affected, although lissencephaly may affect other breeds of dog and cats. The disorder occurs in animals younger than 1 year of age, and signs consist of dementia, aggression, seizures, and visual dysfunction. The lack of gyri and sulci and thin cortex may be visualized on MRI. There is no specific therapy for this condition. Seizures may be controlled with anticonvulsant drugs (Section 3). The prognosis is poor.

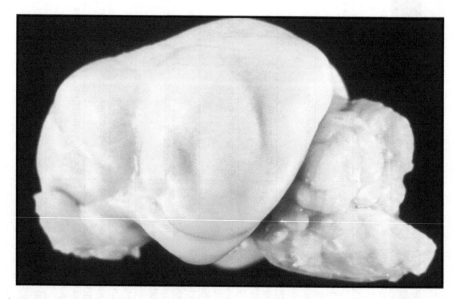

Figure 2-19 The brain of a dog with lissencephaly showing a smooth surface due to the lack of normal gyri and sulci.

Section 3
Seizures

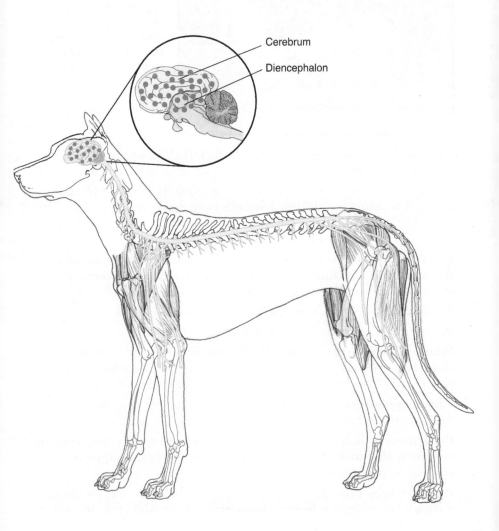

Cerebrum

Diencephalon

Definitions

Seizure (convulsion, ictus, fit): Clinical manifestation of excessive and/or hypersynchronous neuronal discharges in the brain; may manifest as episodic impairment or loss of consciousness; abnormal motor phenomena; psychic or sensory disturbances; or autonomic nervous system signs, such as salivation, vomiting, urination, and defecation (Figures 3-1, 3-3, 3-4, 3-5 and Table 3-1).

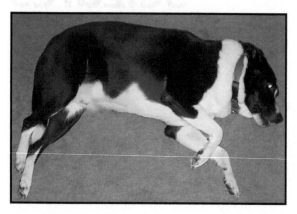

Figure 3-1
Seizures have many clinical manifestations but tonic-clonic limb movements are common.

Epilepsy: A chronic neurologic condition characterized by recurrent seizures.

Tonic: A sustained increase in muscle contraction lasting a few seconds to minutes; during a seizure may result in a facial grimace, opening of the jaws, dorsal extension of the head and neck and extension of the limbs.

Clonic: Regularly repetitive, brief, involuntary muscle contractions; during a seizure may cause facial twitching, chomping of the jaws, and jerking movements of the neck and limbs.

Tonic-clonic: Alternating periods of tonic and clonic activity.

Atonic: Sudden reduction or loss of muscle tone.

Status epilepticus: Continuous seizure activity lasting longer than 10 minutes or the occurrence of multiple seizures without recovery of baseline neurologic function between episodes.

Cluster seizures: Two or more seizures occurring within a 24-hour period.

Prodrome: A behavioral phenomenon that precedes the onset of a seizure; the animal may hide, follow the owner, or appear restless or frightened.

Aura: A subjective sensation that marks the onset of a seizure; difficult to recognize in veterinary medicine unless the animal vomits, salivates, or inappropriately urinates or defecates immediately before onset of the seizure.

Localizing sign: Asymmetric motor involvement of the face or limbs at the onset of a seizure.

Postictal phase: Atypical behavior that immediately follows the seizure; the animal may be restless, delirious, lethargic, confused, blind, thirsty, hungry, inappropriately urinate or defecate; may last from a few seconds to several hours.

Lesion Localization

✓ **Lesions that cause seizures are shown in Figure 3-2** and are located in the:

- Cerebrum
- Diencephalon

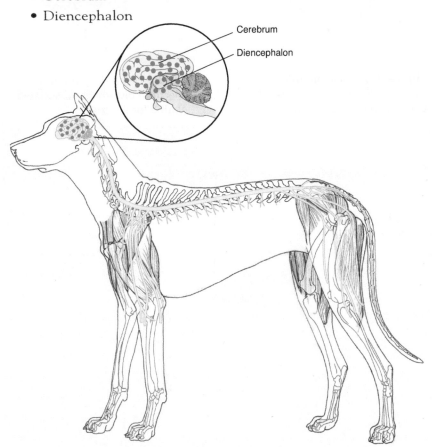

Figure 3-2 Dysfunction of the cerebrum or diencephalon causes seizures (the dots indicate the lesion localization).

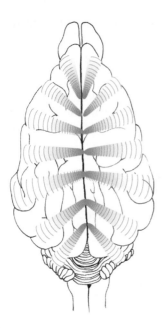

Figure 3-3 A diagram of the electrical disturbance associated with a generalized seizure.

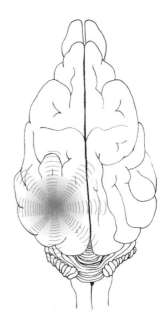

Figure 3-4 A diagram of the electrical disturbance associated with a focal seizure.

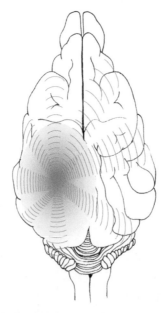

Figure 3-5 A diagram of the electrical disturbance associated with a focal seizure that secondarily generalizes.

Table 3-1
Types of Seizures

Generalized seizures: Abnormal electrical discharges affecting the cerebral hemispheres bilaterally and usually causing symmetric signs (Figure 3-3).

- **Generalized tonic-clonic seizures (grand mal):** Bilaterally symmetric tonic-clonic movements of the face, jaw, and limbs; the animal is unconscious (eyes may be open), in lateral recumbency, and often salivates, urinates, and/or defecates
- **Other variations of generalized motor seizures:** May be exclusively tonic, clonic, or atonic, and the animal may be fully conscious, mentally altered, or unconscious; animal often salivates, urinates, and/or defecates
- **Absence seizures (petit mal):** Impaired consciousness with lack of or minimal motor activity; poorly recognized in animals

Focal (partial) seizures: Abnormal electrical discharges of the neurons in a focal area of the brain (Figure 3-4); may have asymmetric motor or sensory signs, such as twitching of the eyelids, lips, or ears, or pawing at the face on one side; rare manifestations are episodic vomiting or diarrhea; the animal may display bizarre behavior, howling, aimless running, or circling (complex partial or psychomotor seizures or running fits)

Table 3-2
Classification of Epilepsy and Other Causes of Seizures

Type	Former Terms Used in Veterinary Literature	Description
Idiopathic epilepsy	Primary epilepsy or inherited epilepsy	Seizures without an underlying structural lesion of the brain or other neurologic signs; presumed to be genetic and are usually age-dependent
Symptomatic epilepsy	Secondary epilepsy	Seizures caused by an identifiable structural lesion of the brain (head trauma, encephalitis, neoplasia, hydrocephalus, lissencephaly, or lysosomal storage disorder)
Probable symptomatic epilepsy	Cryptogenic epilepsy or acquired epilepsy	Seizures believed to result from a structural lesion of the brain although no cause can be identified; suspected residual brain damage from a previous intracranial or extracranial disorder
Extracranial disorders	Reactive seizures	Disorders, such as hepatic encephalopathy, hypoglycemia, and intoxications, that may cause seizures but are not considered to be epilepsy

Based on the current recommendations of the International League Against Epilepsy. *Epilepsia* 42:796, 2001.

Differential Diagnosis by Age Group

Younger Than 1 Year of Age

✓ Head trauma–common in dogs and cats

✓ Intoxication–common in dogs and cats

✓ Hypoglycemia–common in dogs, occasional in cats

✓ Meningoencephalitis–common in dogs and cats

✓ Hepatic encephalopathy–common in dogs, occasional in cats

✓ Hydrocephalus–common in toy-breed dogs, occasional in others

✓ Probable symptomatic epilepsy–common in dogs older than 6 months of age

✓ Idiopathic epilepsy–occasional in select breeds of dogs older than 6 months of age

✓ Hypocalcemia–occasional in dogs and cats

✓ Thiamine deficiency–rare in dogs and cats

✓ Lysosomal storage disorders–rare in dogs and cats

✓ Lissencephaly–rare in dogs and cats

1 to 5 Years of Age

✓ Probable symptomatic epilepsy–common in dogs, occasional in cats

✓ Hydrocephalus–common in toy breed dogs, occasional in other dogs and cats

✓ Head trauma–common in dogs and cats

✓ Meningoencephalitis–common in dogs and cats

✓ Intoxication–common in dogs and cats

✓ Hepatic encephalopathy–common in dogs, occasional in cats

✓ Idiopathic epilepsy–common in select breeds of dogs

✓ Hypoglycemia–occasional in dogs and cats

✓ Hypocalcemia–occasional in dogs and cats

✓ Cerebrovascular disease–occasional in dogs and cats

✓ Thiamine deficiency–rare in dogs and cats

✓ Neoplasia–rare in dogs and cats

Older Than 5 Years of Age

✓ Probable symptomatic epilepsy–common in dogs, occasional in cats

✓ Meningoencephalitis–common in dogs and cats

✓ Neoplasia–common in dogs and cats

✓ Hypoglycemia–common in dogs and cats

✓ Hepatic encephalopathy–occasional in dogs and cats

✓ Head trauma–occasional in dogs and cats

✓ Intoxication–occasional in dogs and cats

✓ Idiopathic epilepsy–occasional onset in dogs 5 to 7 years of age

✓ Cerebrovascular disease–occasional in dogs and cats

✓ Hypocalcemia–occasional in dogs and cats

✓ Thiamine deficiency–rare in dogs and cats

✓ Uremic encephalopathy–rare in dogs and cats

✓ Polycythemia–rare in dogs and cats

Diagnostic Evaluation

Important Historical Questions

♥ The history is often the most important aspect of evaluating an animal with seizures, as only the owner usually observes seizure events and the neurologic examination is frequently normal. The history is also critical to developing an appropriate diagnostic and therapeutic plan. The following questions will help develop a thorough history and subsequently an appropriate therapeutic plan.

- **Was the first seizure within the past few weeks or months ago?** Extracranial disorders and symptomatic epilepsy may be considered higher on the differential diagnosis list if the seizures began recently; idiopathic and probable symptomatic epilepsy may be more likely in an animal that has had intermittent seizures for many months and is normal between episodes.

- **How frequent are the seizures? Are there episodes of status epilepticus or clusters? Is there a repeatable seizure pattern?** Idiopathic or probable symptomatic epilepsy usually begins with a single seizure and then gradually becomes more frequent, often progressing to cluster seizures or status epilepticus over time. Many dogs with long-term seizures have a predictable pattern when seizures will occur (e.g., every 4 weeks). The seizure frequency and pattern also impact decisions regarding the initiation and type of anticonvulsant therapy.

- **Is there a prodrome?** Describe. If the owner can be warned of an impending seizure by consistent behavioral changes, they might be able to abort or reduce seizure activity by administering rectal, nasal, or oral anticonvulsant drugs. Occasionally, other animals in the household sense the prodrome and can warn the owner.

- **What is the appearance of the seizure?** Generalized seizures are commonly associated with extracranial causes of seizures and inherited epilepsy and occasionally with symptomatic and probable symptomatic epilepsy. Focal seizures and focal seizures that secondarily generalize are associated with an intracranial disorder like symptomatic or probable symptomatic epilepsy. Focal seizures that begin in the facial muscles and then generalize with little motor movement are more common in cats than in dogs.

- **Is a videotape of the seizures available or can the owner obtain one?** A videotape of the episodes can be helpful to differentiate seizures from other disorders and to determine whether the seizures are symmetric or asymmetric.

- **How long are the seizures?** Most seizures last a few seconds or minutes; focal seizures may be brief but can occur in clusters.

- **Is there a postictal phase?** Describe. Identification of a postictal phase can be important to confirm seizures, as such activity is not seen with syncope, narcolepsy, or rapid-eye-movement (REM) behavior disorder. In rare instances, the animal may have to be sedated because of prolonged hyperactivity during the postictal phase and occasionally may become aggressive. Such animals should not be handled until this phase resolves.

- **Is the animal normal between the seizures?** If the animal's behavior is abnormal between well-spaced seizure events, then seizures from extracranial disorders or symptomatic epilepsy is more likely.

- **Are the seizures associated with sleeping, feeding, fasting, exercise or stressful situations**? Some dogs with idiopathic epilepsy or probable symptomatic epilepsy may seize while sleeping but cannot be awakened like animals with REM behavior disorder. Seizures following feeding may be associated with hepatic dysfunction. Seizures during fasting, exercise, or stress may be associated with hypoglycemia. Stressful situations may precipitate seizures in a few dogs with idiopathic or probable symptomatic epilepsy.

- **Do seizures occur after application of pesticides to the animal or environment?** Some epileptic animals will have seizures after exposure to topical or environmental pesticides that do not adversely affect normal animals. The owner should be questioned regarding a relationship between seizures and house or yard spraying or administration of medications for parasite control.

- **Has there been exposure to other drugs or toxins?** Intoxication is a common cause of seizures, and exposure to prescription, over-the counter, illegal drugs, nutriceuticals, and herbal preparations should be questioned. Insulin overdose in diabetic animals frequently causes seizures and altered mentation. Some ceramic products (dishes and bowls), fishing weights, older paint, caulking compounds, golf balls, and other products contain lead that can be toxic to animals. Animals that roam freely may have access to ethylene glycol (antifreeze) especially in the spring and fall.

- **What is the pet's vaccination status?** Incompletely vaccinated animals can have seizures associated with the canine distemper or rabies viruses; animals incompletely vaccinated for rabies that are exposed to wildlife should be handled with appropriate precaution, including use of protective gloves and clothing, quarantine, and limited human contact.

- **Has there been a recent or past illness or neoplasia?** As with the history in other problems, questions regarding recent or past lethargy, anorexia, vomiting, diarrhea, coughing, sneezing, polyuria/polydipsia, or polyphagia are asked to find evidence that might indicate extracranial disorders or symptomatic epilepsy associated with a systemic infection or neoplasia.

- **Was there a recent or past head injury?** Seizures may occur at the time of a head injury or up to 2 years later from residual brain scarring.

- **Is there a familial history of seizures?** If the parents, siblings, or other relatives have epilepsy, an inherited problem should be suspected.

- **What is the diet?** Although rare, thiamine deficiency can cause seizures in dogs and cats. Inadequate nutrition leading to hypoglycemia can cause seizures in toy-breed dogs.

- **What previous medications or treatments have been given for seizures?** Current anticonvulsant medications or other therapies and their effectiveness should be documented to help develop an effective strategy for long-term seizure management if necessary.

- **How frequent can the client administer medications?** The ability of a client to medicate and provide long-term management of an animal with seizures should be discussed, as maintenance anticonvulsant drugs may have to be given every 8 to 12 hours for the life of the animal.

Warning: Some topical products for flea and tick control considered safe in normal animals may precipitate status epilepticus and death in epileptic dogs and cats.

Physical and Neurologic Examinations

✓ Auscultate the chest for evidence of murmurs, arrhythmias, or abnormal lung sounds.

✓ Evaluate body temperature, mucous membrane color, lymph node size, and note evidence of systemic illness.

✓ Carefully palpate the abdomen for evidence of neoplasia.

✓ Examine the retina for evidence of chorioretinitis indicating systemic infections or granulomatous meningoencephalitis (GME).

✓ A thorough neurologic examination is essential to detect abnormalities other than seizures. The animal may be demented or stuporous shortly after the seizure or as a result of anticonvulsant therapy. The neurologic examination should be repeated after recovery from the seizure. Animals with asymmetric neurologic abnormalities most likely have symptomatic or probable symptomatic epilepsy.

Applicable Diagnostic Tests

Diagnostic plans for specific types of seizures are shown in Figure 3-6. An algorithm of seizures, diagnostic tests, and diagnosis is shown in Figure 3-7.

✓ A complete blood count (CBC), serum chemistry profile, and urinalysis are useful to identify extracranial causes of seizures and are often part of the preanesthetic evaluation.

✓ A leukocytosis or leukopenia may be apparent on the CBC in cases of systemic infection, but it is often normal with meningoencephalitis. Polycythemia is obvious on examination of the CBC.

✓ Hypoglycemia, hypocalcemia, other electrolyte abnormalities, elevated liver enzymes, and renal dysfunction may be found on the serum chemistry profile and may be associated with seizures or anticonvulsant therapy.

✓ Urinalysis may detect renal insufficiency or failure, calcium oxalate crystals associated with ethylene glycol intoxication, or ammonium biurate crystals associated with liver dysfunction.

✓ Pre- and post-prandial serum bile acids or blood ammonia assays are useful to detect liver dysfunction.

✓ If organophosphate or lead intoxication is suspected, measurement of serum cholinesterase and blood lead levels might be useful.

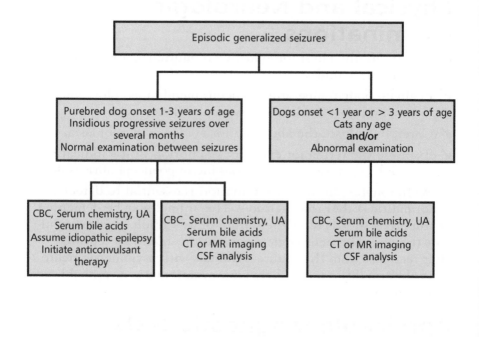

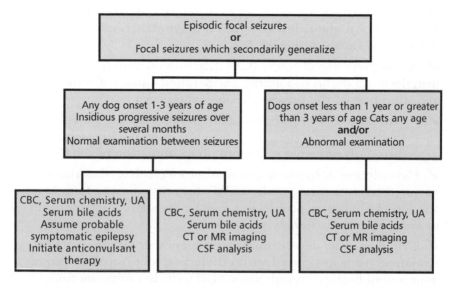

Figure 3-6 Algorithm of diagnostic plans for specific types of seizures. CBC = complete blood count; CSF = cerebrospinal fluid analysis; CT = computed tomography; MRI = magnetic resonance imaging; UA = urinalysis

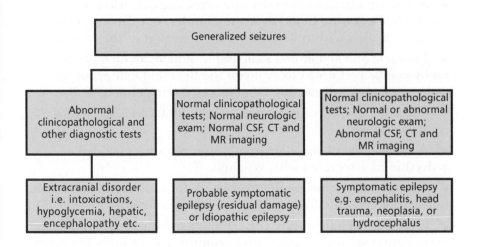

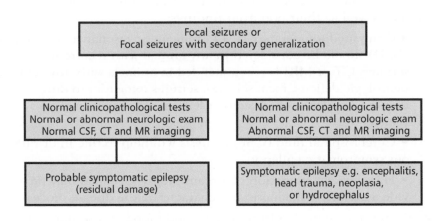

Figure 3-7 Algorithm of seizures, diagnostic tests and diagnosis.

✓ A colorimetric test for ethylene glycol intoxication is available for testing blood or urine samples, but this test is most accurate if used within 24 hours after ingestion of the toxin.

✓ Thoracic and abdominal radiography and abdominal ultrasonography can be performed to evaluate the liver and kidneys or to detect primary or metastatic neoplasia or cardiopulmonary disease.

✓ Ultrasonography of the brain may be useful in some hydrocephalic animals.

✓ A cardiac event recorder or a Holter monitor may detect arrhythmias associated with syncope.

✓ Transcolonic scintigraphy may be useful to detect a portosystemic shunt in animals with hepatic encephalopathy.

✓ Electroencephalography (EEG) may be diffusely abnormal in extracranial seizure disorders and symptomatic or probable symptomatic epilepsy but is often normal in other animals with probable symptomatic and idiopathic epilepsy. Interictal paroxysmal spikes may be seen on EEG in animals with epilepsy that is poorly controlled with anticonvulsant drugs.

✓ The following are tests that are performed under general anesthesia, as well as their potential findings:

• Computed tomography (CT) or magnetic resonance imaging (MRI) should be considered in any animal with recurrent seizures. CT or MRI is recommended in animals with interictal neurologic deficits, focal seizures, seizures refractory to drug therapy, or seizures that begin at less than 1 or greater than 5 years of age.

• Cerebrospinal fluid (CSF) analysis will help to rule in or rule out symptomatic epilepsy.

• Histologic examination of a brain biopsy specimen may provide a definitive diagnosis and characterize the disease process.

✓ Bacterial or fungal culture of CSF and blood and serum and CSF assays for specific organisms are also obtained if an infectious process is suspected.

Seizure Disorders

Head trauma, meningoencephalitis, hydrocephalus, cerebrovascular disorders, cerebral neoplasia, lysosomal storage disorders, and lissencephaly commonly cause seizures and are referred to as symptomatic epilepsy. The seizures and the underlying cause must be treated if possible. Seizures associated with extracranial disorders, such as intoxication, hypoglycemia, hepatic encephalopathy, renal failure, electrolyte disturbances, thiamine deficiency, and polycythemia, must also be treated along with the underlying cause (Figure 3-8). The causes of hypoglycemia are discussed in Section 2, and outlined in Table 2-5. The causes of hepatic encephalopathy are outlined in Table 2-7. An overview of some common toxicants that cause seizures is found in Table 3-3. Many toxicants cause ataxia, tremors, stupor, and coma. When in doubt about a substance, the ASPCA National Animal Poison Control Center (888-426-4435) or other poison control centers can offer assistance. Many extracranial disorders and disorders that cause symptomatic epilepsy also cause dementia, stupor, or coma. The diagnosis, treatment, and prognosis are discussed in Section 2. Hypocalcemia can cause seizures but often produces tremors and is discussed in Section 4.

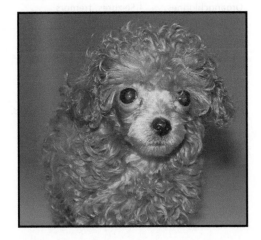

Figure 3-8 A 12-week-old toy poodle with a history of vomiting, anorexia, stupor and seizures from hypoglycemia; correcting the serum glucose resolved the seizure disorder. (Courtesy of Dr. Brian Luria.)

Table 3-3
Toxins That Cause Seizures

TOXIN	CLINICAL SIGNS	ONSET	SPECIFIC ANTIDOTE
Rodenticides			
Alphachloralose	Ataxia, seizures, aggression, coma	Acute	None
Bromethalin	Seizures, paralysis	Delayed	None
Strychnine	Seizures	Acute	None
Zinc phosphide	Seizures	Acute	None
Anticoagulants	Rare seizures, rare paralysis	Delayed	Vitamin K1 (2.5 mg/kg PO or SQ daily)
Cholecalciferol	Rare seizures	Delayed	Calcitonin
Heavy Metals			
Lead	Seizures, hysteria, ataxia, tremors, blindness, megaesophagus	Acute if high dose	Ca-EDTA (25 mg/kg QID SQ for 5 days) and others (see Section 2)
Thallium	Rare seizures, tremors, ataxia, depression, paresis	Acute	Dithizone (50 mg/kg PO TID for 5 days)
Organic mercury	Ataxia, hypermetria, tremors, seizures, blindness	Delayed	D-Penicillimine (10-30 mg/kg PO QID for 1-2 weeks)
Lithium	Tremors, ataxia, coma, seizures	Acute	None
Pesticides			
Organosphosphates or carbamates	Miosis, salivation, lacrimation, tetany, seizures, coma	Acute	Pralidoxime chloride for organophosphates (20-50 mg/kg IM) Atropine for both (0.2 mg/kg IM)
Pyrethroids	Hyperexcitability, tremors, seizures	Acute or delayed	None
Metaldehyde	Seizures, tremors, hyperthemia	Acute	None
Organochlorines	Seizures, tremors	Acute	None
Household products			
Ethylene glycol	Depression, seizures, ataxia, coma	Acute	4-Methylpyrazole, Ethanol (see Section 2)
Methylxanthines—caffeine, chocolate, tea	Hyperactivity, ataxia, rare seizures	Acute	None

IM=intramuscularly; PO=orally; QID=every 6 hours; SQ=subcutaneously; TID=every 8 hours.

Probable Symptomatic Epilepsy

🖐 Animals often have seizures that continue after recovery from a previous head injury, encephalitis, controlled hypoglycemia, surgically excised neoplasia, or surgically corrected extrahepatic portosystemic shunts. In some cases, the seizures may begin up to 2 years after these disorders. Other animals have seizures of no known cause, and inherited epilepsy is not considered likely. These cases are called probable symptomatic epilepsy and residual brain damage from a known or unknown previous process is suspected. Seizures are usually focal or focal with secondary generalization but can also be generalized.

✓ Video documentation of asymmetry during the seizure is important for dog breeders who are concerned about idiopathic (inherited) epilepsy if the physical and neurologic examinations and all diagnostic tests are normal. Some animals with probable symptomatic epilepsy have asymmetric hopping or conscious proprioceptive deficits or other focal neurologic deficits. There may be focal abnormalities on the EEG, but CT, MRI and CSF analysis are normal and differentiates it from symptomatic epilepsy. Although probable symptomatic epilepsy may be difficult to differentiate from idiopathic epilepsy, they both have identical therapies that revolve around control of the seizures.

Idiopathic Epilepsy

🖐 Idiopathic (inherited) epilepsy has been documented in Beagles, German shepherds, Belgian tervurens, Keeshonds, and Dachshunds and is suspected in Saint Bernards, Australian shepherds, Labrador retrievers, Golden retrievers, Irish setters, standard poodles, springer spaniels, cocker spaniels, Lhasa apsos, border collies, and many other purebred dogs (Figure 3-9). Idiopathic epilepsy has not yet been documented in cats. Generalized seizures with loss of consciousness are most common and usually begin between 1 to 3 years of age, but a few dogs begin seizures between 6 months and 1 year or 3 to 7 years of age. The onset of seizures is almost always insidious, beginning with a seizure every few weeks or months but then becoming progressively more frequent. Many dogs eventually develop cluster seizures or status epilepticus. In rare cases, this may be the first known seizure activity. German shepherds, Australian shepherds, Belgian tervurens, springer spaniels, Labrador retrievers, and Saint Bernards are prone to cluster seizures.

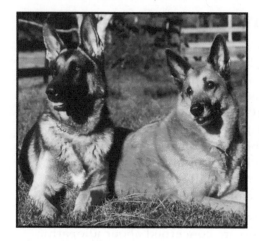

Figure 3-9 Idiopathic epilepsy occurs in German shepherds and is suspected to occur in many other breeds of dogs.

✓ The diagnosis is suspected in a purebred dog with generalized seizures and normal findings on the physical and neurologic examinations between seizures and all diagnostic tests including MRI and CSF analysis. Breeding trials may be needed to confirm the diagnosis if no other dogs in the lineage have had seizures. Unless animals are presented with severe cluster seizures or status epilepticus, therapy is aimed at controlling the seizures with maintenance anticonvulsant therapy.

Status Epilepticus Therapy

💣 Status epilepticus can occur regardless of the cause of seizures and is often precipitated by reduction or discontinuation of maintenance anticonvulsant drug therapy or if serum levels of the drug are affected by a drug interaction. Seizures that last longer than 10 minutes or occur in close succession should be considered a medical emergency. Hypoxia, hypoglycemia, hypertension, tachycardia, metabolic and respiratory acidosis, and hyperthermia associated with seizures can lead to irreversible brain damage or death. Renal failure may develop as a result of rhabdomyolysis and myoglobinuria secondary to prolonged muscle activity. The treatment of status epilepticus is outlined in Tables 3-4, 3-5, and 3-6.

♥ While one person is administering treatment to control the seizures, a second person can provide the supportive emergency monitoring and management of status epilepticus listed in Table 3-6.

Table 3-4
Stop the Seizures!
Drugs for the Treatment of Status Epilepticus

1. If hypoglycemia is suspected in a juvenile toy breed dog or diabetic animal receiving insulin, administer **50% dextrose 1-2 ml/kg IV diluted 1:1 in saline slowly over several minutes.** Oral 50% dextrose 1-2 ml/kg may be used if a vein is not accessible.

2. **Diazepam 0.5-1.0 mg/kg IV up to a maximum dose of 10 mg in dogs and 5 mg in cats** will often stop the seizures. This dose can be repeated twice within a 15-minute period if seizures continue or recur. The anticonvulsant effect lasts 15-30 minutes. Injectable diazepam solution may be administered intranasally at a dose of 0.5-1 mg/kg or rectally 0.5-2.0 mg/kg if a vein is not accessible. Intranasal and rectal absorption are relatively quick and are preferable to subcutaneous, intramuscular, or oral routes.

3. **Diazepam constant-rate infusion (CRI)** (Table 3-5) can be used in animals that are refractory to single injections or as an adjunct for longer-term control. Diazepam CRI is particularly useful in dogs having severe cluster seizures but not actively seizing on admission.

4. **Pentobarbital sodium 3-15 mg/kg IV is given slowly to effect** until seizures are controlled if single injections of diazepam are ineffective, diazepam CRI is unavailable, or rapid control of convulsive activity is critical. Pentobarbital sodium is a general anesthetic without significant anticonvulsant properties, but it controls the physical manifestations of seizures thereby reducing hypoxia, hypoglycemia, and hyperthermia and is neuroprotective. Careful monitoring of respiratory and cardiovascular function is required (Table 3-6). Pentobarbital may be repeated periodically or given as a CRI at 2-5 mg/kg/hr. Animals recovering from pentobarbital often paddle: This is not due to seizure activity and more pentobarbital is not needed.

5. **Animals already receiving oral phenobarbital must continue to receive it at the regular dose and dosing interval;** it may be administered intramuscularly or intravenously if the animal cannot swallow. **Oral anticonvulsants should be used as soon as the animal is able to swallow.**

6. Animals not currently receiving oral phenobarbital therapy may receive a loading dose of phenobarbital 4-5 mg/kg IV every 30 minutes for four doses to achieve rapid blood levels, and dosing should be continued at 2.5 mg/kg every 12 hours. Phenobarbital is usually administered concurrently with diazepam to provide a more sustained anticonvulsant effect in dogs or cats suspected of having intoxication or symptomatic epilepsy or those that have a history of recurrent episodes of status epilepticus. Phenobarbital blood levels should be monitored and should not exceed 35 μg/ml.

7. **If status epilepticus is refractory** to the above treatments, one of the following can be tried, although respiration, heart rate, and blood pressure must be closely monitored:

   • **Propofol** 0.1-0.6 mg/kg/min can be administered by CRI; hypoxemia secondary to apnea and myocardial depression are serious potential side effects.

   • **Isoflurane** inhalation anesthesia may be used but necessitates ventilation and close monitoring. Hypotension may occur during therapy. Avoid enflurane because it may cause seizures.

Table 3-5
Constant-Rate Infusion Diazepam

1. **Administer diazepam as an IV constant-rate infusion** (Figure 3-10) **at a dose of 0.1-2 mg/kg/hr** if seizures are not controlled by single injections. Start at the low end of the range and gradually increase the dose as needed to control the seizures. Most animals respond to 0.25 mg/kg/hr or less.

2. Diazepam can be irritating; a central vein is preferred; avoid the jugular vein if increased intracranial pressure is a concern.

3. Administer with a syringe pump (Figure 3-10) or dilute with 0.9% NaCl or 5% dextrose in a small IV bag or buretrol system.

4. Diazepam is degraded by light and bound by plastic. Run a small amount of the solution through the tubing before administration and prepare only 2-4 hours worth of solution at a time. Cover the line with light resistant brown plastic or aluminum foil.

5. A reasonable goal is to maintain a seizure-free state for 12 hours before attempting to wean the animal from the diazepam. At this time, the infusion rate can be halved every 4-6 hours and then discontinued. If seizures recur, the rate is increased to the previous level and reduced later.

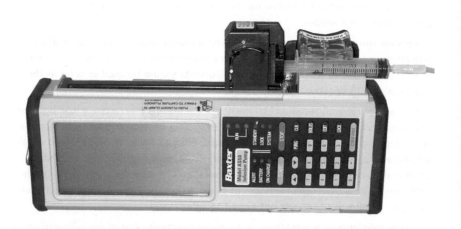

Figure 3-10
A constant-rate infusion pump that can be used for diazepam administration.

Table 3-6
Monitoring and Further Treatment for Status Epilepticus

- **Monitor respiration.** Apnea may occur during a seizure but is usually transient. Drugs may cause respiratory depression and necessitate oxygen or ventilatory therapy. Neurogenic pulmonary edema is a possible sequel of seizures and may necessitate oxygen therapy. In severe cases, animals may have to be maintained on a ventilator. Decisions should ideally be based on the results of arterial blood gas analysis.
- **Monitor cardiac rate and rhythm.** Tachycardia is common during a seizure but the heart rate returns to normal once the seizure has stopped. Bradycardia may result from the medications needed to control the seizures. Bradycardia below 40 beats/minute may have to be treated with atropine sulfate 0.02-0.04 mg/kg or glycopyrrolate 0.01 mg/kg SQ or IV.
- **Monitor body temperature.** Hyperthermia often occurs during a seizure but usually resolves once the seizure has stopped. If body temperature rises above 106°F, ice packs or cool (not ice cold) water and a fan may be used to bring it down. The temperature should be monitored and cooling stopped at 38.9° C (102° F) to prevent hypothermia.
- **Insert an intravenous catheter** for fluid and drug administration. Maintenance fluid therapy should be given in animals unable to drink. Fluid therapy may be increased if the blood pressure is low or myoglobinuria occurs.
- **Monitor blood pressure.** Hypertension associated with seizure activity should resolve once the seizure is stopped. Hypotension may occur from anticonvulsant drug therapy but often improves with intravenous fluid therapy and control of bradycardia. Isotonic saline, with potassium chloride supplementation, may be initiated at a maintenance rate of 2 ml/kg/hr.
- **Monitor serum glucose.** In animals suspected to have hypoglycemia as the cause of their seizures, obtain a serum sample prior to administration of dextrose if possible. Hyperglycemia commonly occurs during seizures due to the release of glycogen stores from the liver. Hyperglycemia resolves once the seizures are stopped and should not be treated with insulin. Fifty percent dextrose 1-2 ml/kg IV diluted 1:1 in saline and administered slowly over 5-10 minutes will correct hypoglycemia if present. Serum glucose is re-evaluated several hours after therapy and later after fasting if it is unclear whether hypoglycemia is the cause or result of the seizures.
- **Monitor arterial blood gases.** Marked respiratory acidosis then metabolic acidosis can occur during prolonged seizures. Once the seizures are controlled, metabolic acidosis should resolve without treatment.
- **Monitor urine for discoloration.** Myoglobinuria can cause kidney damage. Reddish brown urine may be associated with myoglobinuria and intravenous fluids should be increased to 2-3 times maintenance rates to protect the kidneys from damage.
- **Prolonged seizures can result in cerebral edema.** Oxygen therapy will reduce cerebral edema. Mannitol 0.25-1.0 g/kg IV followed by furosemide 0.7 mg/kg IV 15 minutes later can be useful to treat cerebral edema.
- **Initiate therapy for the underlying disease process if possible.**
- **Monitor recovery from sedation.** Paddling of the limbs is common during recovery. Such activity can be differentiated from seizures as seizures usually have tonic, clonic, or tonic-clonic limb movements.

Maintenance Anticonvulsant Therapy

♥ When seizures recur more than once a month, occur in clusters, or last more than 5 minutes, anticonvulsant therapy is recommended. Some seizures may be controlled with acupuncture, herbal therapy, homeopathic remedies, or other alternative therapies. Other animals require one or more anticonvulsant drugs. The most common anticonvulsant drugs used in dogs are phenobarbital and potassium bromide (KBr). Phenobarbital and in some cases diazepam are used for cats. A guide to the use of oral anticonvulsant therapy for epileptic dogs is found in Table 3-7. Oral diazepam is not an effective anticonvulsant in dogs and has been associated with a rare idiosyncratic hepatotoxicity in some cats.

Phenobarbital

✓ Oral phenobarbital often controls seizures within 72 hours. If seizures are not controlled within 7 days, the dosage can be increased. Although 5 mg/kg every 12 hours is the highest suggested phenobarbital dose, some small dogs need 8 mg/kg every 12 hours to reach therapeutic serum levels. Phenobarbital elixir 3 mg/ml may be the easiest way to make small adjustments in the dose for small dogs and cats, although 8-mg phenobarbital tablets are also available. A serum phenobarbital level should be evaluated after the animal has received a consistent dose for 2 weeks to ensure that it does not exceed 35 µg/ml, as hepatotoxicity can occur.

✓ Sedation, ataxia, polyuria/polydipsia, and polyphagia are common side effects of phenobarbital and may necessitate dosage reduction or change to another anticonvulsant. Phenobarbital occasionally causes hyperactivity in dogs and cats, and this may be alleviated by replacing the phenobarbital with mephobarbital (a related drug) at the same dose. Some animals become tolerant to phenobarbital after a few months, and the dose must be increased to maintain the same effective serum level. Alterations of the dose are best made in conjunction with an evaluation of the current serum phenobarbital level.

♥ As hepatotoxicity can occur in dogs on phenobarbital, liver function should be monitored with pre- and post-prandial bile acids every 3 to 6 months for the first year of therapy. Serum alkaline phosphate and alanine aminotransferase levels may be elevated due

Table 3-7
A Guide to the Use of Oral Anticonvulsant Therapy for Idiopathic or Probable Symptomatic Epilepsy in Dogs

1. Evaluate seizure frequency

• If seizures occur once a month or less, may try acupuncture alone or other alternative therapy or KBr 22 mg/kg PO every 12 hours.

• If seizures occur multiple times a month, begin phenobarbital 2-4 mg/kg PO every 12 hours. Control of seizures can occur within a few days. If seizures continue at the same frequency after 7 days, increase the dose of phenobarbital by 10% every 5 to 7 days up to 5 mg/kg every 12 hours if needed.

• If cluster seizures occur, begin phenobarbital 2-4 mg/kg PO every 12 hours combined with KBr 22 mg/kg every 12 hours. Cluster seizures are rarely controlled by phenobarbital alone.

2. If seizures continue at an unacceptable frequency after 14 days, measure peak serum phenobarbital level (2-4 hours after oral phenobarbital is given).

• If the serum phenobarbital level is below 20 μg/ml increase the phenobarbital dose by 10% and repeat serum phenobarbital levels in 10-14 days. Repeat 10% increases of dosage and monitoring serum phenobarbital levels until the serum level is between 30-35 μg/ml or the seizures are controlled at a lower level.

• If the serum phenobarbital level is 30-35 μg/ml and the animal is not on KBR, begin KBr at a dose of 22 mg/kg every 12 hours.

• If the serum phenobarbital level is greater than 35 μg/ml, liver damage may occur, so decrease the dosage by 10% every 10-14 days until a serum level of 30-35 μg/ml is obtained.

3. If the seizures are controlled and the animal is sedated or ataxic on the combined drug regimen, reduce the phenobarbital dose by 10% every 7 days as needed until sedation resolves.

4. If seizures continue, increase the KBr dose by 10% every 7 days until the seizures are controlled; if sedation develops, keep the KBr dose constant and reduce the phenobarbital by 10% every 7 days until sedation resolves.

5. Measure serum bromide levels in 3-4 months. In dogs with poorly controlled cluster seizures, the serum level may have to be 4000-5000 μg/ml before control is achieved. (Most laboratories will report toxic levels). Chloride level will be elevated on a serum chemistry profile (most tests measure bromide ions as chloride).

6. If serum phenobarbital and bromide levels are adequate and the dog is still seizing, consider a diagnosis of active intracranial or extracranial disease or refractory epilepsy. Assistance from a specialist may be required.

7. Adding acupuncture at any phase may assist seizure control.

to enzyme induction, but liver function should remain normal. Hepatotoxicity has not been documented in cats. Idiosyncratic cutaneous hypersensitivities and blood dyscrasias rarely occur. Once seizures are controlled and liver function appears normal, yearly evaluation of the serum phenobarbital level, serum chemistry profile, pre- and post-prandial bile acids measurement, and a CBC should be done. Any dramatic change in results from one year to the next may signal potential intoxication.

💣 **Phenobarbital should never be abruptly discontinued as status epilepticus may result.** Phenothiazines, narcotics, antihistamines, other CNS depressant drugs, valproic acid, and chloramphenicol may increase the effects of phenobarbital and cause severe sedation and respiratory depression. Phenobarbital may decrease the effect of chloramphenicol, doxycycline, metronidazole, theophylline, corticosteroids, ß-blockers, and quinidine. Any drug considered for a dog or cat on phenobarbital therapy should be reviewed for potential drug interactions.

Potassium Bromide

✓ Oral KBr can be the first line of therapy for some dogs (22mg/kg PO every 12 hours), but it may cause inflammatory lung disease in cats and should only be used in this species if liver function is abnormal or if phenobarbital is ineffective. The KBr dose for cats is 15 mg/kg every 12 hours or 30 mg/kg/day. KBr is not metabolized by the liver but is excreted by the kidneys. It must be given with a meal to avoid vomiting from gastrointestinal irritation—dividing the daily dose into two separated doses may result in better tolerance. Because KBr is excreted in the kidneys, it should be used with caution and at reduced doses in animals with renal insufficiency.

✓ KBr is not commercially available and must be made by a compounding pharmacist. KBr crystals readily dissolve in water and can be prepared in any strength, although 250 mg/ml is the most common. The crystals can also be placed in gelatin capsules, but this is not recommended initially because the liquid form of KBr allows for easy dosage adjustments. The owner should wear gloves to avoid skin absorption and place the recommended dose on a piece of bread or small amount of food that the animal will completely eat to ensure that the correct amount is given. Liquid KBr placed directly into the mouth may end up on the owner or the floor, and the correct dose may not be given. Some animals dislike the taste and refuse the drug even in food. KBr can be compounded into corn syrup or chicken stock, which is often readily consumed even by finicky eaters.

♦※ The chloride content of the diet may alter the concentration of KBr in the blood, and the diet should be kept as consistent as possible. A change to salty food or snacks containing high levels of sodium chloride may reduce KBr levels, and seizures may result. Changing the diet may necessitate altering the KBr dose to maintain the serum bromide at effective levels. If renal disease develops, KBr intoxication may occur.

✓ For frequent cluster seizures, KBr may initially be combined with phenobarbital 1–2 mg/kg PO every 12 hours, as KBr may not be effective for several weeks. When KBr begins to take effect, animals often become sedated, at which time the phenobarbital dose can be reduced by 10 % every 7 days until sedation resolves. The phenobarbital dose may be reduced gradually over the months that follow and then discontinued if the seizures remain controlled. Serum KBr levels may be evaluated in 3 to 4 months when they reach a steady state.

♦※ **KBr should never be abruptly discontinued unless in acute respiratory distress of cats as status epilepticus may be precipitated.** The KBr dose may have to be increased to as much as 50 mg/kg every 12 hours to achieve a therapeutic serum bromide concentration. Dose adjustments are best made in conjunction with evaluation of serum levels.

♦※ KBr may cause inflammatory lung disease in cats after a month or more of therapy, and the dose should be tapered and the drug discontinued.

✓ Under special circumstances when seizures cannot be controlled by other means and the patient can be closely monitored, a loading dose of KBr 25 mg/kg every 6 hours may be given over a 5-day period to rapidly increase the serum bromide concentration. As KBr intoxication can cause acute pancreatitis, severe sedation, and death, this technique is not recommended for routine use. If sedation and ataxia develop, the drug is reduced to 22 mg/kg every 12 hours. KBr loading doses should never be given to animals with renal disease.

♥ Polyphagia may occur in some dogs on KBr therapy. A low-calorie diet may have to be instituted to prevent excessive weight gain. If the sodium chloride content differs from the regular diet, the dose of KBr may have to be adjusted to maintain therapeutic levels. Polydipsia/polyuria can occur with KBr therapy but is less common than with phenobarbital therapy. Cutaneous reactions have been observed in some dogs, especially those with a history of dermatitis. Personality changes, such as sedation, irritability, constantly seeking attention, and aimless wandering or pacing, may also occur. KBr may cause pelvic limb stiffness which disappears when the KBr dose is reduced. The adverse effects of KBr are reversible once the dosage is reduced and KBr is generally a very safe drug. When the seizures are controlled, the serum bromide levels, CBC, and serum chemistry should be evaluated annually. Serum chloride levels will appear falsely elevated as most chemistry analyzers mistake the bromide ion for chloride.

Monitoring Therapy

✓ As with any therapeutic drug monitoring, serum samples should be collected in a plain glass tube (red top). Serum separator tubes, which contain silicon, should be avoided because silicon may bind drugs and falsely lower the reported level. In most cases, the serum level of the phenobarbital and KBr do not vary significantly over a 12-hour period once a steady state is achieved, and the serum sample can be collected at any time. In animals whose seizures are difficult to control, peak (2 hours after the pill) and trough (8 to 12 hours after the pill) measurement of serum phenobarbital levels may be useful to detect cases of rapid metabolism. Such animals may benefit from administration every 8 hours. Serum anticonvulsant drugs are monitored for the reasons outlined in Table 3-8.

♥ **Most laboratories report serum phenobarbital concentrations of 15 to 45 μg/ml as therapeutic, although this is highly variable between individual animals.** Some animals may require high levels of phenobarbital for seizure control. However, the risk of hepatotoxicity increases when the serum phenobarbital level exceeds 35 μg/ml. **Serum levels of KBr of 1000–5000 μg/ml (1000–5000 mg/dl or 1–5 mg/ml) are considered therapeutic.** The units of measurement for KBr levels in serum vary from laboratory to laboratory and can be confusing. Many laboratories will indicate that levels over 2000 mg/ml are toxic, which is not the case for dogs.

Table 3-8
Reasons to Monitor Serum Levels of Anticonvulsant Drugs

When seizures are controlled:

- To determine the effective therapeutic level for an individual animal

- To ensure drug levels are below hepatotoxic ranges

If seizures are not controlled:

- To determine if an increased dose or different anticonvulsant is needed
- To determine what changes need to be made if the animal becomes sedated, ataxic, or ill from liver or kidney disease or if it has begun a new drug therapy or diet that may alter serum levels of the anticonvulsant

♥ Maintenance anticonvulsant drugs may have to be continued for years and often for the rest of the animal's life. In some cases, the medications may be reduced after the animal has been free of seizures for 1 year and then slowly tapered over the following several months. The ultimate goal is to reduce the frequency and severity of the seizures with doses of medication that produce minimal side effects and are unlikely to result in toxicity. The animal may still have a few seizures a year. Advice to owners of epileptic dogs is outlined in Table 3-9.

Table 3-9
Advice to Owners of
Epileptic Dogs on Anticonvulsant Therapy

- Administer anticonvulsant drugs at the specific times required. Don't miss doses, as seizures will occur.

- Feed a healthy, balanced diet; encourage regular exercise; try to reduce environmental stress; ensure plenty of rest; and maintain a regular routine.

- Avoid changes in diet or salty snacks in pets receiving KBr.

- Avoid pesticides on the animal and in the environment if possible; if not, closely monitor for increase in seizure frequency and avoid organophosphates.

- If cluster seizures occur in relation to the monthly heartworm prevention treatment in dogs, see your veterinarian about switching to an alternative drug.

- Avoid acepromazine for travel or sedation as it may induce seizures.

- Do not give any other medications without the advice of a veterinarian, as drug interactions can occur.

- Avoid situations that seem to trigger seizures; if such situations cannot be avoided, then see a veterinarian about increasing the anticonvulsant drugs a few days prior to the event.

- Once seizures are controlled, yearly evaluation of the serum anticonvulsant levels, serum chemistry profile, measurement of pre- and post-prandial bile acids, and CBC should be performed.

- Most animals with epilepsy can lead a long and healthy life.

Diazepam

♥ Although intravenous diazepam is effective to control status epilepticus in dogs, it undergoes rapid and extensive hepatic metabolism once in the circulation and has a very short half-life. In addition, dogs build up a tolerance to the anticonvulsant effects of diazepam in 1 to 2 weeks, and it is therefore not a useful oral anticonvulsant for this species. **The half-life of diazepam in cats is nearly 20 hours and therefore it may be used as an oral anticonvulsant in this species at a dose of 0.25–2 mg/kg every 12 hours.** The dose may be increased by 1-mg increments if needed in order to control seizures and avoid sedation. Polyphagia and sedation are common side effects.

💣 Idiosyncratic hepatotoxicity can occur in cats and therefore diazepam is typically used only if phenobarbital is not effective for seizure control. Acute fulminant hepatic necrosis has been seen in cats as early as 5 days after beginning oral diazepam, and therefore liver enzymes should be evaluated every 5 to 7 days initially. Diazepam should be discontinued if liver enzyme elevations are detected or if clinical signs of hepatic disease become evident. Abrupt withdrawal of diazepam following prolonged treatment can cause seizures or signs of withdrawal, such as tremors, anorexia, and weight loss.

Adding a Second Drug

✓ Although the use of one drug is effective in many animals, a significant proportion of dogs with idiopathic or probable symptomatic epilepsy require additional medication for seizure control. Animals that have phenobarbital levels of 35 µg/ml or greater and continue to have an unacceptable number of seizures may have KBr added at 22 mg/kg every 12 hours. Most dogs with cluster seizures cannot be controlled with phenobarbital alone. Within a few days to a week when the KBr begins to take effect, the animal may become sedated and ataxic. The phenobarbital can then be reduced by 10% every 7 days until sedation resolves. The most effective way to manage a dog with severe cluster seizures is to maintain a serum KBr level of 4000–5000 µg/ml with a phenobarbital level of 25–35 µg/ml.

✓ Phenobarbital and KBr used alone or in combination control seizures in over 80% of animals with idiopathic or probable symptomatic epilepsy. When phenobarbital or KBr alone or together are unsuccessful in controlling seizures or their side effects are intolerable, and lowering the dosage results in seizures, other anticonvulsants may be considered. Other drugs rarely used in dogs include primidone, diphenylhydantoin, chlorazepate, felbamate, valproic acid, and gabapentin. Hepatotoxicity and expense limit the use of these agents.

Other Rarely Used Anticonvulsant Drugs

💣 **Primidone** (Mysoline, Athena) can cause irreversible liver damage in dogs and should be used with extreme caution. **Primidone may be administered at 15–22 mg/kg PO every 12 hours for dogs. Primidone is toxic to cats and should not be used.**

Monthly monitoring of liver function with pre- and post-prandial bile acids is essential for the first 6 months and every 3 months thereafter. If liver function becomes abnormal, the dose is reduced over a 3-week period and then discontinued. Much of the anticonvulsant effect of primidone is from phenobarbital, one of its metabolites. Phenobarbital levels are monitored in dogs on primidone as they correlate with anticonvulsant efficacy. Therapeutic serum levels are 15–45 μg/ml of phenobarbital. Some seizures that were not controlled with phenobarbital might be controlled with primidone.

✓ **Diphenylhydantoin** (Dilantin, Parke-Davis) has a short half-life, is poorly absorbed from the gastrointestinal tract, and is not very effective for seizure control in dogs. **Diphenylhydantoin is toxic to cats and should not be used in this species. Diphenylhydantoin 25–30 mg/kg PO every 6 hours may be administered to dogs in an attempt to achieve a therapeutic serum level of 10–20 μg/ml after 2 weeks.** When used in conjunction with phenobarbital or primidone, the risk of hepatotoxicity is increased.

✓ **Chorazepate** (Tranxene, Abbott) has a half-life in dogs of approximately 4 to 6 hours and is not very effective when used alone. **The dose of chlorazepate is 0.6–2 mg/kg PO every 8 hours for dogs.** When used in combination with phenobarbital, a lower dose is suggested as serum phenobarbital levels are increased. Sedation and ataxia may necessitate further dose reduction. The serum phenobarbital and chlorazepate levels may be measured at 2 and 4 weeks, respectively. Generic preparations may reduce the costs of therapy. Chlorazepate may be useful for short-term breakthrough seizure control.

✓ **Felbamate** (Felbatol, Wallace) **5–100 mg/kg PO every 8 hours may be used alone or in conjunction with phenobarbital and KBr for refractory generalized or focal seizures in dogs.** It may be best to start at the lowest dose and then increase the dose in increments of 5 mg/kg every 8 hours. Although the half-life of felbamate is 4.5–6.5 hours in dogs, it may be effective as a single therapy for focal seizures. Excessive sedation may occur when felbamate is administered in conjunction with phenobarbital or primidone. Phenobarbital serum concentrations may increase when felbamate is added, which may increase the risk for hepatotoxicity. The expense of felbamate limits its use in dogs.

✓ **Valproic acid** (Depakene, Abbott) has not proven to be very effective as a single anticonvulsant in dogs. It has been used in combination with phenobarbital but increases the risk of hepatotoxicity. The expense of valproic acid also limits its use in veterinary medicine.

✓ **Gabapentin** (Neurontin, Parke-Davis) has an elimination half-life in dogs of 3 to 4 hours, and effective serum levels may be difficult to achieve even if doses are given every 6 hours. **Some anticonvulsant effect may be achieved in dogs with gabapentin 6–15 mg/kg PO every 6 hours.** The expense of this drug limits its use in veterinary medicine.

✓ Topiramate (Topamax, Ortho-McNeil), zonisimide (Zonegran, Elan), and levitiracetam (Keppra; VCB Inc.) are new anticonvulsant drugs recently developed for use in humans that may be useful in the future for dogs. Many other new drugs are currently under investigation. Other methods for controlling refractory seizures, including vagal nerve stimulation, surgical interventions, and radiation therapy, may play a role in the future treatment of epilepsy in dogs and cats.

Therapy at Home to Control Cluster Seizures

✓ Some dogs have episodes of cluster seizures every few months, which necessitate trips to the emergency room. A compounding pharmacist can make diazepam suppositories (0.5–2 mg/kg each), which the owner can insert rectally when seizures begin. Administration can be repeated for a total of 3 doses within a 24 hour period if seziures continue. Injectable diazepam may also be sent home for rectal or intranasal use but may not be as easy to administer and may have a greater potential for abuse.

Section **4**

Tremors

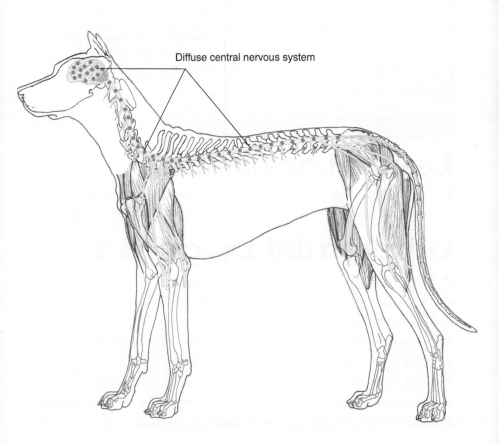

Diffuse central nervous system

Definitions

Tremors: Involuntary trembling or quivering of the head and/or limb muscles, occurring constantly when the animal is awake but disappears during sleep; tremors may worsen with excitement and cold.

"Shaky white dog disease": Frequent occurrence of tremors in white dogs associated with nonsuppurative meningoencephalomyelitis and idiopathic tremors (Figure 4-1).

Meningoencephalitis: Inflammation of the meninges and brain.

Intention tremors: Involuntary head and limb tremors that occur with the initiation of movement resulting from cerebellar disease (Section 8).

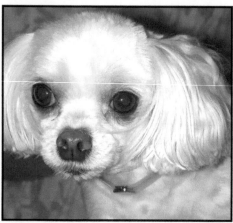

Figure 4-1 Nonsuppurative meningoencephalomyelitis and idiopathic tremors of adult dogs have a high incidence in white dogs, especially Maltese terriers. (Courtesy of Dr. Rita Hanel.)

Lesion Localization

✓ Lesions that cause tremors are found at multifocal sites or diffusely throughout the central nervous system (Figure 4-2).

Differential Diagnosis

✓ Hypocalcemia–common in dogs and cats

✓ Hypoglycemia–common in dogs and cats

✓ Intoxications–common in dogs and cats

✓ Nonsuppurative meningoencephalomyelitis–common in dogs

✓ Idiopathic tremors of adult dogs–common in dogs

✓ Idiopathic tremors of geriatric dogs–common in dogs

✓ Episodic idiopathic head tremors or bobbing–occasional in dogs

✓ Hypomyelination or dysmyelination–rare in dogs

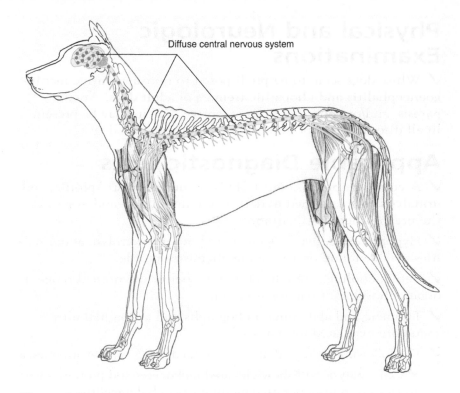

Figure 4-2 The lesions may be multifocal or diffuse.

Diagnostic Evaluation
Important Historical Questions

- Was the onset acute or chronic? Progressive?
- Are tremors absent during sleep?
- Is the animal able to walk, eat, and drink?
- If adult intact female, recent whelping?
- Are other littermates affected?
- Has there been exposure to pesticides, herbicides, heavy metals, prescription drugs, or other toxic substances?
- Has there been recent exposure to prescription, over-the counter, or illegal drugs, nutriceuticals, or herbal preparations?

Physical and Neurologic Examinations

✓ White dogs seem to be predisposed to nonsuppurative meningoencephalitis and idiopathic tremors of adult dogs. Ataxia, paresis, and/or conscious proprioceptive deficits may be present in all disorders except idiopathic tremors of adult dogs.

Applicable Diagnostic Tests

✓ A complete blood count (CBC), serum chemistry profile, and urinalysis are performed to detect systemic illness and as part of the preanesthetic evaluation.

✓ Hypoglycemia, hypocalcemia, and other electrolyte abnormalities may be found on the serum chemistry profile.

✓ Serum cholinesterase levels will be below the normal range if organophosphate toxicosis is present.

✓ Thoracic and abdominal radiographs and abdominal ultrasound are evaluated for masses.

✓ The following are tests that are performed under general anesthesia:

  • CSF analysis will show elevated leukocytes and protein levels in cases of nonsuppurative meningoencephalomyelitis.

  • Electroencephalography (EEG) will often have generalized slow waves and increased amplitude in cases of meningoencephalitis.

✓ Serum and CSF immunoassays for specific organisms are obtained if an infection is suspected.

Tremor Disorders

Hypocalcemia

✓ Hypocalcemia can cause neuronal membrane instability and tremors in dogs and cats. Ataxia and seizures may also occur. Facial pruritis may be present. Hypocalcemia may be associated with many diseases, and an overview is found in Table 4-1. The serum calcium level is usually less than 8 mg/dl. **In an acute hypocalcemic crisis, treatment with 10% calcium gluconate solution 0.5–1.5 ml/kg (up to 20 ml) IV slowly over 20 to 30 minutes will usually stop the tremors.** Respiration and the cardiac rate and rhythm are monitored during administration, preferably with the aid of an electrocardiogram (ECG). If respiratory depression, bradycardia, ST

Table 4-1

Disorders Associated with Hypocalcemia

- Primary hypoparathyroidism
- Inadvertant parathyroidectomy
- Chronic or acute renal failure
- Acute pancreatitis
- Eclampsia
- Hyperphosphatemia
- Intravenous phosphate administration
- Phosphate-containing enema administration (cats)
- Hypomagnesemia
- Hypoalbuminemia
- Ethylene glycol intoxication
- Intestinal malabsorption
- Blood transfusion (citrated blood)
- Vitamin D deficiency
- Tumor lysis syndrome
- Massive soft tissue trauma
- Rhabdomyolysis

segment elevation or Q-T interval shortening are noted, the infusion is temporarily discontinued until the abnormalities resolve and then reinstated at a slower rate. **After the acute crisis, 10% calcium gluconate solution 0.5–1.5 ml/kg IV may be diluted 1:1 with saline and given at a rate of 10–15 ml/kg over a 24-hour period.** Oral therapy is often initiated. The underlying cause should be investigated and addressed. The prognosis varies greatly.

Hypoglycemia

✓ Hypoglycemia is more likely to cause stupor, coma, or seizures rather than tremors. This disorder is discussed in Section 2, and its causes are outlined in Section 2, Table 2-5.

Intoxications

♥ Many toxic substances cause tremors. The possibility of exposure to pyrethrin and pyrethroid insecticides, organophosphates, ivermectin, ethylene glycol, chlorinated hydrocarbons, metaldehyde, hexachlorophene, herbicides, toxic plants, heavy metals, and any prescription, over-the-counter, or illegal drugs should be explored with the client. An overview of the commonly used organophosphates and organocarbamates that can cause intoxication are listed in Table 4-2.

Table 4-2
Commonly Used Organophosphates

- Malathion
- Parathion
- Diazinon
- Carbaryl (Sevin)
- Bendiocarb (Ficam)
- Propoxur (Baygon, Dendran)
- Chlorpyrifos (Dursban)
- Methylcarbamate
- Chlorfenvinphos (Dermaton dip)
- Cythioate (Proban)
- Dichlorvos (Vapona)
- Dioxathion
- Fenthion (ProSpot)
- Ronnel
- Phosmet
- Disulfoton (Di-Syston)
- Golden Malrin (fly bait)

✓ Chlorpyrifos intoxication from improper application of dips or exposure to treated homes and yards is a common cause of tremors. Serum cholinesterase is often less than 500 IU (normal range is 800 to 1200 IU) in dogs and cats with organophosphate intoxication. **Muscle fasciculation associated with organophosphate intoxication can be reduced with pralidoxime chloride (Protopam, Wyeth-Ayerst) 10–15 mg/kg SQ every 8 to 12 hours until recovery occurs.** This therapy is most effective if begun in the first 24 hours after exposure. The animal should be bathed to remove any residual chemicals and reduce further absorption. Supportive care with fluids 2–4 ml/kg/hr IV and quality nutrition is essential. Recovery often occurs within 1 to 4 weeks.

✓ When in doubt about a substance, the ASPCA National Animal Poison Control Center (888-426-4435) or another poison control center can provide additional information on the potential for intoxication and treatment. Emergency management for oral intoxication is outlined in Section 2, Table 2-4. Tremors may be controlled with diazepam 0.5 mg/kg IV up to 10 mg in dogs and 5 mg in cats. A constant-rate infusion of diazepam (Section 3, Table 3-5) 0.1–2 mg/kg/hr IV may be administered with an infusion pump, as tremors may not be controlled by single injections. Respiration, heart rate and rhythm, body temperature, and blood pressure should be monitored and maintained within normal ranges. Many cases of intoxication recover with symptomatic treatment and fluid therapy.

Nonsuppurative Meningoencephalomyelitis and Idiopathic Tremors of Adult Dogs

✓ Nonsuppurative meningoencephalomyelitis and idiopathic tremors of adult dogs are considered together as their clinical appearance, treatment, and prognosis are the same, and they may be the same disease process. The only difference is the presence or absence of other abnormalities on the neurologic examination and CSF. Both cause acute tremors in dogs. White dogs, such as Maltese terriers (Figure 4-1), are often affected. This has lead to their description as "little white shakers" or "shaky white dog disease." Any dog can develop this disorder, so it should not be excluded based on coat color or size of the dog. The tremors may affect only the pelvic limbs or may be diffuse to include thoracic limbs and the head and eyes. In some affected dogs, tremors are the only abnormal clinical sign. Other cases may also have head tilt, ataxia, paraparesis, or quadriparesis.

✓ No history of toxic exposure can be found. The CBC and serum chemistry profile, including calcium levels, are normal. The CSF may be normal or can contain increased leukocytes (primarily lymphocytes and occasionally a mixed cell population) with normal or increased protein. Serum and CSF immunoassays should be obtained in cases where CSF leukocytic pleocytosis is present, but the results of these tests are normal in dogs with nonsuppurative meningoencephalitis. Computed tomography (CT) and magnetic resonance imaging (MRI) are usually normal or may show mild ventricular enlargement.

✋ **If the dog has only tremors and no CSF abnormalities, then a diagnosis of idiopathic tremors of adult dogs is made. If the dog has tremors plus other neurologic signs and/or abnormal CSF, then a diagnosis of nonsuppurative meningoencephalomyelitis is made.**

✓ **Treatment with prednisone 2–4 mg/kg/day PO is given for 2 weeks then reduced to 1–2 mg/kg/day for 2 weeks.** The dosage should then be gradually tapered over the next month, given on alternate days, and then discontinued. Oral famotidine (Pepcid AC, Merck) 0.5–1 mg/kg every 12-24 hours, cimetidine (Tagamet, SmithKline Beecham) 5–10 mg/kg every 8 hours, or misoprostol (Cytotec, Searle) 1–3 µg/kg every 8 hours will reduce the chance of gastrointestinal ulceration and irritation when the dose of prednisone is high.

♥ Tremors are controlled in both nonsuppurative meningoen-cephalomyelitis and idiopathic tremors of adult dogs with diazepam 0.5–2 mg/kg PO every 6 to 8 hours, not to exceed 10 mg every 6 hours, as needed to control tremors. Diazepam is continued for 1 month, and then the dosage is reduced by 25% per week. If tremors reappear, then the lowest effective dose to control the tremors is re-instituted. This is repeated until the tremors completely resolve, which may take 1 to 3 months. Diazepam is never abruptly discontinued as tremors and seizures from withdrawal might occur. The prognosis for both nonsuppura-tive meningoencephalomyelitis and idiopathic tremors of adult dogs is excellent, and most affected dogs eventually return to normal.

Idiopathic Tremors of Geriatric Dogs

✓ Geriatric dogs often develop intermittent or continuous tremors of the pelvic limbs when standing. The cause is unknown, but many tremor syndromes of elderly humans have been associated with neuronal degeneration in the basal nuclei and other specific neuronal regions. A similar process is suspected in dogs. No therapy is recommended, and the tremors do not usually resolve.

Episodic Idiopathic Head Tremors or Bobbing

✓ Doberman pinschers, Shetland sheepdogs, and wired-haired fox terriers may have episodic head bobbing or tremors of unknown cause. Stress or excitement may precipitate the episodes, but affected dogs are usually normal upon presentation. Historically, the episodes occur only periodically and last several minutes. The owner is unable to stop the bobbing or tremors by petting or reassuring the dog. Partial seizures (Section 3) have been suspected in some cases. A CBC, serum chemistry profile (including calcium), CSF analysis, and EEG are normal. No treatment is usually prescribed as the episodes are brief and do not interfere with the dog's normal functions.

Hypomyelination or Dysmyelination

✓ Abnormal myelin development in chow chows, springer spaniels, Weimeraners, and other dogs can result in diffuse, whole-body tremors in puppies from 3 to 12 weeks of age. More than one dog in the litter is often affected to varying degrees. The tremors are absent during rest and sleep and worsen with excitement or cold. Tremors may be so severe that affected puppies find it difficult to walk, eat, or drink. The CBC and serum chemistry profile are normal. The diagnosis is suspected by ruling out other diseases. There is no treatment available, but with supportive care and assistance with eating and drinking, many of these puppies improve over the course of several months and may become normal or acceptable pets. The underlying cause may be genetic or related to viral infection *in utero*.

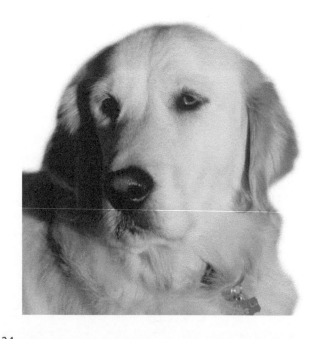

Section 5

Head Tilt, Dysequilibrium, and Nystagmus

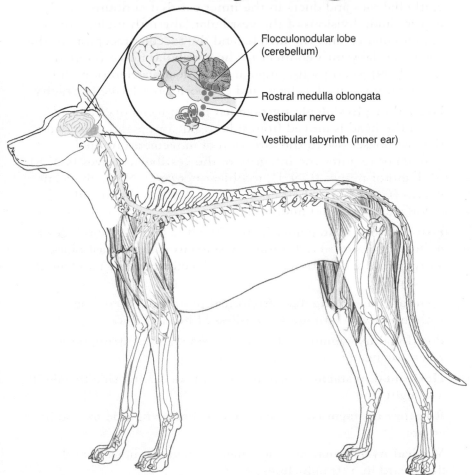

Flocculonodular lobe (cerebellum)

Rostral medulla oblongata

Vestibular nerve

Vestibular labyrinth (inner ear)

Definitions

Head tilt: The head is cocked to one side so that one ear is closer to the ground than the other (Figure 5-1).

Dysequilibrium: Loss of balance to one or both sides characterized by leaning, falling, rolling, or circling with a head tilt.

Nystagmus: Involuntary eye movements characterized by a slow movement in one direction (slow phase) and then a rapid jerk in the opposite direction (fast phase).

Vestibular system: The peripheral nervous system (PNS) and central nervous system (CNS) pathways responsible for maintaining balance and normal head and eye posture.

Vestibular labyrinth: A membranous system of communicating epithelial sacs and ducts in the inner ear that contains endolymphatic fluid; divisions of the vestibular labyrinth include three semicircular canals, the utricle, and the saccule; receptors in the vestibular labyrinth connect to the vestibular nerve (cranial nerve [CN] 8) and sense angular and linear acceleration and deceleration as well as head and eye position relative to gravity.

Normal or physiologic nystagmus: Eye movements induced when the head is moved from side to side or up and down with the fast phase toward the direction of movement; normal nystagmus requires the integrity of the vestibular nerves (CN 8), oculomotor nerves (CN 3), trochlear nerves (CN 4), abducens nerves (CN 6), and their connections through the medulla oblongata, pons, and midbrain.

Post-rotatory nystagmus: If the animal is spun in a circle for a minute or more, a brief normal nystagmus with the fast phase away from the direction turned is induced when the movement is stopped.

Spontaneous nystagmus: Abnormal nystagmus occurring without outward stimulus regardless of head position.

Positional nystagmus: Abnormal nystagmus occurring only when the head is in certain positions.

Horizontal nystagmus: Eye movements occurring side to side in a straight line.

Rotatory nystagmus: Eye movements occurring side to side in an arc.

Vertical nystagmus: Eye movements occurring upward and downward in a straight line.

Positional strabismus: An abnormal position of one eye observed only when the head is in certain positions; when the head is straightened and the nose is elevated, the eye on the side of the head tilt drops below the level of the other eye.

Myringotomy: Puncture of the tympanic membrane for removal of fluid from the middle ear.

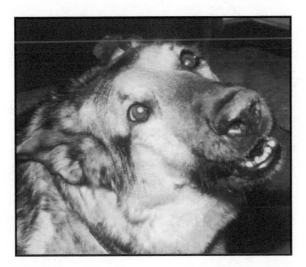

Figure 5-1 Acute onset of a right head tilt associated with an idiopathic vestibular syndrome is common in geriatric dogs.

Lesion Localization

The Vestibular System

✓ The vestibular system is shown in Figures 5-2 and 5-3. Specific locations of lesions that cause head tilt, dysequilibrium, and nystagmus are the:

- Peripheral nervous system (PNS): Sensory receptors in the vestibular labyrinth and the vestibulocochlear nerves (CN 8)

- Central nervous system (CNS): The vestibular nuclei in the medulla oblongata and the flocculonodular lobe of the cerebellum.

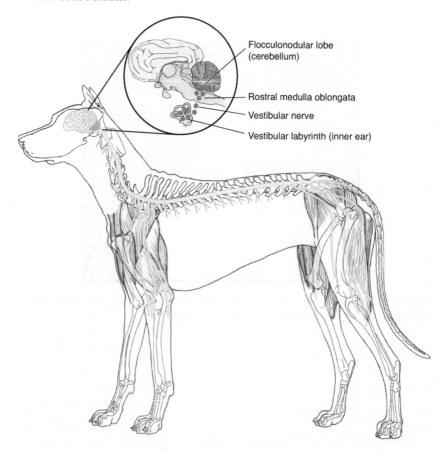

Flocculonodular lobe (cerebellum)

Rostral medulla oblongata

Vestibular nerve

Vestibular labyrinth (inner ear)

Figure 5-2 Dysfunction of the labyrinth, vestibular nerve, rostral medulla oblongata, or cerebellum causes head tilt, dysequilibrium, and nystagmus (the dots indicate the lesion localization).

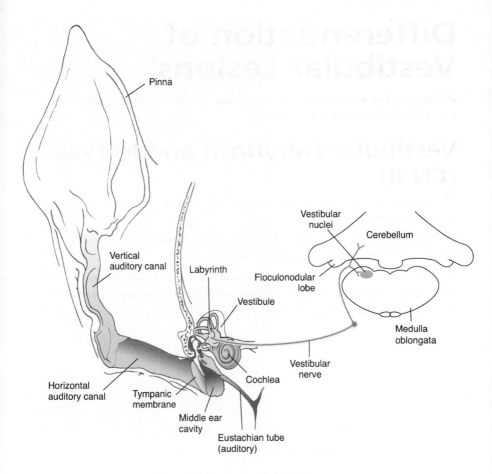

Figure 5-3 The ear and components of the vestibular system.

Differentiation of Vestibular Lesions

✓ Figure 5-4 is an algorithm to assist in differentiating the location of vestibular lesions.

Vestibular Labyrinth and Nerves (CN 8)

✓ Head tilt, circling, falling, or rolling toward the side of the lesion (Figure 5-1)

✓ Nystagmus, if present, is horizontal or rotatory with the fast phase away from the side of the lesion

✓ May have concurrent facial nerve paralysis (CN 7) and Horner's syndrome (ptosis, miosis, and enophthalmos) with middle- and inner-ear lesions

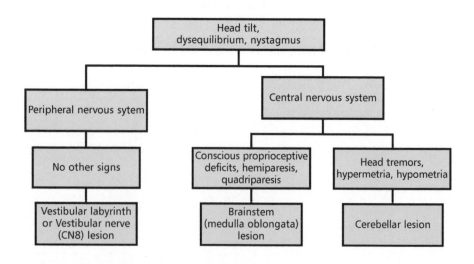

Figure 5-4 Algorithm to assist in differentiating vestibular lesions. CN = cranial nerve

Vestibular Nuclei and the Medulla Oblongata

✓ Head tilt, circling, falling, or rolling toward or away from the side of the lesion

✓ Conscious proprioceptive deficits, hemiparesis, or hemiplegia on the side of the lesion if unilateral or worse on one side if bilateral

✓ Nystagmus, if present, may be horizontal, rotatory, or vertical

✓ May be depressed or stuporous

✓ May have facial paralysis (CN 7), but Horner's syndrome is rare

Flocculonodular Lobe of the Cerebellum

✓ Head tilt, circling, falling, or rolling away from the side of the lesion (Figure 5-5)

✓ Hypermetria of the limbs on the side of the lesion (Figure 5-5)

✓ Nystagmus, if present, may be horizontal, rotatory, or vertical

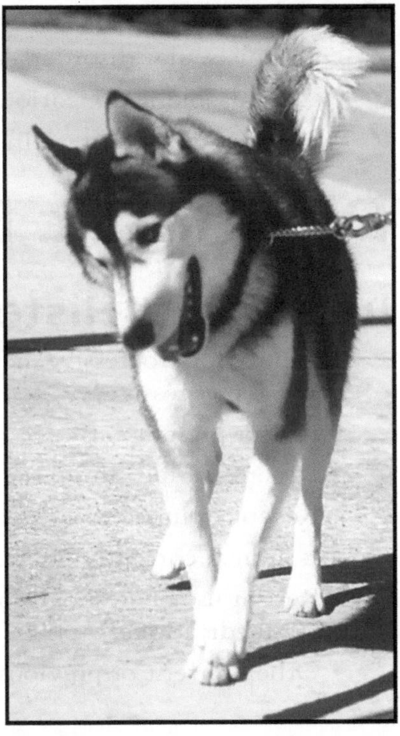

Figure 5-5 A dog with a left-sided cerebellar tumor causing a head tilt to the right and hypermetria on the left.

Differential Diagnosis

Vestibular Labyrinth and Nerve (PNS) Disorders

✓ Idiopathic vestibular syndrome–common in dogs and cats

✓ Otitis interna–common in dogs and cats

✓ Head trauma–common in dogs and cats

✓ Iatrogenic (secondary to ear cleaning)–occasional in dogs and cats

✓ Polyps and neoplasia–occasional in dogs and cats

✓ Hypothyroidism–occasional in dogs

✓ Aminoglycoside intoxication–rare in dogs and cats

Medulla Oblongata and Cerebellar (CNS) Disorders

✓ Meningoencephalitis–common in dogs and cats

✓ Head trauma–common in dogs and cats

✓ Neoplasia–common in dogs and cats

✓ Cerebrovascular disorders–occasional in dogs and cats

✓ Metronidazole intoxication–occasional in dogs and cats

✓ Parasitic migration–rare in dogs and cats

Diagnostic Evaluation

Important Historical Questions

• Acute nonprogressive, acute progressive, or chronic progressive?

• Past or present ear infections?

• Recent ear cleaning?

• Recent trauma?

• Is animal currently on metronidazole?

• Recent use of aminoglycoside antibiotics or other medications?

• Other current or previous illness?

Physical Examination

✓ Examine the external ear canals for evidence of otitis or tumors.

✓ Examine the pharynx for evidence of inflammation or tumors.

✓ Examine the animal for evidence of systemic disease or neoplasia.

Neurologic Examination

✓ The neurologic examination commonly shows unilateral vestibular signs. Affected pets may have one or more of the following signs:

- Head tilt with leaning, falling, rolling, or circling to one side
- Spontaneous nystagmus
- Positional nystagmus
- Positional strabismus

✓ Less commonly, examination will reveal bilateral vestibular signs. One or more of the following signs may be present:

- Absent or mild head tilt but wide swinging head movements side to side
- Leaning, falling, rolling, and loss of balance to both sides
- Circling to both sides
- Loss of normal physiologic nystagmus
- Loss of normal post-rotatory nystagmus
- Neck and thoracic limbs curl ventrally when the animal is held by the pelvis and suspended in air

✓ Determine whether the vestibular lesion is in the PNS or CNS.

Applicable Diagnostic Tests

✓ A complete blood count (CBC), serum chemistry profile, and urinalysis can be useful to detect systemic illness and as part of the preanesthetic evaluation.

✓ Thoracic and abdominal radiographs and abdominal ultrasonography are useful to detect primary or metastatic neoplasia as well as cardiopulmonary disease.

✓ A low serum total thyroxine (T4) and free T4 and an elevated serum thyroid-stimulating hormone (TSH) support the diagnosis of hypothyroidism.

✓ Tests that are performed under general anesthesia, as well as their findings, are as follows:

- Routine or electronic otoscopic examination of the external ear canals and tympanic membranes to detect evidence of infection or masses.

- If a middle ear infection is suspected, myringotomy is attempted for cytologic evaluation and culture of fluid, if obtained.

- Bacterial and fungal cultures of the external or middle ears and antibiotic sensitivity to determine whether infection is present.

- Biopsy or surgical removal and histologic examination of external or middle ear masses.

- Radiographs, computed tomography (CT), or magnetic resonance imaging (MRI) of the osseous bullae, inner ear, medulla oblongata, and cerebellum to determine whether otitis media or interna, traumatic fractures, cerebrovascular disorders, meningoencephalitis, or neoplasia is present.

- CSF analysis to evaluate for leukocytic pleocytosis and increased protein levels in meningoencephalitis, or CNS neoplasia.

- Brainstem auditory-evoked response (BAER) to evaluate the auditory part of CN 8 and the brainstem pathways of hearing; may also differentiate PNS and CNS lesions.

✓ Serum and cerebrospinal fluid (CSF) immunoassays for specific organisms are performed if meningoencephalitis is suspected (Section 2).

> **Warning:** Although recovery from vestibular signs may appear complete, when an animal with a past vestibular problem is placed in water, gravity is altered and dysequilibrium may cause drowning.

Vestibular Labyrinth and Nerve Disorders

Idiopathic Vestibular Syndrome

✓ Sudden onset of head tilt, dysequilibrium, and nystagmus without a known cause may occur in any dog or cat but is most common in geriatric dogs (Figure 5-1) and young cats. The initial signs may be so severe that the animal is unable to stand and rolls whenever handled, making examination difficult.

💣☀ A common misconception in geriatric dogs is that the animal has had a "stroke" and that the prognosis is poor, as the dysequilibrium is so severe that the animal cannot stand or ambulate for several days. Because of their age and severity of the initial signs, dogs with geriatric idiopathic vestibular syndrome are often not given the chance to recover and are euthanized.

✓ Other cranial nerve or other neurologic deficits and Horner's syndrome are absent on the neurologic examination. On rare occasions, bilateral vestibular signs occur, and although there is no head tilt, the equilibrium disturbance is obvious.

✓ The diagnosis is suspected after ruling out other causes of vestibular disease and seeing improvement over the following 72 hours with supportive care only. **In the first 24 to 48 hours, oral meclizine hydrochloride (Antivert, Pfizer) 6.25 mg once daily for cats and 12–25 mg once daily for dogs may be given to reduce the animal's dizziness.** Diazepam 0.1–0.25 mg/kg PO every 8 hours may be given to reduce distress if meclizine is not available but may cause some sedation. Some animals vomit within the first 24 hours after onset of the signs, but this usually resolves without treatment.

✓ An osmolality disturbance of the fluid within the vestibular labyrinth is suspected in cases of idiopathic vestibular syndrome. The prognosis is excellent. Improvement begins within 72 hours, and most animals return to normal in 1 to 3 weeks. Some animals may retain a permanent head tilt. In cases with bilateral vestibular nerve involvement, recovery is often prolonged and incomplete, and permanent hearing loss may result. Recurrence is possible but rare.

Otitis Interna

✓ A unilateral or bilateral inner ear infection or otitis interna is a common cause of vestibular disease in dogs and cats (Figure 5-6). A bacterial infection of the external ear canals or the throat and eustachian tubes may extend into the middle ear and then into the inner ear. The inner ear may less commonly become infected via a hematogenous route. Fungal infections are rare. Onset of vestibular signs may be acute or chronic and progressive. Horner's syndrome from infection of the middle ear (otitis media) may be present. Facial nerve (CN 7) paresis or paralysis causing reduced or absent movement of the eyelids, lip, and ear and reduced or absent tear production commonly occurs with otitis media and interna. Hearing may be obviously affected in bilateral otitis interna.

✓ Otitis externa, inflammation of the external ear canal, may be obvious on physical or otoscopic examination, but the external ear canals can also be normal. An electronic otoscope is most useful to detect bulging, opacity, or tears in the tympanic membrane (Figure 5-7). Myringotomy may be considered to collect samples from the middle ear for cytologic testing, bacterial culture, and antibiotic sensitivity.

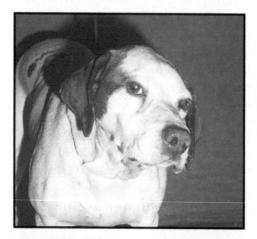

Figure 5-6 A 5-year-old English pointer with a left head tilt associated with an inner ear infection.

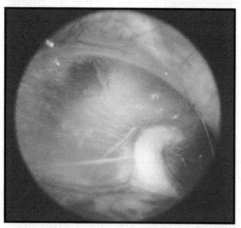

Figure 5-7 The tympanic membrane as viewed with an electronic otoscope.
(Courtesy of Dr. Rosanna Marsella.)

✓ Fluid densities or osteomyelitis may be evident on radiography and CT of the osseous bullae, but MRI is often the best method for visualizing the middle and inner ears (Figure 5-8).

♥ **Appropriate antimicrobial therapy is selected based on the culture and sensitivity results.** If the culture results are negative but bacterial otitis interna is suspected, then enrofloxacin (Baytril, Bayer) 5 mg/kg PO every 12 hours for dogs or cats or a combination of trimethoprim-sulfadiazine 15–30 mg/kg PO every 12 hours and cephalexin (Keflex, Dista) 22 mg/kg PO every 8

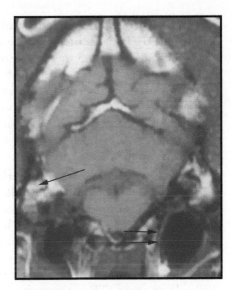

Figure 5-8 A post-contrast transverse T1-weighted MRI of the brain at the level of the medulla oblongata and the osseous bullae; the area of the right (viewer's left) inner ear (arrow) has enhanced with gadolinium indicating inflammation; the left (viewer's right) osseous bulla is indicated by the double arrows.

hours may be administered. **Antibiotic therapy should be continued for 6-8 weeks.** Tear production should be monitored to detect keratoconjunctivitis sicca associated with facial nerve (CN 7) involvement, and antibiotic therapy and artificial tears should be administered if necessary to prevent keratitis and corneal ulceration.

> **Warning:** The owner may prematurely discontinue the antibiotics within the first few weeks of therapy when the signs resolve. This leads to chronic infections, osteomyelitis, and antibiotic-resistant organisms that can be difficult to cure. Owners must be strongly warned of these complications.

♥ In cases of concurrent otitis externa and media with a ruptured tympanic membrane, the external and middle ears are gently flushed with saline or a 2.5% acetic acid solution; caustic ear cleaning substances are avoided if possible. Diluted ear cleaning solutions may be necessary in some cases for debris that cannot be cleared by other means, but thorough rinsing is essential so residual solution does not irritate the vestibular labyrinth. **The external ear canal may be treated topically with small amounts of low-residue, nonirritating antibiotic solutions for a few days, but accumulation of greasy ointments in the middle ear should be avoided.**

✓ Vestibular signs may resolve in 1 to 2 weeks, but if antibiotics are prematurely discontinued, the clinical signs and infection recur and can be more difficult to treat.

✓ **Corticosteroids are usually not required and are avoided if osteomyelitis is present.** In acute cases, prednisone 0.25 mg/kg PO once daily for 1–3 days is sometimes given to reduce inflammation and swelling of the vestibular labyrinth. In animals with recurring otitis, underlying dermatologic problems, such as atopy or hypothyroidism, should be investigated and treated. Ear hygiene should be monitored, but care should be taken when cleaning the external ear canals (see Iatrogenic Vestibular Syndrome, below).

✓ **Some chronic inner ear infections may require surgical removal of debris from the middle ear through bulla osteotomy.** Various surgical procedures to resect the lateral external ear canal may also be beneficial for long-term management of chronic otitis. A rare complication of chronic inner ear infection is an ascending infection into the brainstem region causing bacterial meningitis or abscess formation, which can be very difficult to treat. The treatment of bacterial meningitis is found in Section 2, Table 11.

✓ The prognosis for recovery from otitis interna is good with early and appropriate antibiotic therapy. A residual head tilt, Horner's syndrome, or facial paralysis may result in a few cases but dysequilibrium resolves.

Head Trauma

✓ Acute vestibular dysfunction may be associated with a blow to the head. Blood is often found in the external ear canal, and facial nerve (CN 7) paralysis and Horner's syndrome may also be observed. Diagnosis and treatment of head injuries are discussed in Section 2. Vestibular signs may resolve completely in time, although a residual head tilt is possible.

Iatrogenic Vestibular Syndrome from Ear Cleaning

♥ Acute unilateral and bilateral vestibular dysfunction with or without deafness may occur following routine ear cleaning in both dogs and cats but appears to be more frequent in cats. Rupture of the tympanic membrane and damage to the vestibular labyrinth of the inner ear are suspected. Chlorhexidine and other ear wash preparations suspected to be caustic to the vestibular labyrinth have been incriminated, but attempts to experimentally re-create the problem have failed. A vestibular syndrome may also follow ear cleaning with water alone.

✓ Treatment with corticosteroids as soon as signs appear may reduce any associated inflammation or edema. **Methylprednisolone sodium succinate (Solu-Medrol, Pharmacia & Upjohn) 10 mg/kg IV every 6 to 8 hours for 24 hours followed by prednisone 1 mg/kg PO for 2 to 3 days may improve recovery in some cases.** To protect against gastrointestinal side effects from corticosteroid administration oral famotidine (Pepcid AC, Merck) 0.5–1 mg/kg every 12 to 24 hours, cimetidine (Tagamet, SmithKline Beecham) 5–10 mg/kg every 8 hours, or misoprostol (Cytotec, Searle) 1–3 µg/kg every 8 hours may be administered. Vestibular signs often resolve in 1 to 3 weeks, but some animals may retain dysequilibrium and hearing loss.

Polyps and Neoplasia

✓ Nasopharyngeal polyps and squamous cell carcinoma of the external and middle ears may affect the vestibular labyrinth. Vestibular dysfunction may result, but primary neoplasia of the vestibular nerve is rare. Nasopharyngeal polyps and squamous cell carcinoma can often be visualized on examination of the external ear canal and pharynx and with CT or MRI. **Surgical removal may be attempted.** Removal of squamous cell carcinoma often requires ablation of the external ear canal and bulla osteotomy. **Nasopharyngeal polyps are common in cats and can often be completely removed** (Figures 5-9 and 5-10). Squamous cell carcinoma has a poorer prognosis. Neoplasia affecting the osseous bullae may occur and is often obvious on routine radiography (Figure 5-11). Neurofibroma of CN 8 (acoustic neuroma) can cause a chronic, progressive head tilt. Surgical removal is attempted through bulla osteotomy. A residual head tilt, facial paralysis, and Horner's syndrome may occur.

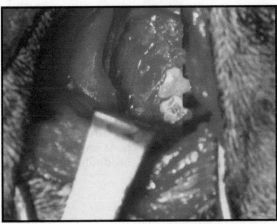

Figure 5-9 A polyp inside the osseous bulla of a cat during bulla osteotomy. (photo courtesy of Dr. Jamie Bellah)

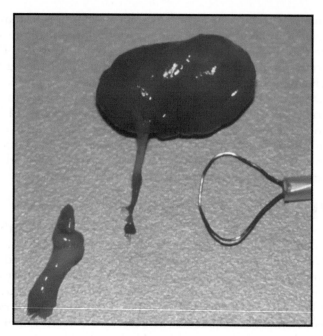

Figure 5-10 The polyp in Figure 5-9 after surgical removal; note the tail that was in the eutstacian tube as a nasopharyngeal polyp was present in the pharynx as well. (photo courtesy of Dr. Jamie Bellah.)

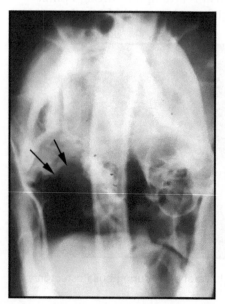

Figure 5-11 Open-mouth skull radiographs of a 6-year-old boxer with a neoplastic process that has obliterated the osseous bulla on the left at the arrows (note the normal osseous bulla on the right); the dog had a left head tilt.

Hypothyroidism

✋ Hypothyroidism may cause acute or chronic unilateral vestibular signs with or without facial nerve paralysis, laryngeal paralysis, or megaesophagus in dogs. Hair coat changes and other signs typical of hypothyroidism are often absent. Microcytic anemia and elevated cholesterol may be found on the CBC and chemistry profile, respectively. The diagnosis is best made through demonstration of a low serum total T4 or free T4 level and elevated serum TSH level. **Levothyroxine sodium** (Soloxine, Daniels Pharmaceuticals) **0.02 mg/kg PO every 12 hours is given.** The serum T4 level is re-evaluated after 4 weeks of therapy, and the levothyroxine dose is adjusted to maintain thyroxine in the normal range. A localized metabolic cranial neuropathy or a cranial polyneuromyopathy is caused by hypothyroidism (Section 6). The prognosis is excellent, as the neurologic signs usually respond to treatment.

Aminoglycoside Intoxication

♥ Systemic or topical gentamicin, amikacin, and streptomycin may cause toxic destruction of receptors in the vestibular labyrinth and cochlea. Animals receiving these antibiotics should be closely monitored for dysequilibrium and deafness. The drugs should be discontinued immediately if signs appear. Dysequilibrium may improve, but some permanent hearing damage may occur.

Medulla Oblongata and Cerebellar Disorders

Meningoencephalitis

✓ Meningoencephalitis can produce acute or chronic progressive vestibular signs with hemiparesis, hypermetria, or both, indicating involvement of the rostral medulla oblongata, cerebellum, or both, respectively. Neurologic deficits associated with other cranial nerves, brainstem segments, and the cerebrum may also occur, indicating a multifocal disease process. Meningoencephalitis has many causes and treatments, and the prognosis varies with each (see Tables 2-8, 2-9, 2-10, and 2-11). The CSF often exhibits leukocytic pleocytosis with or without an elevated protein level. Although CT may show a lesion of the brainstem or cerebellum, MRI is far superior to visualize brainstem and cerebellar lesions (Figure 5-12).

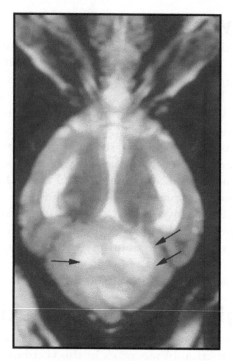

Figure 5-12 Dorsal T2–weighted MRI of granulomatous meningoencephalitis in the cerebellum (arrows) in a 3-year-old poodle with a right head tilt and dysmetria which was worse on the left (the left cerebellum is on the viewer's right, and the right cerebellum is on the viewer's left).

✓ A biopsy with histologic examination may be necessary to differentiate meningoencephalitis from neoplasia, as both may appear as mass lesions on CT or MRI. An overview of the diagnosis and treatment of meningoencephalitis can be found in Section 2.

Trauma

♥ Head injuries may result in trauma to the rostral medulla oblongata and cerebellum, leading to vestibular dysfunction. Brainstem contusion or hemorrhage in the rostral medulla often results in death due to involvement of vital pathways for respiration, cardiac function, and blood pressure. Diagnosis and treatment of head injuries are discussed in Section 2.

Cerebrovascular Disorders

✓ Acute vestibular dysfunction from cerebrovascular disorders (infarction or spontaneous hemorrhage) of the brainstem or cerebellum occur occasionally in animals. CT and MRI are often normal but may occasionally show multifocal abnormalities. CSF analysis is also usually normal but can have increased protein levels. Serial neurologic examinations show slow improvement of neurologic signs over a period of 6 to 8 weeks. Cerebrovascular disorders are discussed in Section 2.

Metronidazole Intoxication

💣※ Animals on metronidazole (Flagyl, SCS) therapy may have acute onset of ataxia, tremors, and vertical nystagmus consistent with CNS vestibular disease. Severe depression and seizures may also occur. Signs of intoxication may develop early or late in the course of metronidazole therapy and may occur at both high and low doses. Metronidazole should be discontinued immediately, and seizures are controlled initially with intravenous anticonvulsant therapy (Section 3, Table 3-4). Signs of intoxication usually improve within 24 to 72 hours of drug discontinuation and usually resolve within a week. Liver function should be evaluated with fasting and 2-hour post-prandial bile acids determinations, as an underlying liver problem may cause intoxication occurring at low doses.

Neoplasia

✓ Adult or geriatric dogs and cats may develop acute or chronic progressive brainstem or cerebellar vestibular dysfunction due to neoplasia. CSF analysis usually shows elevated protein, but leuko-cytic pleocytosis is less common. Neoplasia is best visualized with MRI, but histologic examination of tissue obtained from a biopsy or surgical removal is necessary to confirm the diagnosis. Treatment can be rewarding in some cases, such as with the removal of a cere-bellar meningioma plus adjunctive radiation therapy, which may prolong the animal's survival time by years. Brainstem neoplasia is usually a greater challenge, as the area of involvement is more difficult to reach surgically. The types, diagnosis, and therapy of brain neoplasia are discussed in Section 2.

Parasite Migration

✓ Cuterebra larvae may migrate through the brainstem and cerebellum and cause vestibular dysfunction. Neutrophilic leuko-cytosis and elevated protein may be found on CSF analysis. Prednisone 0.25–0.5mg/kg PO every 12 hours may reduce the inflammation associated with parasite migration and improve function. The disorder is usually diagnosed during necropsy.

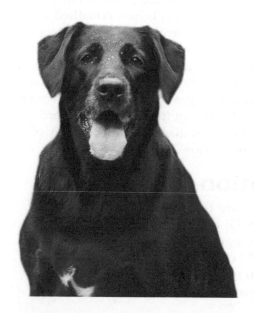

Section 6

Cranial Neuropathies and Myopathies

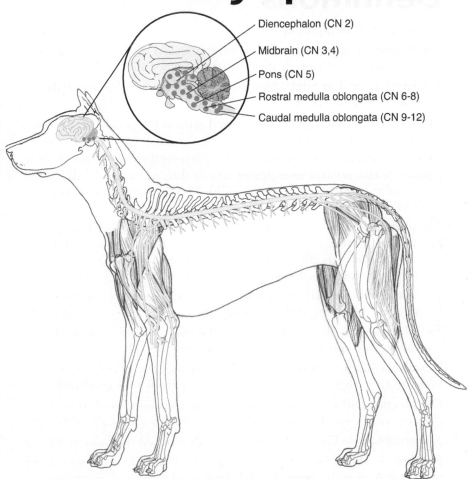

Diencephalon (CN 2)

Midbrain (CN 3,4)

Pons (CN 5)

Rostral medulla oblongata (CN 6-8)

Caudal medulla oblongata (CN 9-12)

Clinical Signs

- ✓ Blindness
- ✓ Strabismus
- ✓ Facial paralysis
- ✓ Dysphagia
- ✓ Stridor
- ✓ Tongue paralysis or atrophy
- ✓ Temporalis and masseter muscle atrophy

- ✓ Anisocoria
- ✓ Jaw paralysis
- ✓ Deafness
- ✓ Megaesophagus
- ✓ Dysphonia
- ✓ Combination of the above signs

Definitions

Anisocoria: Unequal pupil size.

Strabismus: Unilateral or bilateral deviation of the eye or eyes due to paralysis of one or more of the extraocular muscles.

Mydriasis: Dilated pupil associated with fear or a lesion of the oculomotor nerve (CN 3).

Miosis: Constricted pupil associated with a lesion of the sympathetic nerves to the eye.

Ptosis: Reduction in the size of the palpebral fissure secondary to paresis of the levator muscles of the eyelid; associated with a lesion of the oculomotor nerve (CN 3) or sympathetic nerves to the eye.

Enophthalmos: Backward displacement of the eyeball into the orbit that induces passive elevation of the third eyelid and a slight reduction in the diameter of the palpebral fissure; associated with lesions of the sympathetic nerves to the eye.

Jaw paralysis: Inability to close the mouth associated with bilateral dysfunction of the trigeminal nerves (CN 5) (Figure 6-1).

Facial paralysis: Inability to move the eyelid, lip, or ear associated with dysfunction of the facial nerve (CN 7).

Keratoconjunctivitis sicca: Inflammation of the cornea and conjunctiva associated with reduced or absent tear production.

Dysphagia: Difficulty swallowing often associated with dysfunction of the glossopharyngeal (CN 9) or the vagus (CN 10) nerve.

Megaesophagus: Enlarged esophagus with reduced or absent motility.

Stridor: A harsh, high-pitched respiratory sound often associated with inspiration in animals with laryngeal paresis or paralysis.

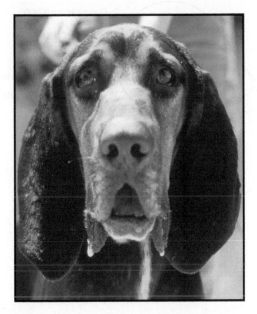

Figure 6-1 A dog with jaw paralysis from idiopathic trigeminal neuropathy; note the dog also had bilateral Horner's syndrome (ptosis, miosis, and enophthalmos).

Dysphonia: A change in voice often associated with laryngeal paresis (CN 10).

Dysautonomia: Dysfunction of the autonomic nervous system.

Lesion Localization

✓ The location of lesions that cause cranial myopathies and neuropathies are shown in Figures 6-2 and 6-3. These lesions are usually found in the:

- Peripheral nervous system (PNS) portion of a cranial nerve
- Central nervous system (CNS) (brainstem) portion of a cranial nerve
- Muscles of the head

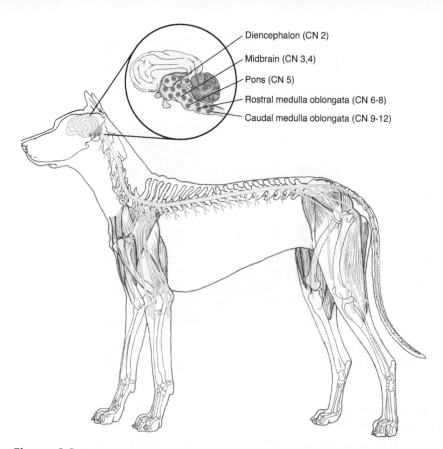

Diencephalon (CN 2)
Midbrain (CN 3,4)
Pons (CN 5)
Rostral medulla oblongata (CN 6-8)
Caudal medulla oblongata (CN 9-12)

Figure 6-2 (above) Lesions may be localized to one or more of the cranial nerves or their associated brainstem segments.

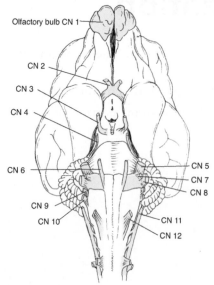

Olfactory bulb CN 1
CN 2
CN 3
CN 4
CN 6
CN 5
CN 7
CN 8
CN 9
CN 10
CN 11
CN 12

Figure 6-3 (left) The ventral surface of the brain showing the location of the cranial nerves and related brainstem segments.

Differentiation of Peripheral and Central Cranial Nerve Lesions

✓ An algorithm to assist in distinguishing peripheral nerve lesions from those of the central cranial nerve lesions is shown in Figure 6-4.

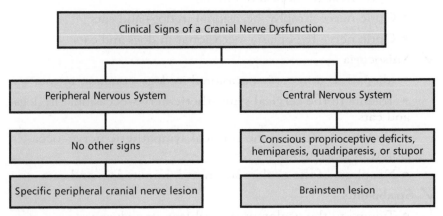

Figure 6-4 Algorithm to assist in distinguishing peripheral nerve lesions from those of the brainstem.

✓ **Peripheral nerve:** Only cranial nerve deficits are present. The rest of the neurologic examination is normal, unless the cranial neuropathy is part of a generalized peripheral nerve disease (Sections 9 and 10).

✓ **Central nervous system:** Cranial nerve signs are present in conjunction with dementia, stupor, unilateral or bilateral conscious proprioceptive deficits, ataxia, hemiparesis, or quadriparesis. Cranial nerves enter or exit the brainstem in the medulla oblongata, pons, midbrain, or diencephalon (Figure 6-3).

✓ **Muscle disease:** Pain on opening the mouth, muscle swelling or atrophy, and inability to open the mouth due to inflammation and fibrosis of the muscles of mastication are found; muscle disorders may be isolated to the head or part of generalized muscle disease (Section 11).

Differential Diagnosis

Peripheral Nerve and Muscle Disorders

✓ **Blindness**

- Sudden acquired retinal degeneration syndrome (SARDS)—common in dogs
- Other ocular and retinal diseases—common in dogs and cats
- Optic neuritis—occasional in dogs
- Optic nerve atrophy—occasional in dogs and cats
- Optic nerve hypoplasia—occasional in dogs and cats

✓ **Anisocoria**

- Idiopathic anisocoria—occasional in dogs, common in cats
- Trauma to the cervical sympathetic nerve—occasional in dogs and cats
- Neoplasia affecting the cervical sympathetic nerve—occasional in dogs and cats
- Neoplasia of the oculomotor nerve—rare in dogs and cats

✓ **Strabismus**

- Trauma to the oculomotor, trochlear, or abducens nerves—common in dogs and cats
- Congenital strabismus—occasional in dogs and cats
- Neoplasia affecting the oculomotor, trochlear, or abducens nerves—rare in dogs and cats
- Extraocular myositis—rare in dogs

✓ **Jaw paralysis**

- Idiopathic trigeminal neuropathy—occasional in dogs
- Bilateral trauma to the trigeminal nerves—rare in dogs and cats

✓ **Temporalis and masseter muscle atrophy**

- Masticatory myositis—common in dogs
- Trigeminal nerve trauma—occasional in dogs and cats
- Neoplasia affecting the trigeminal nerve—rare in dogs and cats

✓ **Facial paresis or paralysis**

- Otitis media or interna—common in dogs and cats
- Idiopathic facial paralysis—common in dogs

- Facial nerve trauma–occasional in dogs and cats
- Hypothyroidism–occasional in dogs
- Myasthenia gravis–occasional in dogs and cats
- Neoplasia affecting the facial nerve–rare in dogs and cats

✓ **Deafness**
- Otitis media or interna–common in dogs and cats
- Senile degeneration–common in dogs and cats
- Congenital deafness–occasional in dogs and cats
- Aminoglycoside intoxication–rare in dogs and cats

✓ **Dysphagia, megaesophagus, stridor, or dysphonia**
- Idiopathic megaesophagus–common in dogs
- Idiopathic laryngeal paresis or paralysis–occasional in dogs and cats
- Trauma to vagus nerves–occasional in dogs and cats
- Polymyositis–occasional in dogs and cats
- Hypothyroidism–occasional in dogs
- Myasthenia gravis–occasional in dogs and cats
- Polyneuropathy–occasional in dogs, rare in cats
- Neoplasia affecting the vagus nerve–rare in dogs and cats

✓ **Tongue paralysis**
- Trauma to the hypoglossal nerve–rare in dogs and cats
- Neoplasia affecting the hypoglossal nerve–rare in dogs and cats
- Polyneuropathy–rare in dogs and cats

✓ **Multiple cranial nerve signs**
- Cranial polyneuropathy–rare in dogs and cats
- Dysautonomia–rare in dogs and cats

Central Nervous System Disorders (Any Cranial Nerve Sign)

✓ Meningoencephalitis–common in dogs and cats
✓ Trauma–common in dogs and cats
✓ Cerebrovascular disorders–occasional in dogs and cats
✓ Neoplasia–common in dogs and cats

Diagnostic Evaluation

Important Historical Questions

- Date of onset?
- Acute or chronic? Nonprogressive or progressive?
- How is vision? Difference in day or night?
- How is hearing?
- Is there a change in the appearance of the face?
- Is there any difficulty drinking, eating, chewing, or swallowing?
- Is there regurgitation or change in voice?
- Any weakness of the limbs or exercise intolerance?
- Seizures, dementia, head tilt, or other neurologic signs?
- Possibility of trauma?
- Concurrent or past illness?
- Concurrent or past neoplastic disease?
- Recent or current medications, nutritional supplements, or exposure to toxins?

Physical Examination

✓ Examine the ocular fundus for evidence of chorioretinitis or other retinal disease.

✓ Examine ears for evidence of otitis externa.

✓ Examine body for evidence of systemic disease.

Neurologic Examination

✓ Determine which cranial nerve or nerves or muscles are involved.

✓ Determine if a PNS or CNS lesion is present.

Applicable Diagnostic Tests

✓ A complete blood count (CBC), serum chemistry profile and urinalysis are performed to detect systemic illness and as part of the preanesthetic evaluation.

✓ Chest and abdominal radiographs with or without abdominal ultrasonography may be performed to check for megaesophagus, aspiration pneumonia, and evidence of neoplasia.

✓ An electroretinogram (ERG) can differentiate retinal disease from optic neuritis.

✓ Serum total thyroxine (T4) or free T4 level may be reduced and thyroid-stimulating hormone (TSH) level elevated with hypothyroidism.

✓ Serum creatine kinase (CK) may be elevated with myositis.

✓ Serum acetylcholine receptor antibody level is often elevated in animals with myasthenia gravis.

✓ Serum 2M-antibody level is often elevated in dogs with masticatory myositis.

✓ The following are tests that are performed under general anesthesia, as well as their findings:

• An electromyogram (EMG) can be useful to determine if there are lesions in more than one cranial nerve or if diffuse polyneuropathy or polymyopathy or myasthenia gravis is present.

• A brainstem auditory-evoked response (BAER) test is used to evaluate hearing and brainstem integrity.

• Computed tomography (CT) or magnetic resonance imaging (MRI) can be abnormal in cases of retrobulbar and ocular disease, inner ear infection and neoplasia, meningoencephalitis, brainstem neoplasia, and trauma.

• The cerebrospinal fluid (CSF) analysis is often abnormal in cases of meningoencephalitis or neoplasia.

• A biopsy of the temporalis and masseter muscles will show inflammation and necrosis in cases of masticatory myositis.

Peripheral Nerve and Muscle Disorders

Blindness

✓ Visual deficits with dilated pupils that do not respond to light are usually associated with diseases of the retina or optic nerves (CN 2). Chorioretinitis, retinal detachment, and some forms of retinal degeneration can be visualized on funduscopic examination. Chorioretinitis may be associated with viral, protozoal, fungal, rickettsial, and other infections as well as granulomatous meningoencephalitis (Section 2). Severe chorioretinitis can result in retinal detachment; this may also be caused by immune-mediated, inherited, neoplastic or idiopathic disorders, and systemic hypertension. Retinal degeneration is a common cause of blindness in dogs but can also occur in cats. Progressive retinal atrophy is usually inherited. Other causes of retinal degeneration are taurine deficiency in cats, enrofloxacin toxicity in cats, vitamin E deficiency, and glaucoma.

🖐 Sudden blindness in dogs with a normal ocular fundus but absent pupillary light reflexes could be due to SARDS, optic neuritis, or toxic optic neuropathy (Figure 6-5). Some cases of optic neuritis show swelling of the optic disk (Figure 6-6), but the disk may also appear normal. Since toxic optic neuropathies have been described in humans, all recent or current medications, nutritional supplements, or exposure to toxic substances should be considered for the potential of neurotoxicity and discontinued if possible. The ERG is abnormal in animals with SARDS but not in optic neuritis, and differentiation of these two diseases is essential, as early diagnosis and treatment of optic neuritis may restore vision. There is no effective treatment for SARDS, and it appears to be a sudden photoreceptor cell death of unknown cause with no associated inflammation.

🖐 Optic neuritis may be associated with an infectious agent (e.g., canine distemper virus, feline infectious peritonitis virus, *Toxoplasma gondii*, and some fungi), granulomatous meningoencephalitis, a paraneoplastic syndrome, trauma, or immune-mediated disorders. It can also be idiopathic. Any enlarged lymph nodes should be aspirated to detect infection or neoplasia. CSF analysis, serum and CSF organism immunoassays,

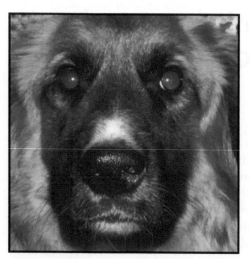

Figure 6-5 A mixed-breed dog with acute blindness and bilateral dilated unresponsive pupils from optic neuritis.

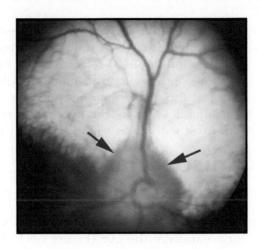

Figure 6-6 Swollen optic disk (arrow) seen on the fundoscopic examination of a dog with optic neuritis.
(Courtesy of Dr. Dennis Brooks).

and MRI may be useful to rule out concurrent meningoencephalitis or neoplasia. Treatment of meningoencephalitis is found in Section 2, Tables 2-10 and 2-11. A thorough examination for neoplasia elsewhere in the body should be performed. If other causes are ruled out, then a diagnosis of idiopathic optic neuritis is made. Since idiopathic optic neuritis is suspected to be immune-mediated, immunosuppressive drugs are given.

✓ **Treatment with prednisone 1–2 mg/kg PO every 12 hours for 2 to 3 weeks with subsequent tapering of the dose often improves vision.** Famotidine (Pepcid AC, Merck) 0.5–1 mg/kg PO every 12 to 24 hours, cimetidine (Tagamet, SmithKline Beecham) 5–10 mg/kg PO every 12 hours, or misoprostol (Cytotec, Searle) 1–3 µg/kg PO every 8 hours is recommended to protect the gastrointesinal tract from upset or ulcers when steroids are administered at high doses.

✓ If there is no response to prednisone alone, the antineoplastic, immunosuppressive drug procarbazine (Matulene, Sigma Tau) may be given at 2–4 mg/kg/day PO for 1 week then increased to 4–6 mg/kg/day. The hemogram and platelet count should be monitored every week initially. If the leukocyte count falls below 4000 cells/µl or platelets are less than 100,000 cells/µl, the drug is discontinued until the leukocyte count returns to normal. Therapy may have to be given for 6 to 12 months to control clinical signs. Periodic drug withdrawal may be used to see if a relapse of visual deficits occurs. In some cases, blindness may be permanent.

✋ If small optic nerves are visualized on funduscopic examination of an animal with reduced or absent vision and reduced or absent pupillary light reflexes, then optic nerve atrophy from a previous optic neuritis, trauma, retrobulbar inflammation or compression, glaucoma, or end stage retinal degeneration are considered. Optic nerve hypoplasia may cause congenital blindness with absent pupillary light reflexes.

Anisocoria

☛ Anisocoria with normal vision and no other ophthalmologic or neurologic signs may be due to a lesion of the parasympathetic portion of the oculomotor nerve (CN 3) or the sympathetic innervation of the eye (Figure 6-7). The sympathetic innervation of the eye is a complex pathway involving three neurons. The first neuron begins in the hypothalamus and descends through the brainstem and cervical spinal cord to the T2 region. A second neuron exits the spinal cord at T2 and passes through the thoracic inlet, traveling cranially with the descending vagus nerve forming the peripheral vagosympathetic nerve. It synapses with a third neuron at the cranial cervical ganglion in the high cervical region. The third neuron goes through the middle ear and into the retrobulbar region to innervate the eye. Lack of parasympathetic innervation causes mydriasis; lack of sympathetic innervation to the eye causes Horner's syndrome (ptosis, miosis, and enophthalmos) (Figure 6-8).

✔ When an animal is presented with anisocoria, the challenge is to determine which is the abnormal eye—the one with the larger or smaller pupil. If vision is normal, the pupil is enlarged, and direct and consensual pupillary light reflexes are absent, then an oculomotor nerve lesion is likely (Figure 6-9). A small pupil that fails to dilate in a darkened room is typical of a sympathetic nerve lesion. Idiopathic anisocoria, which resolves spontaneously, is common in cats and may also occur in dogs. However, other causes should be ruled out. Aniscoria may occur with central nervous system disease but other signs like stupor or coma (Section 2) will be present.

✋ Unilateral oculomotor nerve paralysis may be associated with head trauma and neoplasia (Section 2). CT or MRI of the midbrain area should be considered. Neurofibroma, meningioma, and lymphosarcoma may compress the oculomotor nerve as it exits the brainstem. Neoplasia in this region is very difficult to remove.

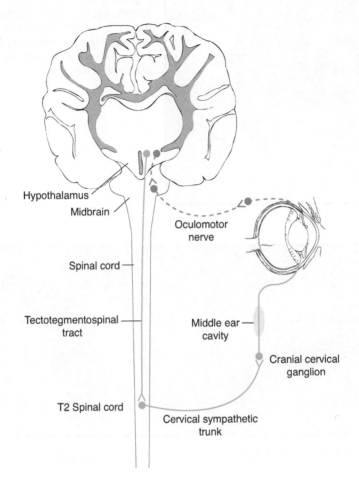

Figure 6-7 Parasympathetic and sympathetic innervation of the eye.

✓ Horner's syndrome with no other neurologic signs is usually associated with trauma or neoplasia affecting the vagosympathetic nerve. Thoracic radiographs may reveal a mass in the thoracic inlet. Horner's syndrome may be associated with inner ear infections (Section 5), brainstem or cervical spinal cord disorders (Sections 9 and 10), and with paralysis of the thoracic limb (Section 14). Retrobulbar masses may also cause anisocoria and affect either sympathetic or parasympathetic innervation to the pupil or both. An idiopathic horner's syndrome may occur.

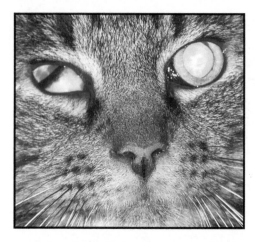

Figure 6-8 Horner's syndrome (ptosis, miosis, and enophthalmos) in the right eye of a cat with a middle ear infection; the cat had a right otitis externa, media, and interna.

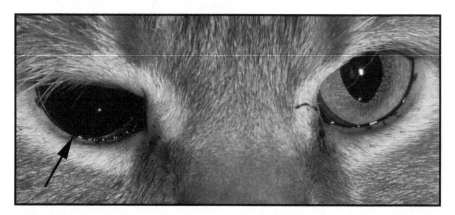

Figure 6-9 A dilated right pupil (arrow) and ptosis from an oculomotor nerve (CN 3) lesion in a cat.

Strabismus

✋ Ventrolateral strabismus may be due to a lesion of the oculomotor nerve (CN 3) (Figure 6-10), while medial strabismus is usually associated with a lesion of the abducens nerve (CN 6). Dysfunction of the trochlear nerve (CN 4) is rare in dogs and cats. Congenital strabismus can be seen in dogs and cats. Strabismus with no other neurologic signs may be due to trauma or neoplasia of the associated peripheral nerve. CT or MRI should be considered if mass lesions of the orbit or cranial nerves are suspected. Neurofibroma or lymphosarcoma of the oculomotor or abducens nerves can occur and are difficult to remove when they are close to the brainstem. Retrobulbar masses may

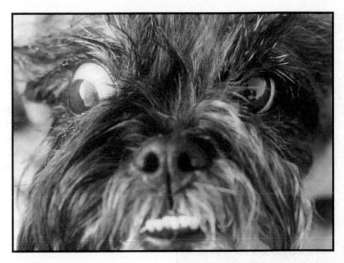

Figure 6-10 Ventrolateral strabismus of the right eye from a right oculomotor nerve (CN 3) lesion in a dog.

cause deviation of the eyeball. Focal extraocular myositis and fibrosis can result in strabismus in Golden Retrievers, Shar-Peis and other dogs, but is rare.

Jaw Paralysis

✓ A syndrome of acute paralysis of the masticatory musculature occurs in dogs and is manifested by an inability to close the mouth (jaw paralysis) (Figure 6-1). The cause is unknown, but neuritis of the trigeminal nerves (CN 5) is suspected. Some dogs also have unilateral or bilateral Horner's syndrome (see Figure 6-1). Most dogs are able to ingest a high-calorie, blended, liquid food or gruel and water to maintain nutrition and hydration. A few dogs may benefit from gastrostomy tube feeding. Jaw function usually returns in 4-6 weeks without specific therapy. Jaw paralysis can also occur from bilateral trauma to the trigeminal nerves, which usually also resolves without treatment (Figure 6-11).

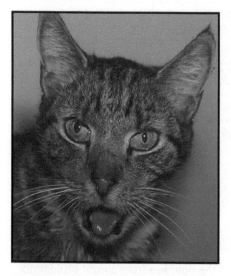

Figure 6-11 A cat with jaw paralysis from trauma; no jaw fractures are present, only bilateral trigeminal nerve (CN 5) paralysis; the cat recovered function of the jaw within 2 weeks.

Temporalis and Masseter Muscle Atrophy

✓ Masticatory myositis is an immune-mediated disease of dogs that can be an acute condition characterized by pain on opening the mouth and muscle swelling or a chronic condition characterized by atrophy of the temporalis and masseter muscle and inability to open the mouth due to muscle fibrosis (Figure 6-12). The immune-mediated response is directed toward the 2M-type fibers of the masticatory muscles. Elevated 2M-antibody levels may be found in the serum of affected dogs. Inflammation and fibrosis are seen on histologic examination of a muscle biopsy. If pain occurs only on opening the mouth, retrobulbar or temporomandibular joint disorders should also be considered.

✓ **If masticatory myositis is confirmed, prednisone 1–2 mg/kg PO every 12 hours is given until jaw mobility returns.** The dosage is then gradually tapered to the level necessary to maintain mobility. Oral famotidine (Pepcid AC) 0.5–1 mg/kg every 12-24 hours, cimetidine (Tagamet) 5–10 mg/kg every 12 hours, or misoprostol (Cytotec) 1–3 µg/kg every 8 hours may reduce gastrointestinal irritation when the dose of steroid therapy is high. If there is no response to prednisone alone, then other immunosuppressive drugs may be considered. Azathioprine (Imuran, Glaxo Wellcome) 2 mg/kg PO once daily may be added to prednisone therapy until improvement is seen and then reduced to every-other-day dosage indefinitely. Hemograms and platelets counts should be closely monitored. Supportive care consists of feeding blended food or gruel and water. Recurrence is common, and alternate-day prednisone therapy may be required indefinitely to control the disease.

♥ Early diagnosis and treatment are essential, as chronic myositis can lead to severe muscle fibrosis and inability to open the mouth, making eating and drinking impossible. Forceful opening of the jaw under anesthesia or surgical excision of fibrosis around the temporomandibular joint may temporarily open the mouth, but the jaw hangs open following surgery, and fibrosis usually recurs.

✓ On rare occasions, masticatory myositis may be asymmetric, but unilateral atrophy of the temporalis and masseter muscles is more commonly associated with a traumatic, inflammatory, or neoplastic disease process affecting the trigeminal nerve (CN 5) (Figure 6-13).

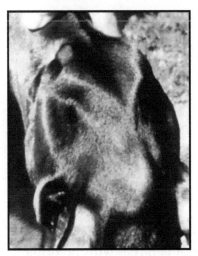

Figure 6-12 A Doberman pinscher with temporalis and masseter muscle atrophy from masticatory myositis.

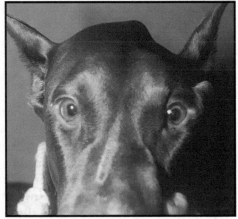

Figure 6-13 A Doberman pinscher with unilateral left temporalis muscle atrophy from a left trigeminal nerve lesion associated with meningoencephalitis of unknown origin.

Facial Nerve Paralysis

✓ Facial nerve paralysis results in inability to move the eyelid, ear, or lip on one or both sides (Figure 6-14). In acute conditions, the ear and the lip on the affected side may be flaccid and hang below the normal side. In chronic paralysis, muscle fibrosis causes the lip and ear to contract and be carried higher than those on the normal side. Inability to close the eyelid is usually obvious on the affected side. The facial nerves innervate the lacrimal and salivary glands, and lesions may cause dryness of the eyes and mouth. Food may collect inside the lips on the affected side. The Schirmer tear test can be useful to evaluate tear production. Administration of artificial tears in the affected eye 3 to 4 times daily may be needed to prevent keratoconjunctivitis sicca and corneal ulceration.

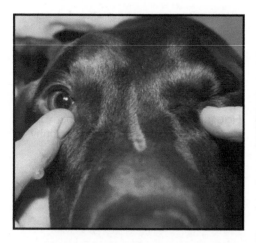

Figure 6-14 A Doberman pinscher with right facial nerve paralysis from an injury.

✓ Otitis media commonly causes facial paralysis with no other signs, especially in dogs with chronic otitis externa. Otitis media and interna may also cause facial paralysis with Horner's syndrome and vestibular signs. The diagnosis and treatment of otitis media and interna are discussed in Section 5.

🖐 Trauma to the facial nerve can cause facial nerve paralysis, which often resolves in time. Hypothyroidism may also cause facial paralysis. Microcytic anemia and elevated cholesterol may be found on the CBC and chemistry profile, respectively, but hypothyroidism is best diagnosed by demonstrating a low serum total T4 or free T4 level in conjunction with an elevated TSH. **Levothyroxine sodium (Soloxine, Daniels Pharmaceuticals) 0.02 mg/kg PO every 12 hours usually results in a resolution of signs.**

✋ An EMG can be evaluated to determine if the facial paralysis is focal or part of a multifocal cranial polyneuropathy.

✓ Idiopathic facial nerve paralysis is diagnosed by ruling out other disease processes and is more common in dogs—especially cocker spaniels—than in cats. Recovery often occurs in 4 to 6 weeks without specific therapy, although paralysis is permanent in some cases.

Deafness

✓ Deafness is associated with bilateral disease of the sensory receptors of the cochlea in the inner ear or the cochlear nerves (CN 8). Congenital deafness may be an inherited disorder in many breeds of dogs, particularly Dalmatians and other breeds with white hair coats and light-colored eyes. Blue-eyed, white cats are also usually deaf at birth. Puppies and kittens can have their hearing tested at 6 to 8 weeks of age using a BAER test. This test can evaluate hearing in each ear individually and detect unilateral deafness, which is important information for breeders. Congenital deafness usually results from lack of development of the receptor organs of the inner ear that are necessary for hearing. There is no treatment.

✋ Any dog or cat with hearing problems should be carefully evaluated for otitis interna, as early diagnosis and treatment may resolve the hearing loss. The diagnosis and treatment of otitis interna is found in Section 5. Intoxication with aminoglycoside antibiotics—especially amikacin, kanamycin, and tobramycin—can cause deafness in dogs and cats. Thus, animals receiving these drugs should have their hearing monitored. Senile degeneration of the inner ear structures may occur with age. The use of hearing aid devices has been attempted but most animals will not tolerate them.

Dysphagia, Megaesophagus, Dysphonia, and Stridor

✓ Dysphagia, megaesophagus, dysphonia, and stridor may all be associated with dysfunction of vagus nerves (CN 10). Dysphagia due to pharyngeal muscle paresis or paralysis can be observed when the animal attempts to swallow food. Megaesophagus associated with paresis or paralysis of the esophageal muscles results in regurgitation shortly after eating. Dysphonia may be witnessed as the animal attempts to bark or meow. It may be a historical complaint and is associated with dysfunction of the laryngeal muscles. Stridor is usually audible and is often associated with unilateral or bilateral paresis or paralysis of the laryngeal muscles. Bilateral laryngeal paralysis can result in severe dyspnea and cyanosis, and emergency measures may have to be taken to establish a patent airway.

🖐 Trauma to the vagus nerves can cause these signs, and the diagnosis is usually obvious from the history or physical examination. Serum diagnostic tests to consider include a serum CK level for polymyositis; T4, free T4, and TSH for hypothyroidism; and serum acetylcholine receptor antibodies for myasthenia gravis. All of these disorders can cause one or more signs of vagus nerve dysfunction. On rare occasions, lead intoxication can cause megaesophagus and laryngeal paralysis, so measuring levels of lead in the blood may be indicated. Hypoadrenocorticism may occasionally be associated with megaesophagus, so adrenal function tests may be considered. Thoracic radiographs usually show megaesophagus, although fluoroscopy with contrast administration may occasionally be necessary. Evidence of aspiration pneumonia may be apparent on thoracic radiographs of animals with dysphagia. Reduced or absent mobility of one or both of the laryngeal folds are observed with laryngeal ultrasonography and upon laryngoscopic examination.

✓ The EMG may be used to detect diffuse or focal nerve involvement. Laryngeal paralysis associated with polyneuropathy has been described in Dalmatians, Rottweilers, and other dogs. Treatment of the underlying polymyositis, hypothyroidism, hypoadrenocorticism, myasthenia gravis, or polyneuropathy often improves the clinical signs (Sections 10 and 11). In laryngeal paresis, mild sedation may control stridor, but in some cases a temporary tracheostomy may be needed to maintain a patent airway. Laryngeal surgery is avoided if possible with these disorders because the animal may recover once the underlying problem is controlled, and if the protective function of the larynx becomes compromised, aspiration pneumonia can be a serious complication.

✓ Congenital megaesophagus occurs in pure- and mixed-breed dogs and cats, including miniature schnauzers, wirehaired fox terriers, Newfoundland terriers, Labrador retrievers, Shar-Peis, Irish setters, and Siamese cats. Idiopathic megaesophagus occurs in Germans shepherds, golden retrievers, Irish setters, Great

Danes, and other dogs and cats between 5 and 12 years of age. There is no specific treatment for congenital or idiopathic megaesophagus. Supportive care consists of feeding small amounts of moist food formed into small balls 2-3 times daily from an elevated surface and then holding the animal vertical for 10-15 minutes after meals to prevent regurgitation. In severe cases, a gastrostomy tube may be necessary for feeding. About 20% to 40% of dogs with congenital megaesophagus may improve as they get older, but spontaneous recovery of idiopathic megaesophagus is rare.

✓ Congenital laryngeal paralysis occurs in young Bouvier des Flandres, Siberian huskies, and other dog breeds. Idiopathic laryngeal paresis or paralysis may occur in adult Labrador retrievers, Afghan hounds, Irish setters, and other dog breeds and cats. Treatment usually involves some surgical intervention, such as unilateral thyroarytenoid lateralization, to distract the vocal folds or partial laryngectomy to open the airway. The most frequent complication of dysphagia, megaesophagus, and surgery for laryngeal paralysis is aspiration pneumonia, which can be fatal.

Tongue Paralysis or Atrophy

✓ Unilateral tongue paralysis or atrophy from a hypoglossal nerve (CN 12) lesion with no other neurologic signs is relatively rare but may be associated with peripheral nerve trauma or neoplasia. If the animal has no known history of trauma, MRI of the caudal brainstem area should be considered to rule out neoplasia, such as neurofibroma, meningioma, and lymphosarcoma affecting the hypoglossal nerve as it exits the brainstem.

Cranial Polyneuropathies

🖐 Multiple cranial nerves may be dysfunctional in dogs with acute polyneuropathies (Section 9), chronic polyneuropathies (Section 10), meningoencephalitis or neoplasia affecting the brainstem (Section 2), and cranial polyneuropathies (Figure 6-15). In animals with cranial polyneuropathies, only muscles associated with cranial nerves are abnormal on the neurologic examination and EMG. No other underlying polymyopathy, hypothyroidism, myasthenia gravis, or polyneuropathy is detected. CSF analysis and MRI are normal and help to rule out brainstem inflammation or multifocal peripheral nerve neoplasias, such as lymphosarcoma. Chronic immune-mediated or paraneoplastic cranial polyneuritis is suspected. Treatment with prednisone with or without azathioprine and gastrointestinal protectants as described above for masticatory myositis can be tried. In some cases, there is no response to therapy and the prognosis is grave.

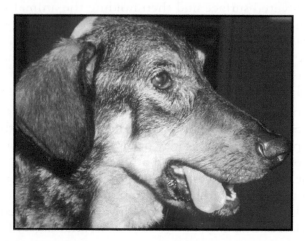

Figure 6-15 A mixed-breed dog with paralysis of the tongue, unilateral atrophy of the temporalis and masseter muscles, and facial nerve paralysis on the right side from granulomatous meningoencephalitis of the pons and medulla; the dog also had hemiparesis and conscious proprioceptive deficits on the right thoracic and pelvic limbs.

Dysautonomia

✓ Dysautonomia is an idiopathic dysfunction of the autonomic nervous system of dogs and cats that causes dilated pupils that do not respond to light with normal vision, anisocoria, prolapsed third eyelids, reduced tear and saliva production, megaesophagus, bradycardia, constipation, and urinary incontinence. A Shirmer tear test is reduced (<15 mm/min). No increased heart rate is observed when atropine 0.02 mg/kg IV is administered. One drop of dilute pilocarpine (0.1%) will constrict the pupils of an animal with dysautonomia but not a normal animal. Affected animals may also have anorexia, weight loss, weakness, and tremors. Reported cases are primarily from the United Kingdom; sporadic cases have been reported in the United States in Kansas and Missouri. The diagnosis is primarily based on the typical clinical signs. Urinary catecholamines are reduced. Treatment is symptomatic and supportive. Initially fluid administration and electrolyte replacement therapy may be necessary. Gastrostomy feeding may be needed to maintain nutrition. The bladder may have to be expressed every 8 hours, and laxatives may be given to assist defecation.

✓ Administration of parasympathomimetic drugs, such as bethanechol hydrochloride (Urecholine, Merck) 5 to 25 mg PO every 8 hours in dogs and 2.5 to 5 mg every 8 to 12 hours in cats, may relieve some of the symptoms. One or two drops of 0.5% physostigmine or 1% pilocarpine ophthalmic preparations in both eyes every 12 hours may have some systemic effect. Aspiration pneumonia secondary to megaesophagus and urinary tract infections require antibiotic therapy. The demeanor and appetite of cats may improve with prednisone 1 to 5 mg every other day. Affected animals may recover after several months, but the nursing care is so intensive that many owners elect euthanasia. A diffuse degeneration of the autonomic ganglia of unknown etiology is found on necropsy.

Central Nervous System Disorders

✓ Cranial nerve signs plus unilateral or bilateral conscious proprioceptive deficits, hemiparesis, or quadriparesis suggests brainstem disease. Meningoencephalitis, head trauma, cerebrovascular disorders, and neoplasia are possibilities and are discussed in Section 2.

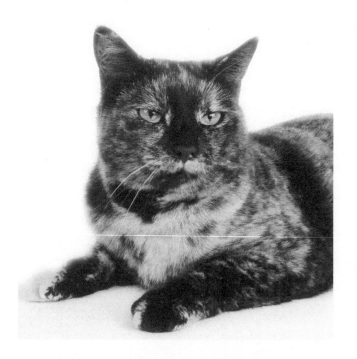

Section 7

Neck or Back Pain

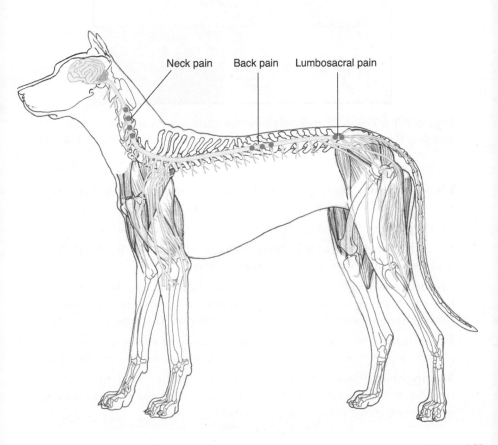

Neck pain   Back pain   Lumbosacral pain

Definitions

Pain: An aversive sensory and emotional experience, which elicits protective motor actions and results in learned avoidance (Figure 7-1).

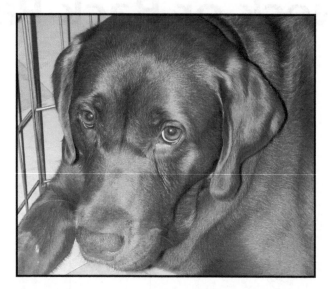

Figure 7-1 A 7-year-old chocolate Labrador retriever with an anxious look, guarding the neck because of pain from an intervertebral disk protrusion at C5-6.

Hyperesthesia: Increased sensitivity to stimulation resulting in a negative behavioral reaction from the animal.

Hyperpathia: An exaggerated response to painful stimuli.

Paresthesia: Abnormal burning or tingling; often affects limbs and feet and manifests as self-mutilation.

"Root signature": A sign that a lesion is irritating the nerve roots to a limb; manifests as reluctance to bear weight on the limb when standing and lameness or pain of the limb.

Fenestration: A surgical procedure to remove the nucleus pulposus of the intervertebral disk to prevent future extrusions.

Meningitis: Inflammation of the meninges (i.e., the three membranes that surround the spinal cord and brain: dura mater, arachnoid membrane, and pia mater).

Lesion Localization

✓ The location of lesions that cause neck and back pain are shown in Figure 7-2. These lesions usually originate in the:

- Cervical, thoracic, lumbar, or sacral regions
- Referred cervical pain may originate from an intracranial lesion (rare)

✓ The following structures can be sources of pain:

- Meninges
- Nerve roots
- Vertebrae
- Intervertebral disks
- Spinal ligaments
- Muscles

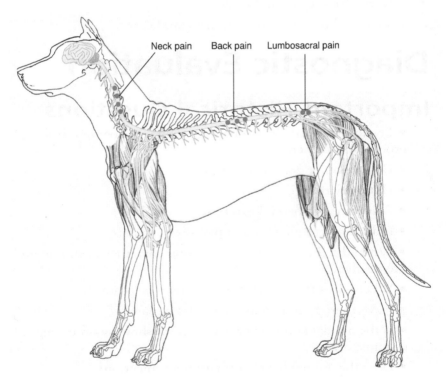

Neck pain   Back pain   Lumbosacral pain

Figure 7-2 The lesion is usually at the site of the pain in animals with neck or back pain.

Differential Diagnosis

Neck and back pain with no other associated neurologic signs:

✓ Degenerative intervertebral disk disease (IVDD)—common in dogs, rare in cats

✓ Diskospondylitis or osteomyelitis—common in dogs, rare in cats

✓ Meningitis—common in dogs, occasional in cats

✓ Vertebral fracture —common in dogs and cats

✓ Lumbosacral degeneration—common in dogs

✓ Atlantoaxial subluxation—occasional in dogs

✓ Caudal cervical spondylomyelopathy—occasional in dogs

✓ Spondylosis deformans—occasional in dogs and cats

✓ Vertebral neoplasia—occasional in dogs and cats

✓ Nerve root or spinal cord neoplasia—occasional in dogs and cats

✓ Polymyositis or other polymyopathy—occasional in dogs and cats

✓ Polyarthritis—occasional in dogs

✓ Intracranial neoplasia—rare in dogs and cats

Diagnostic Evaluation

Important Historical Questions

• Possible trauma? (If so, obtain vertebral radiographs before proceeding further.)

• Depression or decreased activity?

• Difficulty rising?

• Reluctance to bend down to eat or drink?

• Reluctance to jump or go up or down stairs?

• When did the signs start? How long have they been present? Progressive?

• Where does the owner think the pain is located?

• Have there been previous episodes of pain?

• Is the animal anorexic or depressed or showing other signs of systemic disease?

• Does the animal have a urinary tract infection?

• Are there any previous or current medications or other treatments for the pain?

Physical and Neurologic Examinations

✓ The body temperature may be elevated in diskospondylitis, spondylitis, and meningitis, but it can also be normal.

✓ A heart murmur may be auscultated in animals with bacterial endocarditis that has become a systemic infection and caused diskospondylitis, spondylitis, or meningitis.

✓ If the animal is in extreme pain, a complete neurologic examination may be impossible, but neurologic deficits may be detected by observing the animal.

✓ The evaluation of neck and back pain is outlined in Table 7-1.

✓ Once the painful area has been localized, the pain should be controlled as outlined in Table 7-2.

Table 7-1.
Evaluation for Neck or Back Pain

Evidence of pain that can be observed

- Depression
- Decreased activity
- Episodes of yelping or loud vocalization
- Head held toward the ground (neck pain)
- Reluctance to move the neck (eyes move without moving the neck)
- Holding one limb flexed when standing (root signature)
- Visible spasms of the neck or back musculature
- Arched back
- Difficulty rising
- Reluctance to jump or climb
- Reluctance to go up or down stairs
- Lameness or stiff gait

Palpation to detect pain

- The patient's neck or back should only be manipulated if a vertebral fracture or luxation is unlikely
- Pressing on the dorsal spinous processes and squeezing across the transverse processes or the articular facets may elicit pain in abnormal or very sensitive animals
- Placing one hand on the abdomen of the animal while palpating the paravertebral muscles may help detect tension in the abdominal muscles as painful areas are approached
- Palpation through the rectum can evaluate for pain of the ventral surface of the lumbosacral region
- When palpated, the animal may cry out or try to bite, or the paravertebral musculature may become rigid
- Spasms of the musculature can often be felt

Manipulation

If pain was not found on palpation, the vertebral column may be manipulated.

- Flexion, extension, and turning of the head and neck often elicit increased resistance, pain, and palpable muscle spasms when there are problems in the cervical region; a normal young animal can touch its nose to its flank without discomfort
- Extension of the lumbosacral region by dorsal extension of the tail or the pelvic limbs can elicit pain in animals with lumbosacral disease
- Lumbosacral pain must be differentiated from hip pain

Table 7-2:*
Stop the Pain!

Regardless of the cause, pain relief is provided as soon as possible. The type of pain relief varies with the cause and severity:

Muscle spasms

- Intravenous diazepam 0.5 mg/kg (not to exceed 10 mg in dogs and 5 mg in cats) once, then give orally

- Oral diazepam 0.5 mg/kg (not to exceed 10 mg in dogs and 5 mg in cats) every 6-8 hours

Nerve root and meningeal irritation

- Oral prednisone 0.25-1 mg/kg every 12 hours; taper doses over 7-14 days (strict crate rest is essential!)

- Acupuncture: Dogs and cats may need 6 or more treatments (prednisone therapy may interfere with the effectiveness of acupuncture)

Mild bone pain

- Oral carprofen (Rimadyl, Pfizer) 2.2 mg/kg every 12 hours for dogs

- Oral etodolac (Etogesic, Fort Dodge) 15 mg/kg once daily for dogs

- Oral buffered aspirin 10-25 mg/kg every 8-12 hours for dogs and 10-15 mg/kg every 24-72 hours for cats

- Acupuncture: Dogs and cats may need 6 or more treatments (NSAIDS may interfere with the effectiveness of acupuncture)

Warning: Never use caprofen, etodolac or aspirin in combination with prednisone or other corticosteroids as gastrointestinal ulcers and perforation can lead to death!

Mild to moderate pain

- Intravenous or subcutaneous buprenorphine (Buprenex) 0.005-0.02 mg/kg for dogs and 0.005-0.015 mg/kg for cats every 3-8 hours

Moderate to severe acute pain

- Intravenous or subcutaneous hydromorphone 0.05-0.2 mg/kg for dogs and 0.05-0.1 mg/kg for cats every 3-6 hours

- Intravenous morphine 0.05-0.4mg/kg for dogs; give slowly over 1 minute as it may cause histamine release

- Subcutaneous morphine 0.05-0.2 mg/kg every 3-4 hours for dogs

Mild to moderate chronic pain

- Transdermal fentanyl patch (0.005 mg/kg/hr) for dogs and cats; takes up to 24 hours in dogs and12 hours in cats to reach therapeutic plasma levels; lasts up to 72 hours in dogs and 100 hours in cats (not all animals reach therapeutic levels and may require additional opioid therapy, such as hydromorphone, if they are still in pain)

- Acupuncture: Dogs and cats may need 6 or more treatments

* Table formulated in conjunction with Dr. Sheilah Robertson.

Applicable Diagnostic Tests

✓ Vertebal column radiographs if fracture is suspected.

✓ A complete blood count (CBC) may show neutrophilic leukocytosis in cases of diskospondylitis, spondylitis, and some cases of meningitis. Fibrinogen levels may be elevated as well.

✓ Urinalysis may show evidence of a urinary tract infection in cases of diskospondylitis, and urine culture and antibiotic sensitivity should be performed.

✓ Blood culture and antibiotic sensitivity may be indicated in cases of diskospondylitis, spondylitis, and bacterial meningitis.

✓ A serum chemistry profile may be performed to detect systemic illness and as part of the preanesthetic evaluation.

✓ The serum creatine kinase (CK) may be elevated in animals with polymyositis and other polymyopathies.

✓ Cytologic evaluation and culture of joint fluid may be useful to confirm a polyarthritis.

✓ Thoracic and abdominal radiographs and abdominal ultrasound are indicated if neoplasia is suspected or abnormalities are found on the physical examination.

✓ The following are tests that are performed under general anesthesia; potential findings are also listed:

• Cerebrospinal fluid (CSF) analysis may show leukocytosis with or without elevated protein in animals with acute intervertebral disc disease (IVDD), meningitis, and some neoplastic processes; only elevated protein is noted in cases of IVDD, trauma, and neoplasia.

• An electromyogram (EMG) may show positive sharp waves and fibrillation potentials in the paravertebral muscles in the area of a lesion that affects ventral nerve roots.

• Vertebral column radiographs may show vertebral fractures and luxations, calcified intervertebral disks, diskospondylitis, spondylitis, atlantoaxial subluxation, spondylosis deformans, and vertebral neoplasia.

• A myelogram may demonstrate spinal cord compression in animals with caudal cervical spondylomyelopathy, IVDD, or some spinal cord neoplasia. Primary spinal cord neoplasia may cause the spinal cord to appear swollen on the myelogram.

• Computed tomography (CT) and magnetic resonance imaging (MRI) can be useful to demonstrate intervertebral disk disease, diskospondylitis, and vertebral and spinal cord neoplasia.

✓ Serum and CSF immunoassays for specific organisms are indicated if CSF analysis shows evidence of inflammation.

Disorders That Cause Neck or Back Pain

Degenerative Intervertebral Disk Disease

✓ Degeneration of the intervertebral disk with extrusion or protrusion of the disk material into the spinal canal is one of the most common causes of neck and back pain in dogs. The intervertebral disk is situated ventral to the spinal cord and consists of an inner gelatinous portion, the nucleus pulposus, surrounded by an outer fibrous ring, the anulus fibrosus (Figure 7-3). Hansen Type I and Hansen Type II IVDD affect different types of dogs and often have a different clinical course. In Hansen Type I IVDD, the nucleus pulposus ruptures through the anulus fibrosus, extrudes into the vertebral canal or compresses nerve roots, and causes acute neck or back pain (Figure 7-4). A "root signature," which is caused by compression of the C6-T2 or L4-S2 nerve roots by a lateralized disk extrusion, causes lameness or pain in one thoracic or pelvic limb. The disk may herniate to one side of the dorsal longitudinal ligament, which lines the floor of the vertebral canal, causing the limb or limbs of one side to be more affected than the other.

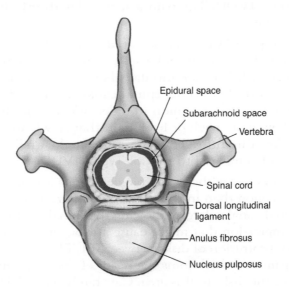

Epidural space

Subarachnoid space

Vertebra

Spinal cord

Dorsal longitudinal ligament

Anulus fibrosus

Nucleus pulposus

Figure 7-3 The relationship of the intervertebral disk to the spinal cord.

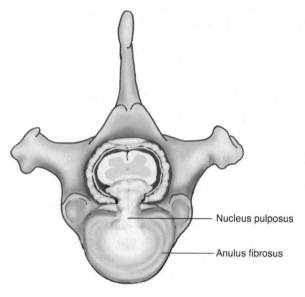

Figure 7-4
Type I intervertebral
disk extrusion.

Nucleus pulposus

Anulus fibrosus

✓ Hansen Type I IVDD is usually caused by chondroid degeneration of the disk. It often affects chondrodystrophic dogs but can affect other dogs. Dachshunds, Pekingese, pugs, Lhasa apsos, Shih Tzus, beagles, cocker spaniels, and many other small-breed dogs are commonly presented for neck and back pain from Hansen Type I IVDD. The pain associated with this disorder can be excruciating.

✓ Hansen Type II IVDD is associated with a fibroid type of disk degeneration. The nucleus pulposus protrudes through some annular fibers, while other annular fibers remain intact, hypertrophy, and protrude into the spinal canal (Figure 7-5). Hansen Type II IVDD is more common in older nonchondrodystrophic dogs with low-grade neck or back pain that slowly worsens over several weeks or months. The pain associated with Type II IVDD is usually mild compared to that of Type I IVDD.

✓ Pain from IVDD without neurologic deficits is more common in the cervical region than in the thoracolumbar region as the cervical spinal canal is larger, allowing the spinal cord more space to avoid compression that might cause ataxia, paresis, or paralysis. Extrusion or protrusion of disks between T1-T10 is rare, as the conjugal ligament, which joins the heads of the ribs, reinforces the region above the disks in this area. Cats rarely have IVDD, but older cats can have chronic Type II disk protrusion.

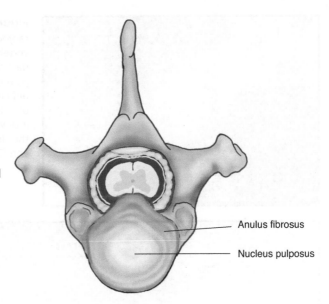

Figure 7-5
Type II intervertebral disk protrusion.

Anulus fibrosus

Nucleus pulposus

✍ Calcified disks, narrowed disk spaces, and calcified disk material in the vertebral canal are often seen on routine vertebral radiographs in Type I IVDD (Figures 7-6 and 7-7). However, radiographic abnormalities are rare in type II IVDD. CSF analysis may be normal or have elevated protein levels with or without mild leukocytic pleocytosis. Spinal cord compression is usually absent or minimal on the myelogram of animals with pain only, but some animals can have significant spinal cord compression and pain with minimal neurologic dysfunction. Degenerated disks and disk material in the vertebral canal is best visualized with CT or MRI (Figures 7-8, 7-9, and 7-10).

✓ Acute neck or back pain often responds to medical management as outlined in Table 7-3. **Crate rest for 4 weeks is the most important part of therapy** because if the dog is kept quiet during the healing process, the extruded disk material can contract away from nerve roots, relieving the pain without surgical intervention.

✓ Prednisone can often be discontinued after a few days, but diazepam may be continued longer. If diazepam is continued for more than 2 weeks, it should be tapered over several days as opposed to being discontinued abruptly. Failure to improve with rest, recurrent episodes of pain, and development of paresis or paralysis are indications for surgical intervention. Most dogs with cervical IVDD require surgical removal of the extruded disk material because of intractable pain.

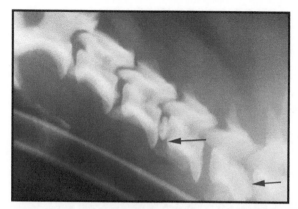

Figure 7-6 A lateral radiograph of the cervical vertebrae in a 5-year-old dachshund with neck pain and no neurologic deficits shows evidence of calcified degenerated intervertebral disks within the disk spaces at C4-5 and C6-7 (arrows).

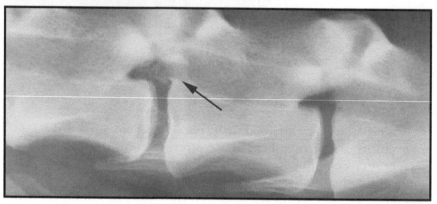

Figure 7-7 Lateral radiographs of the lumbar vertebral column in a 5-year-old German shepherd with chronic back pain and intermittent paraparesis for the past 8 months; signs were controlled with prednisone but would return when the prednisone was discontinued; calcified disk material can be seen in the disk space as well as in the intervertebral canal at L2-3 (arrow).

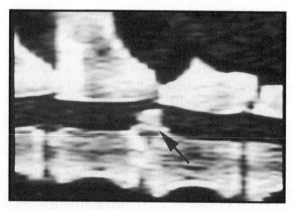

Figure 7-8 Reconstructed sagittal CT of Type I intervertebral disk extrusion at L2-3 (arrow) from the dog in Figure 7-7.

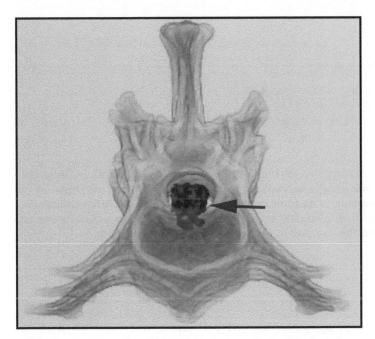

Figure 7-9 Reconstructed transverse CT of a Type I intervertebral disk extrusion at L2-3 from the dog in Figure 7-7; surgical removal of the disk resulted in complete recovery even when prednisone therapy was discontinued.

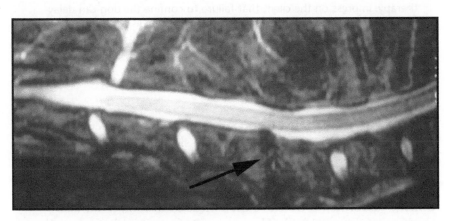

Figure 7-10 Sagital T2-weighted MRI of a 2-year-old Doberman pinscher with neck pain only from intervertebral disk degeneration at C6-C7 shown by the arrow (T2-weighted image with CSF surrounding the spinal cord and the nucleus pulposus of the normal disks are white); this dog had been attack-trained and had done much "bite work," which may have been stressful to the cervical disks and contributed to the degenerative process.

Table 7-3
Medical Management of Neck and Back Pain from Intervertebral Disk Disease

1. **Strict crate confinement** for 4 weeks. Activity is limited to short leash walks with a harness for urination and defecation; dog can be held on the owner's lap. Collars and neck restraint are avoided if cervical IVDD is present.

2. **Oral diazepam 0.5-2 mg/kg every 6-8 hours as needed, not to exceed 10 mg every 6 hours** to relieve painful muscle spasms.

Warning: If the dog is still in pain or has any weakness, then give prednisone, which will reduce nerve root and spinal cord irritation or swelling. Crate confinement is even more critical when prednisone is given, as pain relief is so complete that the dog may become overactive, and this can lead to acute paraplegia or quadriparesis.

3. **Oral prednisone 0.25-1 mg/kg every 12 hours for 3 days, then reduced to every other day for** three doses.

4. **Oral famotidine** (Pepcid AC, Merck) **0.5-1 mg/kg every 12-24 hours, cimetidine** (Tagamet, SmithKline Beecham) **5-10 mg/kg every 8 hours, or misoprostol** (Cytotec, Searle) **1-3 μg/kg every 8 hours** may be given to reduce gastrointestinal upset.

5. If further pain control is needed, see Table 7-2

Warning: Owners may try to discontinue crate confinement after a few days especially when pain is controlled by the diazepam and prednisone therapy. Impress on the client that failure to confine the dog can delay healing, cause paralysis from the extrusion of more disk material, and necessitate expensive surgery.

♥ With cervical IVDD, the dog is placed in dorsal recumbency and the disk material is removed through a slot drilled into the two adjacent vertebral bodies at the site of the extruded disk material (ventral slot technique, Figure 7-11). With thoracolumbar disk disease, dogs are placed in sternal recumbency and hemilaminectomy is performed to retrieve the extruded disk material (see Section 12, Figure 12-6). The prognosis for pain relief is usually excellent. Since other disks may be in various stages of degeneration and cause future problems, prophylactic fenestration of other disks near the surgical site is often performed in small dogs. Other strategies to reduce the chances or effects of future intervertebral disk herniation are outlined in Table 7-4.

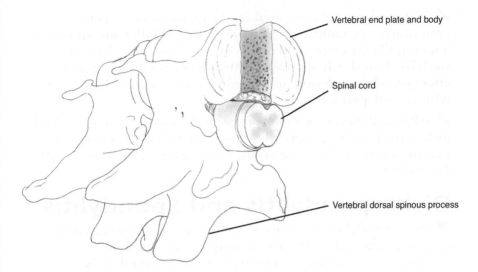

Vertebral end plate and body

Spinal cord

Vertebral dorsal spinous process

Figure 7-11 The ventral slot technique for surgical removal of inter-vertebral disk material. (Dog is in dorsal recumbency)

Table 7-4
Advice to Dog Owners: Strategies to Reduce the Chances or
Effects of Future Intervertebral Disk Herniation

Do's

- Reduce weight if obese.
- Feed a well-balanced diet.
- Give a daily antioxidant supplementation of vitamin E 10-25 IU/kg and vitamin C 15 mg/kg.
- Use a harness instead of a collar.
- Can go for daily walks on a leash (when recovered).
- Can do obedience training (no jumping).

Don'ts

- No jumping on and off furniture, running down stairs, sitting up to beg, or dancing on the hind legs.
- No playing frisbee, "tug of war," chase the ball, shake the toys, or other activities that cause quick sharp turns of the neck or back.
- No rough play with other dogs.
- No agility training that necessitates jumping or climbing.
- No jogging and "road work" behind a vehicle.

✓ Antioxidants reduce spinal cord damage from oxygen containing free radicals, which are produced following an injury. Vitamin C may cause diarrhea, so a lower dose may be used initially then slowly increased. High doses of vitamin E may affect blood coagulation and should be used cautiously in animals with coagulopathies.

✓ Although pain is often a feature of the disease, intervertebral disk extrusion also commonly causes ataxia, hemiparesis, quadriparesis, quadriplegia, paraparesis, or paraplegia (Sections 8, 9,10, 12, and 13).

Diskospondylitis and Spondylitis

♥ Diskospondylitis is a painful infection of the intervertebral disk and vertebral endplates. Spondylitis, or vertebral osteomyelitis, is a painful infection of the vertebral body. Diskospondylitis is more common than spondylitis, and both are usually caused by a bacterial infection. Fungal infections, such as aspergillosis, foreign-body migrations (such as grass awns), and aberrant parasite migrations (such as spirocercosis) occur infrequently. *Staphylococcus (S) aureus* and *S. intermedius* that arrive via a hematogenous route are the most frequent bacteria isolated, although *Streptococcus canis, Escherichia coli, Brucella canis*, and other organisms are also cultured. Preexisting or concurrent skin, urinary tract, or cardiorespiratory infections are often present. The lumbosacral, thoracolumbar, cervicothoracic, and mid-thoracic regions are frequently affected. Involvement of multiple sites is common.

✋ On examination, pyrexia may or may not be present. Sites of systemic infection should be investigated by performing a thorough clinical examination accompanied by a CBC, serum chemistry profile, and urinalysis and urine culture. The CBC may be normal or show neutrophilic leukocytosis, but fibrinogen is usually elevated. Cystitis is common, and the bacterial organism isolated from the urine often also infects the disk and vertebrae. Fungal hyphae associated with *Aspergillus spp.* may occasionally be seen on examination of the urine sediment. Several bacterial cultures of the blood taken at different intervals may also help identify the causal organism but are negative more than half of the time. Serologic testing for *Brucella canis* is often performed because of the public health significance of this infection. Radiographs are used to confirm the diagnosis of diskospondylitis and spondylitis. Characteristic routine radiographic changes may only be present 1 to 2 weeks after the onset of signs, and repeated radiographs may be necessary to demonstrate the lesions in some cases. Radiographic abnormalities include lysis of adjacent vertebral endplates with collapsed intervertebral disk spaces or vertebrae. CT or MRI may show lesions earlier and detail the changes better than routine radiographs (Figures 7-12, 7-13, and 7-14).

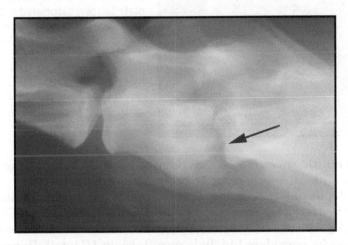

Figure 7-12 Lateral radiograph of diskospondylitis at the lumbosacral intervertebral disk space from a dog with severe lumbosacral pain.

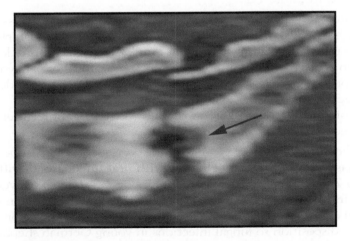

Figure 7-13 Reconstructed sagittal CT showing endplate lysis of L7 and S1 (arrow) of the dog in Figure 7-12.

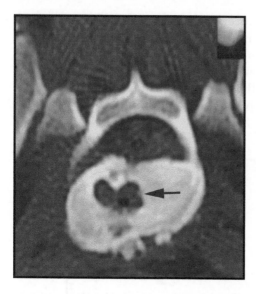

Figure 7-14
Transverse CT showing a hole in the center of the vertebral end plate (arrow) associated with the diskospondylitis at L7-S1 in the dog in Figures 7-12 and 7-13.

♥ Antibiotic therapy is selected based on the results of the culture and antibiotic sensitivity. **If no culture results are available, antibiotic combinations of oral trimethoprim-sulfadiazine 15–30 mg/kg every 12 hrs and cephalexin (Keflex, Dista) 30 mg/kg every 8 hours may be administered. Other antibiotics that may be considered include enrofloxacin (Baytril, Bayer) 5mg/kg PO every 12 hours, ciprofloxacin (Cipro, Bayer) 2.5–5 mg/kg every 12 hours, and clindamycin (Antirobe, Pharmacia & Upjohn) 5.5–11 mg/kg every 12 hours. Antibiotic therapy should be continued for 6 to 8 weeks.** Pain can be controlled as described in Table 7-2.

✓ In animals that are unresponsive to initial therapy, aspirates of the intervertebral disk space guided by fluoroscopy or ultrasonography may be useful in deciding treatment. Surgical debridement or decompression is rarely needed unless the animal has paresis or paralysis and does not respond to therapy. A myelogram, CT, or MRI is needed to visualize a lesion causing spinal cord compression. The overall prognosis for bacterial diskospondylitis is very good, but recurrences have been reported.

✓ Diskospondylitis due to a fungal infection, such as with *Aspergillus spp.*, has a grave prognosis. **Therapy with oral fluconazole (Diflucan, Pfizer) 2.5–5.0 mg/kg once daily in dogs or 2.5–10 mg/kg every 12 hours in cats for a minimum of 6 weeks may cause remission of the clinical signs.** An underlying immune deficiency may be responsible for a predisposition to fungal infections in young German shepherds and other dogs. As a result, recurrence is likely when antifungal medications are discontinued.

Meningitis

🖐 Meningitis can cause neck or back pain in dogs and cats that have no other neurologic deficits. Pain may be worse in the cervical region, but can be multifocal or extend along the entire vertebral column. Dogs with meningitis are often lethargic, anorexic, and may or may not be febrile. Neutrophilic leukocytosis may be evident on the CBC, but it may also be normal. Meningitis is suspected when leukocytic pleocytosis is found on a CSF analysis. Bacteria, viruses, fungi, protozoa, rickettsial organisms and immune-mediated processes may cause meningitis. Specific immunoassays may be performed for many organisms (Section 2). Bacterial meningitis is suspected if the CSF contains an increased number of degenerative neutrophils. A gram stain of the CSF and bacterial culture with antibiotic sensitivity may assist in confirming the diagnosis and indicate the appropriate antibiotic therapy. Bacterial meningitis can result from hematogenous spread of infections located in the endocardium, uterus, bladder, prostate, or elsewhere in the body or from direct extension of bacteria from sinus or ear infections, animal bites, and neurosurgical procedures. Antibiotic therapy for bacterial infections is discussed in Section 2. The prognosis is often poor, and epidural abscesses can form. It is rare for other organisms aside from bacteria to produce only meningitis with neck pain and no neurologic deficit.

✓ Neutrophilic leukocytosis (often greater than 1000 cells/µl) noted on CSF analysis can also be associated with immune-mediated meningitis. Necrotizing vasculitis or steroid-responsive meningitis-arteritis (SRMA) is an immune-mediated necrosis of meningeal arteries that causes neck pain in beagles, boxers, Bernese mountain dogs, German shorthaired pointers, and other dogs younger than 2 years of age. Immune-mediated meningitis has also been described in older dogs. A few dogs may have impaired mental status, cranial nerve deficits, seizures, blindness, ataxia, and paresis (Sections 2,3,5,6 and 8). In some cases of steroid-responsive meningitis, CSF leukocytosis consists of a mixture of neutrophils, lymphocytes, and macrophages. Serum and CSF organism titers should be evaluated to rule out other causes of meningitis but are usually normal (Section 2).

♥ **Long-term treatment with oral prednisone 2 mg/kg every 12 hours for 2 days, then reduced to 1 mg/kg every 12 hours for 2 weeks, then 0.5 mg/kg every 12 hours for 1 month, and then tapered to alternate-day therapy for 4 to 20 months usually results in remission.** Oral famotidine (Pepcid AC) 0.5–1 mg/kg every 12 to 24 hours, cimetidine (Tagamet) 5–10 mg/kg every

12 hours, or misoprostol (Cytotec) 1–3 µg/kg every 8 hours may be given to protect the gastrointestinal tract from irritation or ulceration when the steroid dose is high. Pain may be controlled as indicated in Table 7-2. Diazepam often relieves muscle spasms associated with meningitis. With aggressive immunosuppressive therapy, dogs with SRMA often have a good prognosis for recovery. Recurrence can occur and may necessitate long-term, alternate-day therapy once remission has been achieved.

Vertebral Fractures

✓ Animals with vertebral fractures may present with pain and no neurologic deficits, but this is more likely in the cervical region than in the thoracolumbar region. Diagnosis and management of vertebral fractures are discussed in Sections 9 and 12.

Lumbosacral Degeneration

✋ Lumbosacral degeneration, also known as lumbosacral stenosis, lumbosacral disease, and cauda equina syndrome, causes pain at the L7-S1 region in German shepherds, German shepherd mixes, and other large-breed dogs. The degenerative changes include proliferation of the interarcuate ligament (*i.e.*, the ligament connecting the vertebrae dorsal to the cauda equina),vertebral facet osteophyte formation, Type II IVDD and spondylosis deformans at L7-S1. These degenerative changes cause stenosis of the vertebral canal and compression of the L7-Cd nerve roots.

✓ Pain is manifested as low tail carriage; reluctance to wag the tail; and difficulty rising, climbing stairs, or jumping on furniture or into the car. Signs of pain may increase after exercise. A flaccid tail and urinary and fecal incontinence can occur as stenosis and nerve root compression worsen (Section 15). Proprioceptive deficits and weakness of one or both pelvic limbs can rarely occur (Section 13).

♥ Many dogs have concurrent orthopedic disease of the hips that causes pain, and careful palpation of the lumbosacral joint alone is essential. Placing the thumbs on the midline, with fingers on each ileum, allows the examiner to exert direct pressure over the lumbosacral articulation without placing stress on the hip joints. Dorsal flexion of the tail usually elicits pain. Palpation of the ventral lumbosacral region through the rectum may also be painful.

✓ Early diagnosis and treatment will help prevent irreversible urinary and fecal incontinence. Positive waves and fibrillation potentials may be found on EMG examination of the caudal lumbar muscles, tail, and anal sphincter. Plain radiographs are often normal (Figure 7-15), or they may show spondylosis deformans and narrowing of the lumbosacral intervertebral disk space. Type II IVDD and cauda equina and lateral nerve root compression are best documented with CT or MRI of the lumbosacral region (Figure 7-16).

✓ Acute pain is controlled as described in Table 7-2 for IVDD. **Dorsal laminectomy (see Figure 12-7) and diskectomy are recommended if pain recurs when medical therapy is discontinued or to avoid progressive compression of nerve roots, which may result in urinary and fecal incontinence.** Crate confinement as described for IVDD is essential with or without surgery to prevent pain from recurring. Dogs with pain alone have an excellent prognosis for recovery with surgery.

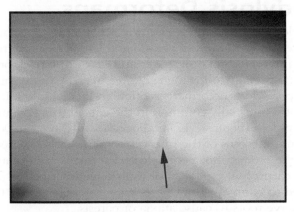

Figure 7-15 Lateral radiographs of a 5-year-old mixed-breed large dog with lumbosacral pain showing little evidence of abnormalities.

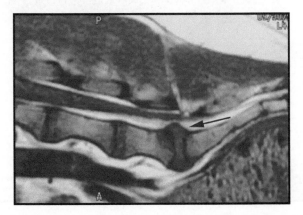

Figure 7-16 Sagital T-1 weighted MRI of the dog in Figure 7-15 clearly showing a Type II intervertebral disk protrusion, which may be associated with early lumbosacral degeneration (arrow).

Atlantoaxial Subluxation

✓ Small dogs with atlantoaxial subluxation due to congenital abnormalities of the dens and ligaments of C1-2 may be presented for neck pain alone but are more often presented for acute quadriparesis or quadriplegia (Section 9).

Caudal Cervical Spondylomyelopathy

✓ Caudal cervical spondylomyelopathy may cause neck pain in Great Danes and Doberman pinschers and other large-breed dogs, but ataxia and quadriparesis are the most common clinical signs (Section 8).

Spondylosis Deformans

✓ Spondylosis deformans, also known as hypertrophic spondylosis, is characterized by formation of ventral and lateral osteophytes that bridge the intervertebral disk spaces and may cause neck or back discomfort, especially following excessive exercise or during cold weather. Spondylosis deformans is often an incidental radiographic finding that is especially common in the caudal thoracic and lumbar vertebrae in dogs (Figure 7-17) and occasionally in cats. Degeneration of the annulus fibrosus of the intervertebral disk is suspected to result in osteophyte production. Spondylosis deformans rarely causes severe pain. **Oral carprofen, etodolac, or aspirin as described in Table 7-2 can be used to control pain.** Osteophytes rarely compress the spinal cord and nerve roots to cause ataxia or paresis.

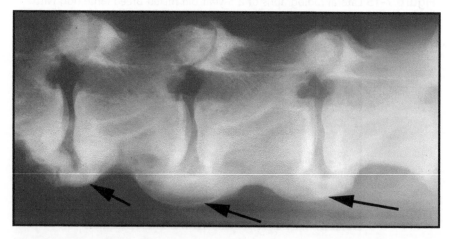

Figure 7-17 Lateral radiograph of the ventrolateral bony proliferation known as spondylosis deformans (arrows), which may cause some intermittent discomfort but rarely causes severe pain; usually an incidental radiographic finding.

Vertebral Neoplasia

✓ Osteochondromatosis, also known as multiple cartilaginous exostoses, is the development of proliferative benign masses of cartilage and bone that arise from metaphyseal growth plates, often at multiple sites in young animals. Vertebral osteochondromas may cause neck and back discomfort, but most animals are not presented to a veterinarian until chronic progressive ataxia, paresis, or paralysis develops (Sections 8, 10, and 13).

✓ Most neoplasms of the vertebrae are extremely painful. Osteosarcoma, chondrosarcoma, fibrosarcoma, hemangiosarcoma, myeloma, and metastatic prostatic or mammary adenocarcinomas are the most common types. Vertebral neoplasia often compresses the spinal cord and causes chronic ataxia and paresis. A pathologic fracture of the neoplastic vertebrae occasionally causes acute quadriparesis, quadriplegia, paraparesis, or paraplegia.

✓ Bony lysis with or without bony proliferation can usually be seen on plain radiographs of the vertebral column (Figure 7-18), but CT is superior (Figure 7-19) to visualize vertebral neoplasia. A myelogram or MRI may show spinal cord compression. A fluoroscopic-guided needle aspirate or biopsy of the affected vertebra may assist in differentiating spondylitis and neoplasia and establishing a definitive diagnosis.

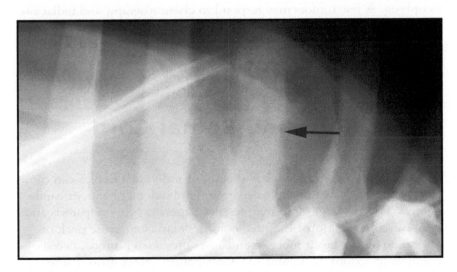

Figure 7-18 Lateral radiograph of the thoracic vertebral column showing proliferative bony changes on the dorsal spinous process of T3 (arrow) in a 6-year-old boxer with back pain.

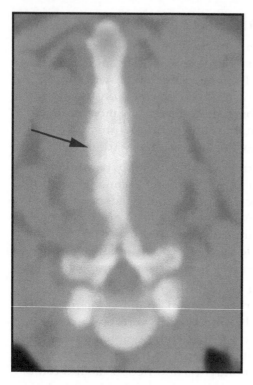

Figure 7-19 Transverse CT of the T3 vertebra from Figure 7-18 demonstrates the bony proliferation (arrow) in more detail than routine radiographs; metastatic carcinoma was suspected from the histopathologic examination of a vertebral biopsy, but the primary tumor could not be located.

✓ A limited number of therapeutic options exist for vertebral neoplasia. A few tumors may respond to chemotherapy, and radiation therapy may be useful in others. Removal of the affected vertebra may be attempted in select cases, but for the most part treatment is palliative. Pain is controlled as outlined in Table 7-2. Dogs and cats with a vertebral neoplasm generally have a poor prognosis, and increased, uncontrollable pain often necessitates euthanasia.

Nerve Root and Spinal Cord Neoplasia

✓ Neoplasia of the nerve roots, plexus, or individual nerves can cause pain of the neck, brachial plexus, back, lumbosacral plexus, or cauda equina. This disorder often manifests as lameness or monoparesis and is discussed in Section 14. Spinal cord neoplasia can cause neck or back pain alone, but it more often causes progressive ataxia, paresis, or paralysis (Sections 8, 10, and 13). Gabapentin (Neurontin, Parke-Davis) 6–15 mg/kg PO every 6 hours may be tried for nerve pain in dogs if pain is not controllable by other means. The expense of gabapentin prohibits its use in many cases.

Polymyositis and Other Polymyopathies

✓ Polymyositis and other myopathies, such as carnitine polymyopathy, are diffuse muscle diseases that may cause neck and back pain. Concurrent pain is usually found in limb and head muscles. The diagnosis is confirmed on histologic examination of a muscle biopsy. Muscle diseases are discussed in Section 11.

Polyarthritis

✓ Animals with polyarthritis may have neck and back pain but are usually presented for a stiff and stilted gait. Pain with or without swelling is found on palpation and manipulation of the joints of the limbs. The diagnosis is made by demonstration of inflammatory cells in fluid collected from the joints. Pain may be controlled with oral carprofen, etodolac, or aspirin as described in Table 7-2.

✓ **If immune-mediated polyarthritis is suspected, treatment with oral prednisone 2 mg/kg every 12 hours for 2 days, then reduced to 1 mg/kg every 12 hours for 2 weeks, then 0.5 mg/kg every 12 hours for 1 month, and then tapered to alternate-day therapy for several months may resolve the clinical signs.** Oral famotidine (Pepcid AC) 0.5-1 mg/kg every 12 to 24 hours, cimetidine (Tagamet) 5-10 mg/kg every 12 hours, or misoprostol (Cytotec) 1-3 µg/kg every 8 hours may be given to protect the gastrointestinal tract from irritation or ulceration when the steroid dose is high. Recurrence of immune-mediated polyarthritis is common, and long-term, alternate-day prednisone may be necessary.

Intracranial Disease

✓ Brain tumors or other intracranial mass lesions may cause signs of neck pain. Elevated intracranial pressure, which stretches small nerve endings in the meninges and blood vessels, is suspected to radiate pain into the cervical region. CT or MRI of the brain should be considered in animals with unexplained cervical pain. Brain tumors are discussed further in Section 2.

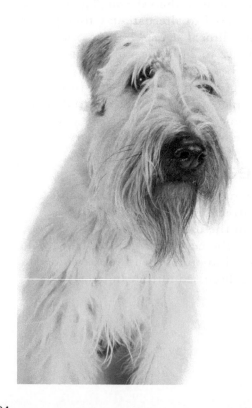

Section 8

Ataxia

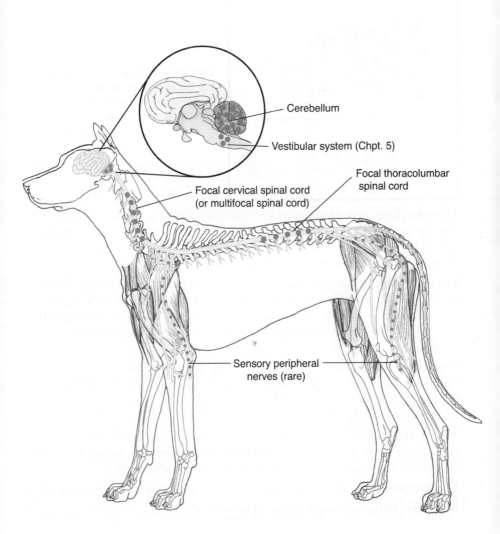

Cerebellum

Vestibular system (Chpt. 5)

Focal cervical spinal cord
(or multifocal spinal cord)

Focal thoracolumbar
spinal cord

Sensory peripheral
nerves (rare)

Definitions

Ataxia: Failure of muscle coordination.

Intention tremors: Tremors seen with initiation of movements.

Dysmetria: Improper degrees of limb flexion and extension during movement.

Hypermetria: Exaggerated flexion when walking, trotting, and turning; over-reaching (Figure 8-1).

Hypometria: Reduced flexion and exaggerated extension when walking, trotting, or turning; under-reaching.

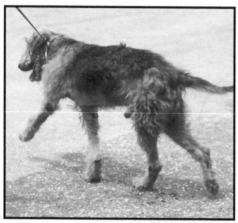

Figure 8-1 Hypermetria of the left thoracic limb in an 8-year-old Airedale terrier with cerebellar neoplasia.

Unconscious proprioception: Sensory information concerning limb position that reaches the cerebellum via the spinocerebellar tracts to provide coordinated movements; tested by observing coordination of the head and gait.

Conscious proprioception: Sensory information concerning limb position that travels to the thalamus and parietal cortex to give conscious perception of position in space; tested by standing with the toes knuckled over and observing whether the abnormal posture is corrected.

Opisthotonus: Dorsal extension of the head and neck with extension of the thoracic limbs and flexion of the pelvic limbs; usually associated with acute cerebellar lesions (decerebellate rigidity).

"Root signature": A sign that a lesion is irritating the nerve roots to a limb; manifests as reluctance to bear weight on the limb when standing and lameness or pain of the limb.

Meningomyelitis: Inflammation of the meninges and spinal cord.

Myelitis: Inflammation of the spinal cord.

Hypesthesia (hypoesthesia): Reduced sensation to touch or noxious stimuli.

Paresthesia: Abnormal burning or tingling; often affects limbs and feet and manifests as self-mutilation.

Lesion Localization

✓ The location of lesions that cause ataxia are shown in Figure 8-2. These locations are:

- Cerebellum
- Spinal cord
- Sensory peripheral nerves
- Vestibular system (Section 5)

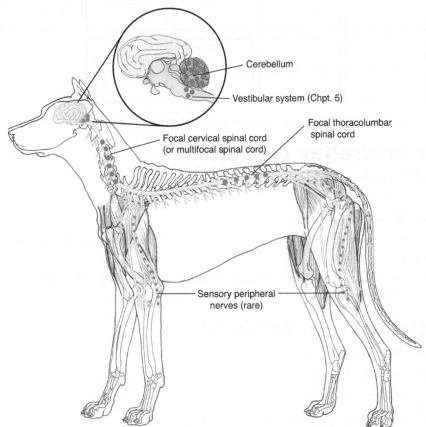

Figure 8-2 Dysfunction of the cerebellum, vestibular system, spinal cord, or sensory nerves causes ataxia (the dots indicate the lesion localization).

Differentiation of Lesions Causing Ataxia

✓ An algorithm to differentiate lesions that cause ataxia is shown in Figure 8-3.

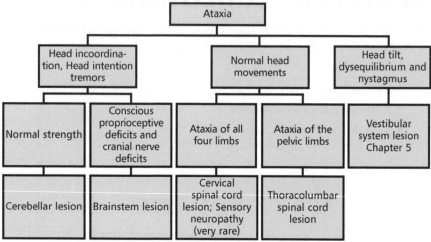

Figure 8-3 Algorithm showing how to differentiate lesions that cause ataxia.

Cerebellar Lesions

✓ Ataxia of the head and limbs

✓ Intention tremors of the head

✓ Wide-base stance

✓ Severe ataxia with no evidence of weakness or conscious proprioceptive deficits

✓ Head tilt, dysequilibrium, and nystagmus (Section 5) if the vestibular portion of the cerebellum is affected

Brainstem Lesions

✓ Ataxia of the head and limbs

✓ Intention tremors of the head

✓ Wide-base stance

✓ Conscious proprioceptive deficits

✓ Quadriparesis

✓ Cranial nerve deficits

✓ Stupor (possible)

✓ Head tilt, dysequilibrium, and nystagmus (Section 5) if the vestibular nuclei are affected

Spinal Cord Lesions

✓ Ataxia of the limbs with normal head coordination

✓ Cervical lesions affect thoracic and pelvic limbs

✓ Thoracolumbar lesions affect pelvic limbs only

✓ May have neck or back pain

✓ May have conscious proprioceptive deficits and paresis

Sensory Nerve Lesions

✓ Ataxia of the limbs only

✓ Conscious proprioceptive deficits

✓ Loss of superficial and deep pain sensation

✓ Self-mutilation (Section 16)

✓ Lesions of the sensory nerves are very rare

Vestibular System Lesions

✓ Head tilt

✓ Ataxia with dysequilibrium

✓ Nystagmus

✓ For a comprehensive discussion of these signs, see Section 5

Differential Diagnosis

Cerebellar Disorders

✓ Trauma—common in dogs and cats

✓ Meningoencephalitis—common in dogs and cats

✓ Cerebrovascular disorders—occasional in dogs and cats

✓ Intoxication—occasional in dogs and cats

✓ Neoplasia—occasional in dogs and cats

✓ In-utero cerebellar degeneration and hypoplasia—occasional in dogs and cats

✓ Cerebellar abiotrophy and other degenerations–rare in dogs and cats

✓ Neuroaxonal dystrophy–rare in dogs

✓ Cerebellar cysts–rare in dogs and cats

Spinal Cord Disorders

✓ Degenerative intervertebral disk disease–common in dogs, rare in cats

✓ Caudal cervical spondylomyelopathy–common in large dogs

✓ Trauma–common in dogs and cats

✓ Meningomyelitis–common in dogs and cats

✓ Diskospondylitis–common in dogs, rare in cats

✓ Atlantoaxial subluxation–occasional in dogs

✓ Neoplasia–occasional in dogs and cats

✓ Spinal cord cysts–rare in dogs and cats

Sensory Nerve Disorders

✓ Toxic sensory polyneuropathy–rare in dogs and cats

✓ Idiopathic sensory polyganglioneuritis–rare in dogs and cats

✓ Congenital sensory polyneuropathy–rare in dogs and cats

Diagnostic Evaluation

Important Historical Questions

• Possible trauma? If so, obtain vertebral radiographs before proceeding.

• Acute or chronic?

• Progressive or nonprogressive?

• Other signs of illness?

• Exposure to toxic substances?

• Recent medications, nutriceuticals, or herbal supplements?

• Ataxia since birth?

• Painful neck or back?

• Signs of self-mutilation?

• Relunctance to jump or go up or down stairs?

• Blood in the urine or straining to urinate?

Physical and Neurologic Examinations

✓ Examine the animal carefully for evidence of a systemic disease process. A careful evaluation is especially important to differentiate cerebellar and spinal cord disease.

Applicable Diagnostic Tests

✓ A complete blood count (CBC), serum chemistry profile, and urinalysis are performed to detect systemic illness and as part of the preanesthetic evaluation.

✓ Thoracic and abdominal radiographs and abdominal ultrasonography are indicated if neoplasia is suspected or abnormalities are found on the physical examination.

✓ The following are tests that are performed under general anesthesia, as well as their potential findings:

- Cerebrospinal fluid (CSF) analysis may show increased leukocytes and/or protein levels in meningoencephalitis, meningomyelitis, or central nervous system (CNS) neoplasia and other spinal cord compressions.

- An electromyogram may show positive sharp waves and fibrillation potentials in the paravertebral muscles in spinal cord lesions that affect ventral nerve roots.

- Vertebral column radiographs may show vertebral fractures and luxations, calcified intervertebral disks, diskospondylitis, spondylitis, atlantoaxial subluxation, spondylosis deformans, and vertebral neoplasia.

- A myelogram with dynamic views is useful to evaluate the instability and ligamentous hypertrophy associated with caudal cervical spondylomyelopathy.

- A myelogram may also demonstrate spinal cord compression in animals with intervertebral disk disease, vertebral fracture or subluxation, diskospondylitis, spinal cord cysts or neoplasia. The spinal cord may appear swollen on the myelogram in cases of primary spinal cord neoplasia.

- Computed tomography (CT) and magnetic resonance imaging (MRI) can be useful to demonstrate cerebellar inflammation, infarction, cysts, neoplasia, or hypoplasia as well as some degenerative diseases.

- Cerebellar biopsy with histopathologic examination may be necessary for a definitive diagnosis.

- CT and MRI can be useful to demonstrate intervertebral disk disease, diskospondylitis, cysts and vertebral and spinal cord neoplasia.

✓ Serum and CSF immunoassays for infectious diseases are indicated if there is evidence of inflammation on the CSF analysis.

Cerebellar Disorders

Trauma

✓ Acute cerebellar trauma is often associated with opisthotonus (decerebellate rigidity) (Figure 8-4) and preserved consciousness. If the animal is ambulatory, ataxia of the limbs and head may be noted. Ataxia often improves over the next 6 to 9 months. Diagnosis and management of head trauma are discussed in Section 2.

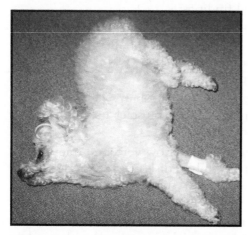

Figure 8-4 A 3-year-old Poodle with opisthotonus.

Meningoencephalitis

🖐 Inflammation of the cerebellum associated with infectious organisms or of unknown causes is considered in dogs and cats of any age presenting with progressive ataxia of the head and limbs. Organisms that may cause CNS inflammation in dogs include canine distemper virus, *Ehrlichia canis*, *Rickettsia rickettsii*, *Toxoplasma gondii*, *Neospora caninum*, *Cryptococcus neoformans*, *Aspergillus spp.*, and aerobic or anaerobic bacteria (Section 2, Table 2-8). Organisms that cause encephalitis in cats include feline infectious peritonitis (FIP) virus, *Toxoplasma gondii*, *Cryptococcus neoformans*, and aerobic or anaerobic bacteria (Section 2, Table 2-8). Steroid-responsive meningoencephalitis, granulomatous meningoencephalomyelitis, and unclassified viral meningoencephalomyelitis may also produce cerebellar signs in dogs and cats. CSF analysis and MRI can potentially support the diagnosis, although a biopsy of the cerebellum may be necessary in some cases for a definitive diagnosis. Serum and CSF immunoassays for specific organisms may be performed. Meningoencephalitis is discussed in Section 2.

Cerebrovascular Disorders

✓ Hemorrhage or infarction of the cerebellum may be considered in dogs with acute onset of nonprogressive ataxia and head tremor. CT or MRI may show the cerebellar lesion or might be normal. The diagnosis is often suspected but not proven. Improvement of ataxia often occurs over the following 6 to 9 months. Cerebrovascular accidents are further described in Section 2.

Intoxication

✓ Ataxia can occur with most intoxicants that affect the CNS, such as ethylene glycol, ivermectin, organophosphates, and pyrethroids, as well as with overdoses of anticonvulsant and other drugs (Section 2). A thorough history should discuss possible contact with a toxin, the owner's prescription medications, illegal substances, and toxic plants. All current medications or nutritional supplements and herbs should be evaluated for the potential for toxicity. In humans, cerebellar degeneration has been associated with overdoses of tricyclic antidepressants, diphenylhydantoin, and toxic plants. When in doubt about whether a substance is poisonous, contact ASPCA National Animal Poison Control Center (888-426-4435) or another poison control center.

Neoplasia

✓ Chronic progressive ataxia of the limbs and head may be associated with cerebellar neoplasia, especially if asymmetric signs are present. Neoplasia may occasionally produce acute signs related to hemorrhage or mass effect. Cerebellar neoplasia may obstruct CSF flow and cause secondary hydrocephalus and signs of cerebral dysfunction (Section 2). The diagnosis of neoplasia is made from CSF analysis, MRI, and histologic examination of tissue obtained from a cerebellar biopsy. Options for treatment of brain neoplasia are found in Section 2.

In-Utero Cerebellar Degeneration and Hypoplasia

⚷ In-utero degeneration of the cerebellum occurs in both dogs and cats. The cerebellum continues to develop throughout gestation and is not completely formed until several days after birth. An infection or toxic exposure during a critical phase of development can lead to a loss of neurons in all three layers of the cerebellum. The signs are apparent when the animal begins to ambulate. Panleukopenia virus and herpes virus infections are the most common causes of in-utero cerebellar degeneration in cats and dogs, respectively. Other dogs and cats may have an incompletely developed cerebellum or cerebellar hypoplasia that is unassociated with an infection.

✓ Ataxia and intention tremors of the head and body are seen as neonates begin to move. Some cases are mild while others are severe. In severe cases, walking and eating may be very difficult. The signs do not change or progress over time. Mildly affected animals may be acceptable pets but do not improve. CT or MRI may demonstrate a small cerebellum; a small cerebellum is also found on necropsy (Figure 8-5). **No treatment is available,** but appropriate panleukopenia vaccination of nonpregnant queens is an effective prevention. Vaccination of pregnant cats with modified live-virus panleukopenia vaccines has been incriminated as a cause of the disorder in some cats.

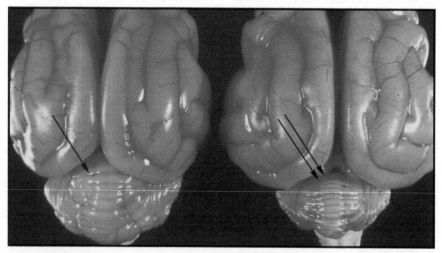

Figure 8-5 A normal-sized cerebellum in a kitten (left, single arrow), and a small cerebellum from in-utero cerebellar degeneration in another kitten (right, double arrows).

Cerebellar Abiotrophy, and Other Degenerations

✓ Cerebellar abiotrophy is an inherited disorder associated with premature death of neurons, which may affect all layers of the cerebellum. Kerry blue terriers, Gordon setters, collies, and other purebred dogs and very rarely cats usually develop progressive ataxia at a young age. The age of onset and speed of progression varies with each breed. Kerry blue terriers are severely affected by 1 year of age, but Gordon setters develop signs later. In this breed, the disease progresses more slowly and they may be acceptable pets for a longer period. These disorders have traditionally been diagnosed by histologic examination at necropsy or with cerebellar biopsy. However, characteristic changes may be seen on MRI, allowing a presumptive diagnosis in the appropriate breed. There is no treatment, and most animals progress to a point where they are incapacitated and have a poor quality of life.

✓ Various forms of spongiform degeneration affect the cerebellum and cause progressive ataxia and episodic opisthotonus in Labrador retrievers, Samoyeds, silky terriers, and Egyptian mau cats younger than 1 year of age. Involvement of other regions of the CNS is often seen. There is no treatment. The clinical signs may worsen in Labrador retrievers but improve over time in Egyptian mau cats.

✓ Several lysosomal storage disorders, such as GM-2 gangliosidosis and sphingomyelinosis, cause progressive ataxia. Lysosomal storage disorders are outlined in Section 2, Table 2-15. As with abiotrophies, spongiform degeneration and lysosomal storage disorders may show characteristic changes on MRI of the brain.

✓ Late-onset cerebellar degeneration occurs in adult dogs and progresses slowly over several months to years. Initially, the signs are restricted to mild ataxia of the pelvic limbs, but all four limbs and the head become affected insidiously over time. Most diagnostic tests are within normal limits, although CT or MRI may demonstrate a small cerebellum. Histologic examination of a cerebellar biopsy shows degeneration. The cause is unknown. Antioxidant therapy with N-acetylcysteine 25 mg/kg PO every 8 hours every other day may delay progression of signs, but affected dogs ultimately become severely incapacitated. Such animals are unable to walk without the assistance of a harness and must be hand fed and watered because head movements are so uncoordinated. Many animals are euthanized because their quality of life becomes so poor.

Neuroaxonal Dystrophy

✓ Neuroaxonal dystrophy (NAD) has been described in Rottweilers, collies, and cats. Affected Rottweilers develop insidious progressive ataxia that begins within the first 1 to 2 years of life. Severe ataxia, intention tremors, nystagmus, and menace deficits eventually develop. The diagnosis is suspected based on the signalment, clinical signs, and absence of abnormal findings on CSF analysis and MRI. **There is no known treatment, and the prognosis is poor.** Most affected dogs are incapacitated by 6 years of age. Finding axonal spheroids in the vestibular nuclei and nuclei of the dorsal spinocerebellar tracts on necropsy supports the diagnosis of NAD. Collies with NAD show similar signs, but onset occurs at 2 to 4 months of age. At 5 to 6 weeks of age, tricolor cats begin with head tremors and progress to ataxia. An autosomal recessive inheritance is suspected in dogs.

Brain Cysts

✓ Epidermoid, dermoid, and arachnoid cysts may rarely affect the cerebellum and produce progressive neurologic signs. The cysts are visualized on CT and MRI. Surgical removal or drainage of the cyst from the cerebellum can be attempted. These cysts can also cause progressive compression of the spinal cord and are discussed in Section 13.

Spinal Cord Disorders

Degenerative Intervertebral Disk Disease

✓ Ataxia of all four limbs or the pelvic limbs only is commonly caused by Type I and Type II degenerative intervertebral disk disease (IVDD) (Section 7). Some degree of quadriparesis is also usually present, and this is discussed further in Section 9. The diagnosis and medical treatment of IVDD are described in Sections 7 and 9.

✓ Ataxia associated with Type I IVDD may resolve with crate rest, diazepam, and prednisone (Section 7, Table 7-3). Ataxia associated with Type II IVDD often improves with prednisone but recurs when medication is reduced or discontinued. If quadriparesis develops or ataxia returns when the medication is discontinued, then surgical decompression via a ventral slot (Section 7, Figure 7-11), dorsal laminectomy, or hemilaminectomy (Section 12, Figures 12-6 and 12-7) is performed.

Caudal Cervical Spondylomyelopathy

✓ Caudal cervical spondylomyelopathy (CCSM), also known as cervical vertebral malformation, cervical vertebral instability, and wobbler's syndrome, occurs in both young and old large-breed dogs. A malformation and malarticulation of the cervical vertebrae, which can be exacerbated by a high-protein diet, causes stenosis of the vertebral canal in young dogs. In older dogs, joint instability with hypertrophy of the associated ligaments and Type II IVDD cause stenosis of the vertebral canal. CCSM affects the caudal cervical vertebrae from C4-C7. Although many large-breed dogs are affected, 1 to 2-year-old Great Danes and 5 to 10-year-old Doberman pinchers are most commonly affected.

✓ Onset of clinical signs can be acute or slow and insidious. Ataxia is present in all four limbs, although the pelvic limbs often seem affected to a greater extent. The pelvic limbs circumduct during ambulation, and the hips wobble from side to side. The thoracic limb deficits are often misconstrued as compensation for the pelvic limb ataxia, and a lesion below T2 may be initially suspected. However, on closer examination, a stiff, stilted, short-strided gait is observed on the thoracic limbs. Atrophy or fasciculation of the deltoideus, biceps, and infraspinatus and supraspinatus muscles may be present. A "root signature" may be apparent. Conscious proprioceptive deficits may be seen in the pelvic limbs alone or in all four limbs. One side may be more affected than the other. Some degree of neck pain can usually be elicited by palpation and neck manipulation, although this is often subtle. Some dogs are presented for acute nonambulatory quadriparesis (Section 9).

✋ In young dogs, vertebral malformation and a stenotic vertebral canal may be obvious on routine cervical radiographs, but a myelogram with lateral and ventrodorsal views is essential to appreciate the location and extent of the spinal cord compression. Narrowed disk spaces, calcified disks, a narrowed vertebral canal, spondylosis deformans, and arthritis in the dorsal articular facets may be seen on routine cervical radiographs in older dogs. CSF analysis is usually within normal limits, although some cases have mild leukocytosis (7–10 cells/μl; normal = 6 cells or less) or elevated protein (25–35 mg/ml; normal = less than 20).

Diagnosis of CCSM is confirmed with myelography. Lateral compression may be obvious on ventrodorsal views. Dorsal spinal cord compression from hypertrophy of the ligamentum flavum and dorsal articular facets may be found. Ventral compression from Type II IVDD and hypertrophy of the dorsal longitudinal ligament is seen on a lateral myelogram without traction (Figure 8-6). If traction is applied, ventral compression may be reduced (Figure 8-7). As CCSM is a dynamic lesion, mildly flexed and extended views are important to appreciate the effects of different neck postures on the spinal cord compression. If spinal cord compression is alleviated with flexion and accentuated on extension, the problem is partially caused by ligamentous hypertrophy ventrally. If flexion and extension do not affect the lesion, Type II IVDD alone is most likely. Compression may be found at more than one site.

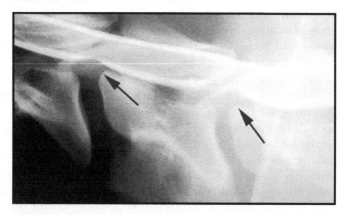

Figure 8-6 Lateral myelogram showing ventral compression of the spinal cord at C5-C6 and C6-C7 in a 7-year-old Doberman pinscher with caudal cervical spondylomyelopathy (arrows).

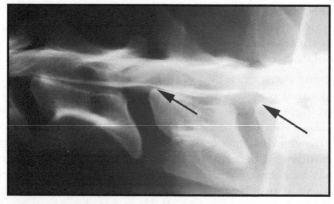

Figure 8-7 Lateral myelogram with neck traction of the dog in Figure 8-6 showing reduction of the compression at both sites (arrows).

✓ Dynamic studies using MRI are more difficult than with myelography. Myelography accompanied by CT imaging can provide more information about some lesions, particularly those in young dogs with bony malformations and encroachment of the facets into the neural canal. The degree of spinal cord atrophy may be assessed with CT or MRI.

✓ **Mildly affected dogs will improve on prednisone 0.25 mg/kg PO every 12 hours and oral muscle relaxants, such as diazepam 0.5–2 mg/kg PO every 6 to 8 hours as needed (not to exceed 10 mg every 6 hours).** Acupuncture may also help relieve the pain. Ataxia often returns if prednisone is discontinued.

♥ **Surgical decompression and stabilization surgery are necessary in most cases.** The type of surgery depends on whether the spinal cord compression is dorsal, lateral, or ventral and if hypertrophy of the dorsal longitudinal ligament is present. If dorsal or lateral spinal cord compression is present, then a dorsal laminectomy (Section 12, Figure 12-7) over one or more sites may be necessary.

♥ A ventral slot technique may achieve decompression if only a Type II IVDD is present (Section 7, Figure 7-11). If dorsal longitudinal ligamentous hypertrophy and vertebral instability are present, then a ventral decompression with vertebral distraction and fusion are recommended. The distraction-fusion technique (Figure 8-8) involves separation of the vertebrae with an implant device (polypropylene ring or metal washer) and fixation in this distracted position with orthopedic screws, wires, or pins. If more than one site of compression is seen on the myelogram, the distraction-fusion technique may be performed at several sites at the same time.

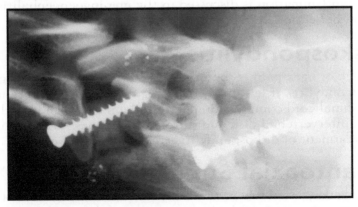

Figure 8-8 Radiographs of the distraction fusion technique with polypropylene spacers and screws for caudal cervical spondylomyelopathy in the same dog as in Figures 8-6 and 8-7.

✓ Following surgery, the patient is confined to a crate or small room for 4 weeks, and the neck is supported with a light brace and bandage. The dog's activity level is then gradually returned to normal. The prognosis for most dogs with surgical intervention is very good. Most patients will recover to 80% of normal in the first 3 months but will continue to improve for 9 to 12 months. Because of increased stress on the vertebrae adjacent to the fused vertebrae, Type II IVDD may occur on either side of the surgical site several months or years following the initial surgery (the "domino effect").

Trauma

✓ Spinal cord trauma most commonly causes acute quadriparesis, paraparesis or paraplegia along with ataxia and is discussed in Section 9.

Meningomyelitis

✓ Most of the inflammatory diseases of the brain discussed in Section 2 can also cause focal cervical or thoracolumbar lesions, or multifocal spinal cord disease. Meningomyelitis or myelitis can occasionally present as ataxia with or without pain and paresis. Diagnosis is based on finding leukocytic pleocytosis and elevated protein levels in the CSF. CSF collected from the lumbar subarachnoid space may have higher leukocyte counts and protein levels than that of the cerebellomedullary cistern due to the caudal flow of CSF. Serum and CSF immunoassays for specific organisms may help to identify causative agents. An inflammatory focus may be visible on MRI. Treatment of nervous system inflammation is discussed in the meningoencephalitis section of Section 2, Tables 2-10 and 2-11.

Diskospondylitis

✓ Neck or back pain is the most common initial clinical sign of diskospondylitis. If left untreated, progressive ataxia can result from spinal cord compression due to inflammation and swelling of the intervertebral disk and surrounding tissues. The diagnosis and treatment of diskospondylitis are discussed in Section 7.

Atlantoaxial Subluxation

✓ Mild atlantoaxial subluxation from agenesis or hypogenesis of the dens may cause ataxia of the limbs in toy breed dogs younger than 1 year of age, but acute quadriparesis is most common. Atlantoaxial subluxation is discussed in Section 9.

Neoplasia

✓ Vertebral osteochondromas are proliferative benign masses of cartilage and bone at metaphyseal growth plates; these masses compress the spinal cord in dogs and cats, causing chronic progressive ataxia and paresis. Other types of vertebral and spinal cord neoplasia occasionally produce ataxia of all four limbs or only the pelvic limbs. Spinal cord tumors often cause chronic progressive quadriparesis and paraparesis along with ataxia, and diagnosis and treatment of such tumors are discussed in Sections 10 and 13.

Spinal Cord Cysts

✓ Depending on their location, epidermoid and arachnoid cysts may compress the spinal cord and cause progressive ataxia of all four limbs or only the pelvic limbs in dogs and cats. Progressive quadriparesis or paraparesis usually occurs. These cysts are discussed in Section 13.

Sensory Nerve Disorders

Sensory Polyneuropathy

✓ Ataxia may be caused by a generalized disorder of sensory peripheral nerves. Conscious proprioceptive deficits, hypesthesia, paresthesia, anesthesia, and self-mutilation may also be present due to the involvement of other senses. Sensory polyneuropathy may be suspected after other causes of ataxia have been ruled out, as these disorders are very rare. No response to electrical stimulation of sensory nerves is found on an EMG examination. The possibility of toxicity should be explored historically. An idiopathic sensory ganglioneuritis and congenital sensory polyneuropathy have been described in dogs.

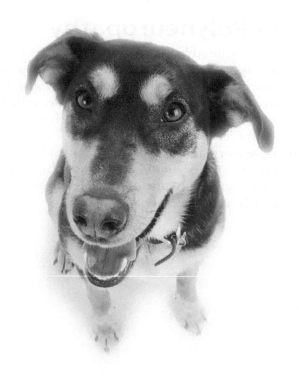

Acute Quadriparesis, Quadriplegia, Hemiparesis, and Hemiplegia

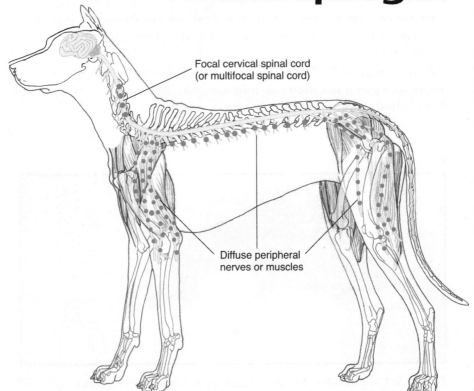

Focal cervical spinal cord
(or multifocal spinal cord)

Diffuse peripheral
nerves or muscles

Definitions

Acute quadriparesis, quadriplegia, hemiparesis, and hemiplegia: Onset of signs over a 24 to 72-hour period.

Quadriparesis (tetraparesis): Weakness (paresis) in all four limbs, which can be mild (ambulatory), moderate (nonambulatory, sternal recumbency) (Figure 9-1), or severe (nonambulatory, lateral recumbency), but some voluntary limb movement is retained; most ambulatory animals with quadriparesis from spinal cord lesions also show ataxia and conscious proprioceptive deficits.

Quadriplegia (tetraplegia): Loss of voluntary movements in all four limbs.

Hemiparesis: Weakness of the thoracic and pelvic limbs on one side.

Hemiplegia: Loss of voluntary movements of the thoracic and pelvic limbs on one side.

Flaccid or lower motor neuron paresis or paralysis: Paresis or paralysis with reduced or absent spinal reflexes in one or more limbs.

Spastic or upper motor neuron paresis or paralysis: Paresis or paralysis with normal or increased spinal reflexes in one or more limbs.

"Root signature": A sign that a lesion is irritating the nerve roots to a limb; manifests as reluctance to bear weight on the limb when standing and lameness or pain of the limb.

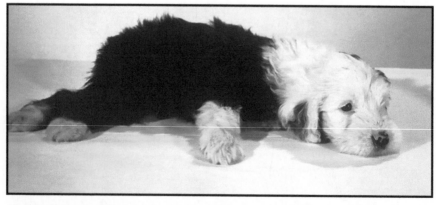

Figure 9-1 A 3-month-old English sheepdog with acute quadriparesis.

Fenestration: A surgical procedure to remove the nucleus pulposus of the intervertebral disk to prevent future extrusions.

Neuromuscular system: The peripheral nerves, neuromuscular junctions, and muscles.

Polyradiculoneuritis: Inflammation of many nerve roots and peripheral nerves.

Decubital ulcer: A deep wound with sloughing skin and muscle; occurs over bony prominences due to constant pressure from lying in one position too long; often the bone is exposed.

Syringomyelia: Fluid-filled cavitation of the spinal cord resulting from trauma, infarction, or unknown cause (most often causes chronic quadriparesis).

Meningomyelitis: Inflammation of the meninges and spinal cord.

Myelitis: Inflammation of the spinal cord.

Lesion Localization

✓ The location of lesions that cause acute quadriparesis, quadriplegia, hemiparesis or hemiplegia is shown in Figure 9-2. These lesions are usually found in the:

- Focal cervical and cranial thoracic spinal cord (C1-T2)
- Multifocal cervical, thoracic, and lumbar spinal cord (C1- L7)
- Generalized neuromuscular system (peripheral nerves, neuromuscular junctions and muscles)

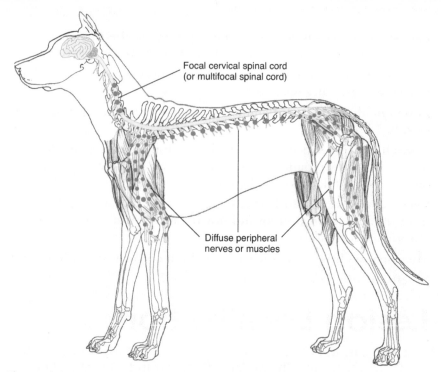

Figure 9-2 Acute quadriparesis, quadriplegia, hemiparesis, or hemiplegia can be associated with a focal cervical lesion, a multifocal spinal cord lesion, or a generalized neuromuscular lesion (dots indicate lesion localization).

Labels in figure:
Focal cervical spinal cord (or multifocal spinal cord)
Diffuse peripheral nerves or muscles

Differentiation of Spinal Cord and Neuromuscular Lesions

✓ Figure 9-3 is an algorithm to assist in differentiating spinal cord and neuromuscular lesions.

C1-C5 Spinal Cord Lesions

✓ If crossed extensor reflexes are present in the thoracic limbs and pelvic limb spinal reflexes are normal or hyperactive, then the lesion is localized to C1-C5.

✓ If the spinal reflexes of all four limbs are normal or if thoracic limb spinal reflexes are normal and the pelvic limb spinal reflexes are hyperactive, the lesion could be at either C1-C5 or C6-T2.

✓ May have unilateral Horner's syndrome on the side of the lesion.

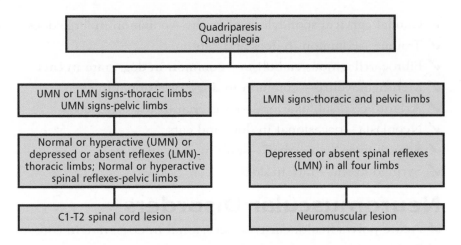

Figure 9-3 Algorithm to assist in differentiating spinal cord and neuromuscular lesions. LMN = lower motor neuron; UMN = upper motor neuron.

C6-T2 Spinal Cord Lesions

✓ If the lesion affects most of the C6-T2 region, the flexor reflexes of the thoracic limbs are reduced or absent, and the spinal reflexes in the pelvic limbs are normal or exaggerated.

✓ If the lesion affects only part of the C6-T2 region, the flexor reflexes of the thoracic limbs may still be normal, and this lesion cannot be distinguished from a C1-C5 lesion.

✓ May have unilateral Horner's syndrome on the side of the lesion.

✓ May have loss of cutaneous trunci response on the side of the lesion.

Neuromuscular Lesions

✓ Decreased or absent thoracic and pelvic limb spinal reflexes.

✓ Decreased or absent muscle tone in all four limbs.

✓ Loss of the cutaneous trunci response.

Differential Diagnosis

Spinal Cord Disorders

✓ Degenerative intervertebral disk disease (IVDD) —common in dogs, rare in cats

✓ Caudal cervical spondylomyelopathy—common in large dogs

✓ Trauma—common in dogs and cats

✓ Fibrocartilaginous embolism—common in dogs, rare in cats

✓ Meningomyelitis—common in dogs, occasional in cats

✓ Atlantoaxial subluxation—occasional in toy breed dogs

✓ Neoplasia—occasional in dogs and cats

✓ Spontaneous hemorrhage—rare in dogs and cats

✓ Syringomyelia—rare in dogs

Neuromuscular Disorders

✓ Acute polyradiculoneuritis—occasional in dogs, rare in cats

✓ Tick paralysis—occasional in dogs, rare in cats

✓ Snake envenomation—occasional in dogs and cats in specific geographic locations

✓ Myasthenia gravis—rare in dogs and cats

✓ Botulism—rare in dogs

✓ Other acute polyneuropathy—rare in dogs and cats

✓ Aminoglycoside intoxication—rare in dogs and cats

Diagnostic Evaluation

Important Historical Questions

- Acute onset (i.e., over 24 to 72 hours)?

- Progressive or nonprogressive?

- Possibility of recent trauma? If so, obtain vertebral radiographs before proceeding further.

- Is the neck painful?

- Have there been past episodes of quadriparesis?

- Past or present urinary or fecal incontinence?

- Can the animal urinate voluntarily?

- Are there signs of anorexia, depression, regurgitation, coughing, respiratory distress, or other systemic illness?

- Possible exposure to ticks, raccoons, snakes or dead carrion?

- Recent vaccination?

- Current or recent medications?

Physical and Neurologic Examinations

✓ Evaluate respiration; mucous membrane color; heart rate, rhythm, and pulse; and give emergency treatment if needed.

✓ Examine the ocular fundus for chorioretinitis.

✓ Examine for evidence of other systemic disease or neoplasia.

✓ Differentiate spinal cord from neuromuscular lesions.

✓ Examine the animal for a tick or a bite wound if a neuromuscular lesion suspected.

✓ Is Horner's syndrome present? (suggests a C_1–T_2 spinal cord disorder)

✓ Are one or more cranial nerves affected? (suggests a neuromuscular disorder)

✓ Determine whether the animal is in pain.

Applicable Diagnostic Tests

✓ A complete blood count (CBC), serum chemistry profile, and urinalysis are performed to detect systemic illness and as part of the preanesthetic evaluation.

✓ Serum acetylcholine receptor antibody test will be elevated in mysthenia gravis.

✓ Thoracic and abdominal radiographs and abdominal ultrasonography are indicated if neoplasia is suspected or abnormalities are found on the physical examination.

✓ The following are tests that are performed under general anesthesia, as well as their potential findings:

- Cerebrospinal fluid (CSF) analysis may show leukocytosis with or without elevated protein in acute intervertebral disk disease, meningitis, and some neoplastic processes, or elevated protein may be present only in intervertebral disk disease, fibrocartilaginous embolism trauma, and neoplasia.

- Vertebral column radiographs may show vertebral fractures and luxations, calcified intervertebral disks, atlantoaxial subluxation, and vertebral neoplasia.

- A myelogram with dynamic views is useful to evaluate the instability and ligamentous hypertrophy associated with caudal cervical spondylomyelopathy.

- A myelogram may also demonstrate spinal cord compression in animals with intervertebral disk disease, vertebral fracture or subluxation or spinal cord neoplasia. Primary spinal cord neoplasia may cause the spinal cord to appear swollen on the myelogram.

• Computed tomography (CT) and magnetic resonance imaging (MRI) can be useful to demonstrate intervertebral disk disease, hemorrhage, syringomyelia and vertebral and spinal cord neoplasia.

• An electromyogram (EMG), including needle EMG, motor nerve conduction velocity, repetitive nerve stimulation, and F-waves, is performed to determine if a diffuse neuromuscular disease is present and if the lesion is in the peripheral nerve, neuromuscular junction, or muscle.

• Histologic examination of a muscle and nerve biopsy can confirm and characterize lesions.

✓ Serum and CSF immunoassays for infectious diseases are indicated if CSF analysis shows evidence of inflammation.

Spinal Cord Disorders

Degenerative Intervertebral Disk Disease

✓ Acute quadriparesis or quadriplegia commonly occurs in dachshunds, Pekingese, Lhaso apsos, beagles, cocker spaniels, Shih Tzus, and many other small-breed dogs and some large-breed dogs from acute Type I intervertebral disk extrusion. Degenerated nucleus pulposus ruptures through the anulus fibrosus of the intervertebral disk into the vertebral canal, traumatizing and compressing the spinal cord (Section 7, Figure 7-4). Dogs that are ambulatory often have a "root signature" in one thoracic limb caused by compression of the C6-T2 nerve roots by a lateralized disk extrusion.

✓ A narrowed disk space and calcified disk material in the vertebral canal are often found on cervical vertebral radiographs (Figure 9-4). Increased protein levels and occasionally mild leukocytic pleocytosis are found on CSF analysis. Cervical myelography with or without CT can be performed to confirm the site of spinal cord compression.

✓ MRI can also be useful to visualize degenerating disks and spinal cord compression (Figures 9-5 and 9-6). Common sites of disk extrusion include C2-C3 in small-breed dogs and C5-C6 or C6-C7 in Doberman pinschers, Rottweilers, German shepherds, boxers, and other large-breed dogs, although involvement of any cervical disk is possible.

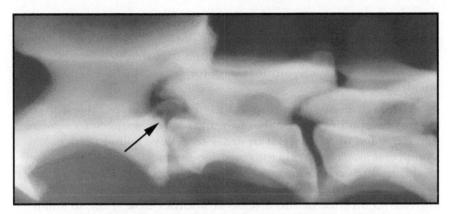

Figure 9-4 Lateral radiograph of a 3-year-old dachshund with acute quadriparesis associated with a herniated intervertebral disk at C2-3; note the narrowed intervertebral disk space and calcified material in the intervertebral foramen (arrow).

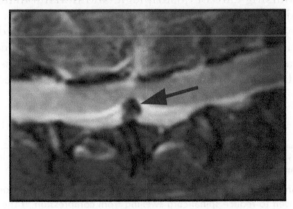

Figure 9-5 Sagittal T2-weighted MRI of the cervical spine of a 4-year-old English bulldog with acute onset of neck pain and ambulatory quadriparesis (right side worse than left); a Type I intervertebral disk extrusion at C4-5 can be seen compressing the spinal cord (arrow).

Figure 9-6 A transverse T2-weighted MRI of the dog in Figure 9-5 showing a Type I disk extrusion that is more prominent on the right than on the left (arrow).

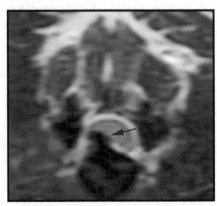

✔ If quadriparesis is mild and the dog is ambulatory, then medical management can be tried as outlined in Table 9-1. Aggressive steroid therapy as described in Table 9-3 for spinal cord injuries is usually unnecessary for cervical disk extrusion, as quadriplegia is rare.

♥ **Although many dogs respond to medical therapy, those that do not respond or are unable to walk require surgery to remove the extruded disk material in order to relieve spinal cord compression.** A ventral slot technique is most commonly performed (Section 7, Figure 7-11). Prophylactic fenestration of other disks in the area at the time of surgery may help to prevent further recurrence of the disease at another disk space in small dogs. The prognosis for return to normal function with surgery is usually excellent.

✔ Proper nursing care of quadriplegic and nonambulatory hemiparetic and quadriparetic dogs is outlined in Table 9-2. Such care can be very time-consuming and difficult in large-breed dogs, but it is essential to prevent complications and assist in recovery. Pneumonia can be a fatal complication, so the dog must be turned and respiration and body temperature monitored.

Table 9-1
Medical Management of Ambulatory Dogs with Mild Quadriparesis from Cervical Disk Disease

- **Strict crate confinement** for 4 weeks (activity is limited to short leash walks with a harness for urinating and defecating).

- **Oral prednisone 0.25–1 mg/kg every 12 hours with tapered doses over 7-14 days** is given to reduce spinal cord swelling from compression. If the animal improves then relapses as the dose is reduced, increase prednisone dose again and recommend surgery.

- **Oral famotidine** (Pepcid AC, Merck) **0.5–1 mg/kg every 12-24 hours, cimetidine** (Tagamet, SmithKline Beecham) **5-10 mg/kg every 8 hours, or misoprostol** (Cytotec, Searle) **1–3 µg/kg every 8 hours** may be given to reduce gastrointestinal upset when the prednisone dose is high.

- **Oral diazepam 0.5–2 mg/kg every 6-8 hours as needed (not to exceed 10 mg every 6 hours)** may help relieve painful muscle spasms.

- **If pain is severe, see Section 7, Table 7-2.**

Warning: Prednisone therapy often causes polyuria/polydipsia, polyphagia, and panting. Give extra water, and feed smaller amounts of a high-quality, low-calorie diet, as quadriparetic dogs can only minimally exercise. Long term corticosteriod therapy can cause gastrointestinal ulcers, hepatopathy, and myopathy

✓ Decubital ulcers are avoided by turning and keeping the dogs on a clean, padded surface. Dermatitis can occur secondary to irritation from urine and contamination from feces so cleanliness is essential. The bladder should be expressed so excessive distention does not damage the bladder wall. Most dogs will defecate reflexively, but an enema or stool softener may be needed if they become constipated.

✓ Assistance in drinking is important to avoid dehydration, and a balanced diet ensures good nutritional support and subsequent healing. Physical therapy is needed to reduce muscle atrophy and tendon contracture. The prognosis for recovery of quadriparetic dogs following surgery is usually excellent, but recovery may take several weeks or months. Advice to owners concerning strategies to prevent recurrence of problems associated with cervical disk disease is outlined in Section 7, Table 7-4.

Table 9-2
Nursing Care and Physical Therapy for Quadriplegic and Nonambulatory Hemiparetic and Quadriparetic Dogs

- Keep on a clean, padded surface, and turn to the opposite side every 4-6 hours.

- Monitor for cough, increased lung sounds, and respiratory distress twice daily (pneumonia).

- Monitor for fever twice daily.

- Express bladder every 6-8 hours if unable to urinate.

- Use enemas or stool softeners to assist with defecation if necessary.

- Keep skin dry and free of urine and feces (apply water-repellent ointment to perineal and caudal abdominal areas).

- Artificial tears or ophthalmic lubricant ointment may be needed if the palpebral reflex is absent.

- Hand-feed high-quality food, and hand-water until the dog can maintain sternal recumbency.

- Massage and perform passive range-of-motion exercises of limbs for 15 minutes 3-4 times a day.

- Give whirlpool baths, and allow to swim daily.

- Assist attempts to stand and support weight 3-4 times a day.

- Sling walks can begin when some movement returns.

Table 9-3
Methylprednisolone Sodium Succinate Therapy
for Acute Quadriplegia

Acute quadriplegia presented within 8 hours of onset:

- Methylprednisolone sodium succinate (MPSS) 30 mg/kg IV. (Refer immediately for emergency surgical decompression if the animal is stable.)

- Two hours after the initial dose, MPSS 15 mg/kg IV is given and repeated every 6 hours for 24-48 hours if voluntary movement is still absent.

- To prevent gastrointestinal complications, give IV famotidine (Pepcid AC) 0.5–1 mg/kg every 12-24 hours or cimetidine (Tagamet) 5-10 mg/kg every 8 hours.

Acute quadriplegia presented after 8 hours but within 24 hours of onset:

- MPSS 15 mg/kg IV every 6 hours for 24 hours. (Refer for emergency surgical decompression after the first dose if the animal is stable.)

Warnings

- Do not use MPSS at higher doses, in ambulatory animals, or if the patient presents more than 24 hours after the onset of injury, as the pathologic condition may be worsened.
- Stop treatment if melena or vomiting occurs.

Caudal Cervical Spondylomyelopathy

✓ Dogs with caudal cervical spondylomyelopathy (CCSM) may occasionally present with acute quadriparesis or quadriplegia associated with rapid extrusion of an intervertebral disk. Most dogs with CCSM are initially presented because of ataxia or chronic progressive quadriparesis (Sections 8 and 10).

Trauma

💣⁜ Cervical vertebral fractures, subluxation or luxation, and traumatic intervertebral disk herniation can cause acute quadriparesis or quadriplegia due to hemorrhage and compression of the cervical spinal cord. If trauma is known or suspected, manipulation of the cervical vertebrae and head during physical and neurologic examinations is avoided. It should not be assumed that animals with minimal neurologic deficits do not have serious spinal injuries. Dogs and cats with spinal fractures or luxations may be ambulatory and have neck pain with little or no neurologic impairment (Section 7), but manipulation of the neck can cause the vertebrae to collapse, resulting in subsequent quadriplegia.

♥ Acute quadriplegia is an emergency situation, as involvement of neurons controlling respiration can lead to hypoventilation, respiratory paralysis, hypoxia or death. Assisted ventilation and oxygen therapy may be needed. Aside from the immediate traumatic damage to the spinal cord, induction of secondary neurotoxic processes results in formation of oxygen containing free radicals and a cycle of progressive spinal cord destruction that continues over 24 to 48 hours. Methylprednisolone sodium succinate (MPSS) may be given to dogs and cats with quadriplegia to attempt to reduce spinal cord damage as outlined in Table 9-3. The antioxidant properties of this agent have been shown in experimental animals to reduce spinal cord destruction if given intravenously in a specific dose range within 8 hours of the onset of paralysis.

💣 The MPSS regimen is not given to dogs that can move voluntarily. Giving a higher-than-recommended dose of MPSS or beginning treatment more than 24 hours after the onset of quadriplegia may worsen the spinal cord damage. Surgical decompression within the first 24 hours has the optimal effect, so emergency referral after the first initial dose of MPSS is recommended if the animal is stable. A few dogs and cats with severe spinal cord injury can develop ascending myelomalacia and die from respiratory paralysis regardless of therapy.

💣 Corticosteroids at high doses can cause gastrointestinal (GI) irritation and lead to life-threatening ulceration and pancreatitis, so the use of drugs to protect the GI tract is highly recommended.

✓ Dexamethasone has not been shown to have the same neuroprotective effects as MPSS.

✋ Radiographs of the vertebral column should be obtained as soon as possible with the animal immobilized on a rigid surface, such as a radiolucent plastic board, to prevent movement and further spinal cord injury. Radiographs of the cervical, thoracic, and lumbar vertebrae should be obtained to identify multiple fracture sites. Fractures and luxations are usually obvious on plain radiographs, although occasionally an unstable subluxation may be viewed in the normal position. Fractures of the axis (C2) are seen most commonly, and this region should be evaluated carefully. The degree of spinal cord compression and swelling can be seen with a myelogram. CT and MRI can be useful to visualize hemorrhage within the spinal canal, additional compression remote from the obvious injury, and spinal cord edema; they may be especially helpful when no radiographic lesions are seen.

♥ If there is significant hemorrhage, bone fragments, or other space-occupying lesions within the spinal canal, then surgical decompression of the spinal cord through a ventral slot or dorsal laminectomy may be necessary. Vertebral fractures or luxations are stabilized with Steinmann pins or orthopedic screws and poly-methyl methacrylate (Section 12, Figures 12-9 and 12-10). Pain is controlled as outlined in Section 7, Table 7-2. Postoperative nursing care and physical therapy are outlined in Table 9-2.

✓ Trauma can damage vertebral arteries causing hemiparesis, quadri-paresis, or quadriplegia with no vertebral fractures or instability or spinal cord compression. Recovery is possible with strict crate confinement for a minimum of 4 weeks and nursing care as outlined in Tables 9-1 and 9-2. Animals with cervical spinal cord trauma often have a good chance of making a functional recovery and usually have a better prognosis than those with thoracolumbar injuries. Caudal cervical spinal cord injury can cause damage to neuronal cell bodies and nerve roots, and recovery can be slow and incomplete in one or both thoracic limbs.

Fibrocartilaginous Embolism

☞ Fibrocartilaginous embolism (FCE) and infarction of the spinal cord is the most common vascular disorder of dogs. Young, large-breed dogs, miniature schnauzers, and very rarely cats are presented with acute asymmetric quadriparesis, hemiparesis, or hemiplegia. Asymmetric paraparesis with paralysis of one pelvic limb is also common with FCE of the thoracic and lumbar spinal cord (Section 12). Infarction of the spinal cord results from occlusion of either spinal arteries or veins with fibrocartilage. The origin of the fibrocartilage is unknown, although most theories suggest that it arises from degenerating intervertebral disk material, which gains entrance to the spinal cord vascula-ture. The route of entrance is still speculative.

✋ A history of acute collapse with or without vigorous exercise is common. The clinical signs may worsen within the first few hours but are usually nonprogressive by the time veterinary help is obtained. Initially, the animal may be painful, but this usually passes in a few hours and pain is usually not evident on palpation of the neck. If the lesion involves the caudal cervical region, hyporeflexia or areflexia of one or both thoracic limbs and possibly Horner's syndrome or loss of the cutaneous trunci reflex may be observed. With severe infarctions, respiratory compro-mise may be evident. The diagnosis is typically one of exclusion, although an acute, nonprogressive, nonpainful, asymmetric paresis or paralysis in a young, large-breed dog is highly suggestive of FCE. An overview of the diagnostic criteria and treatment for FCE in dogs is outlined in Table 9-4.

♥ In severe cases of quadriparesis, ventilatory support and oxygen therapy may be needed. After 24 hours, prednisone 0.25 to 1 mg/kg PO every 12 hours with doses tapered doses over 7 to 14 days may be given.

🖐 If quadriparesis is symmetric or remains severe, CSF analysis can rule out meningomyelitis, while myelography and other imaging techniques may demonstrate spinal cord swelling or are normal with no evidence of spinal cord compression. MRI may show evidence of intramedullary edema. Evaluation of appropriate blood tests can help to rule out coagulopathy or other factors predisposing to thrombus formation. The prognosis for this disease is excellent, and functional recovery can usually be achieved in all but the most severely affected dogs. One thoracic limb may remain weaker than the other.

Table 9-4
Diagnostic Criteria and Treatment for Cervical Fibrocartilaginous Embolism in Dogs

- Acute onset of nonpainful quadriparesis or quadriplegia (one side is often worse than the other) with no history of trauma, especially in large-breed dogs

- Pelvic limb spinal reflexes are normal or hyperactive; thoracic limb reflexes are normal, hyperactive, depressed, or absent

- Horner's syndrome may be present on the same side as the most-affected limbs

- **Treatment is with IV methylprednisolone sodium succinate 15 mg/kg every 6 hours for 24 hours and IV famotidine (Pepcid AC) 0.5-1 mg/kg every 12-24 hours or cimetidine (Tagamet) 5-10 mg/kg every 8 hours for 24 hours**

- On re-evaluation in 12-24 hours, the dog may be ambulatory with assistance with hemiplegia or hemiparesis still present

- If improvement is significant, may opt for serial neurologic examinations and nursing care (Table 9-2)

- May opt for myelography or MRI which is normal or shows mild spinal cord swelling and edema

- Most dogs become functional pets again in 2-6 weeks

Meningomyelitis

✓ The same inflammatory diseases of the brain discussed in Section 2 can affect the spinal cord. Meningomyelitis or myelitis can cause acute quadriparesis with or without cervical pain. The diagnosis is suspected by finding leukocytic pleocytosis and elevated protein levels on CSF analysis. CSF from the lumbar subarachnoid space may have a higher leukocyte count and protein content than that of the cerebellomedullary cistern due to the caudal flow of CSF. An inflammatory focus may be visible on MRI. Serum and CSF immunoassays for specific organisms may be performed. The diagnosis and treatment of infections and other inflammations are discussed in the meningoencephalitis section of Section 2 (Tables 2-8, 2-9, 2-10, and 2-11).

Atlantoaxial Subluxation

✓ Atlantoaxial (C1-C2) subluxation is usually associated with agenesis or hypogenesis of the dens and surrounding ligaments in toy-breed dogs younger than 1 year of age. On occasion, a seemingly insignificant traumatic event, such as falling off the furniture or playing with another animal, will cause subluxation in dogs that are a few years old. Periodic syncope-like episodes have been noted, presumably from an abnormal dens compressing the ventrally located basilar artery, which reduces the blood flow to the brain. Acute subluxation can cause severe spinal cord injury.

✓ Pain is usually elicited in the high cervical region on cervical palpation. Ataxia of all four limbs, quadriparesis of varying degrees, or quadriplegia is present, and the thoracic limbs are often worse than the pelvic limbs. Spinal reflexes are normal to hyperactive, and crossed extensor reflexes may be present in all four limbs. The diagnosis can usually be made with a lateral radiograph of the cervical spine, which shows an abnormal separation of the dorsal arch of the atlas and the dorsal spinous process of the axis (Figure 9-7). Slight flexion of the neck can occasionally facilitate this observation, although this must be done with extreme caution in anesthetized animals with an intact dens to avoid further spinal cord injury. Myelography can confirm the compression but is usually not necessary. Syringomyelia may occur secondarily and can be seen with MRI.

♥ **The treatment of choice is ventral surgical fusion of the atlantoaxial joint.** Stabilization with Steinmann pins or orthopedic

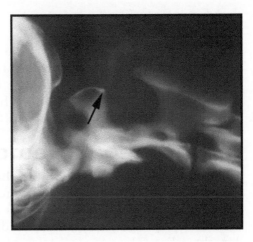

Figure 9-7 Lateral radiograph of a 1-year-old poodle with acute quadriparesis from atlantoaxial subluxation; note the wide separation between the dorsal spinous process of C1 (arrow) and C2.

screws and polymethylmethacrylate is usually effective (Figures 9-8 and 9-9). A neck brace is also used for 4 to 6 weeks in dogs after surgery and in those with pain and ataxia only. Crate confinement and the treatment outlined in Table 9-1 for cervical disk disease are also suggested. Postoperative nursing care is easier with toy-breed dogs and is outlined in Table 9-2. The prognosis for functional recovery following surgery is usually fair to good.

💣 Without surgical fusion, recurrence of quadriparesis and potentially severe spinal cord injury is common.

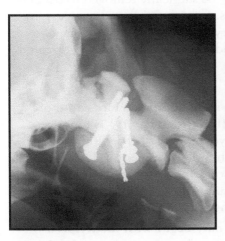
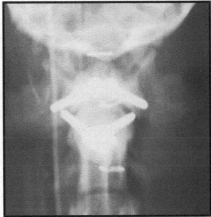

Figure 9-8 (left) Lateral radiograph of a surgical repair of atlantoaxial subluxation; pins, screws, and polymethylmethacrylate were placed ventrally to fuse vertebrae C1-C2.

Figure 9-9 (right) Ventrodorsal radiograph of the surgical repair of the atlantoaxial subluxation in Figure 9-8.

Neoplasia

✓ Neoplasia of the vertebrae, nerve roots, meninges, or spinal cord can result in acute quadriplegia if these conditions cause hemorrhage, ischemia or pathologic fractures. However, most animals with neoplastic conditions have neck pain or chronic progressive ataxia and quadriparesis (Sections 7, 8, and 10).

Spontaneous Hemorrhage

✓ Spontaneous hemorrhage within the spinal canal or spinal cord causing acute quadriparesis unassociated with trauma, intervertebral disk extrusion, or neoplasia is rare but may occur secondary to thrombocytopenia, von Willebrand's disease, or other coagulopathies. For unknown reasons, greyhounds seem to be at increased risk for spontaneous spinal cord hemorrhage. Evaluation of platelet counts, coagulation parameters, and bleeding function tests may identify an underlying disorder. Thrombocytopenia and other coagulopathies must be treated before invasive tests or surgery are performed. If it is safe to collect CSF, hemorrhage, xanthochromia, or erythrophagocytosis by neutrophils or macrophages may be observed. Spinal cord compression from a suspected hematoma may be observed on myelography, CT, or MRI; however, the imaging characteristics of hemorrhage are complex, and definitive diagnosis can be difficult. A hematoma may be surgically removed to decompress the spinal cord in some cases. Improvement and recovery are often possible even without surgery, although the recurrence of hemorrhage is a concern if the underlying problem is not corrected.

Syringomyelia

✓ Syringomyelia of the cervical spinal cord is a rare cause of acute quadriplegia. The syrinx (fluid-filled cavity) is found within the spinal cord on the myelogram or MRI. Primary syrinx formation may be associated with a developmental defect like hydrocephalus. A syrinx may also form secondary to atlantoaxial subluxation or other injury, vascular disorder, infection, or neoplasia. Sometimes the inciting cause is unclear.

Treatment of acute quadriplegia may begin with methylprednisolone sodium succinate IV 15 mg/kg every 6 hours for 24 hours and famotidine (Pepcid AC, Merck) IV 0.5–1 mg/kg every 12–24 hours or cimetidine (Tagamet, SmithKline Beecham) 5–10 mg/kg every 8 hours for 24 hours. After 24 hours, prednisone 0.25–1 mg/kg PO every 12 hours with doses

tapered over 7 to 14 days may be given along with oral doses of one of the gastrointestinal protectants. The underlying cause if found should be addressed accordingly. Nursing care and physical therapy are performed as outlined in Table 9-2. Affected dogs may recover, but the long-term prognosis depends on the inciting cause. Syringomyelia is most commonly associated with chronic progressive quadriparesis.

Neuromuscular Disorders

Acute Polyradiculoneuritis

✓ Acute polyradiculoneuritis causes acute, flaccid quadriparesis or quadriplegia. In dogs, the condition was originally called "coonhound paralysis," as it was first described in coonhounds 7 to 10 days after exposure to an antigen in raccoon saliva. The inciting cause is often unknown, although recent vaccination or illness can be documented in some cases. Some evidence has suggested the involvement of clostridial organisms in the intestine as a source of antigen. These external antigens are apparently similar to proteins that make up part of the ventral nerve roots and motor nerves, and clinical signs are caused by an immune-mediated attack of these structures with the invasion of inflammatory cells.

✓ Animals present with acute, progressive, flaccid quadriparesis that often ascends from the pelvic limbs to the thoracic limbs over a 12 to 24-hour period. On rare occasions, the thoracic limbs are more involved than the pelvic limbs. The palpebral reflex may be depressed or absent in both eyes due to involvement of the facial nerve (CN 7), and dysphagia may be present due to dysfunction of the vagus nerve (CN 10). If respiratory involvement is severe, abdominal respiration, hypoventilation, and hypoxia occur. Hyporeflexia or areflexia with hypotonicity is usually present in all four limbs. Some tail movement may be preserved. Sensation remains intact, and some animals have generalized hyperesthesia.

✓ Diffuse positive waves and fibrillation potentials with normal or reduced motor nerve conduction velocity are often found on the EMG, suggesting diffuse polyneuropathy. Motor nerve conduction velocity may be normal or slowed. The F-wave is abnormal, suggesting ventral root disease. CSF protein levels can be normal or elevated, but the leukocyte count is usually normal. If the animal presents within 24 hours of the onset of paralysis, intravenous methylprednisolone sodium succinate may be given as outlined in Table 9-3.

♥ Affected dogs should be closely monitored, as they may worsen over a 7-day period before they stabilize and begin to slowly improve. Paresis then paralysis of intercostal and diaphragmatic muscles can occur, so respiration should be monitored to detect hypoventilation and hypoxia. Blood gas determinations should be evaluated if possible to detect increased pCO_2 and decreased pO_2. Oxygen therapy or assisted ventilation may be necessary for a few days in some cases. The nursing care and physical therapy required are outlined in Table 9-2. Severe generalized muscle atrophy may occur, making physical therapy essential. The prognosis is usually good with adequate support, and most dogs recover in 4 to 12 weeks. Avoidance of known antigenic stimuli, such as vaccinations, should be considered to prevent recurrence of signs. Recurrence with no known stimulus has been documented in some dogs and cats.

Tick Paralysis

Tick paralysis is caused by a neurotoxin secreted by female ticks of the genus *Dermacentor* (North America) or *Ixodes* (Australia). The toxin causes inhibition of acetylcholine release at the neuromuscular junction or impairs depolarization of the distal lower motor neurons and is released as long as the tick is embedded and feeding. Dogs are most frequently affected. This disease is rarely seen in cats except in Australia.

✓ An ascending acute, flaccid quadriparesis develops over a 12 to 24-hour period and is clinically identical to acute polyradiculoneuritis. Severely depressed or absent spinal reflexes in all four limbs with preserved sensation is typically found on the neurologic examination. Some tail movement may be preserved. Respiratory distress from paresis of intercostal muscles and the diaphragm can be seen in advanced cases. Reduced or absent palpebral reflexes due to facial nerve (CN 7) dysfunction may be present, but involvement of other cranial nerves is rare in North America. Laryngeal and pharyngeal paresis may occur in cases in Australia.

✓ The EMG can be used to differentiate tick paralysis and acute polyradiculoneuritis. In tick paralysis, no fibrillation potentials or positive sharp waves are seen to indicate denervation, and there is little or no response to nerve stimulation. The EMG abnormalities of dogs with tick paralysis, coral snake envenomation, and botulism are similar as they all affect neuromuscular transmission.

♥ Any dog or cat with acute flaccid quadriplegia should be carefully examined for an engorged tick, including in and around the ears and between the toes. Care should be taken to remove the whole tick if found. Removal of ticks with topical pesticides should be done with caution, as organophosphates may further compromise neuromuscular function. Cases in Australia have been documented to become progressively worse even after tick removal, but this has not been documented in North America. Respiration should be monitored, as a few cases may require oxygen therapy or ventilatory assistance. Supportive nursing care as outlined in Table 9-2 is given, but in North America, once the tick is removed full recovery occurs within 24 to 72 hours.

Snake Envenomation

☖┱ The Elapidae family of snakes includes cobras, mambas, and tiger snakes and is represented in the United States by the eastern coral snake (*Micrurus fulvius fulvius*) in the southeastern states and the Texas coral snake (*M. f. tenere*) in Texas, Louisiana, and Arkansas. The toxin in the venom is thought to cause a postsynaptic, nondepolarizing blockade of the neuromuscular junction, similar to curare.

✓ There may be a history of playing with a snake, or a dead snake may be found in the yard where the animal has been. The bite wounds are usually not obvious, as there is typically minimal tissue reaction. However, a small, red mark may sometimes be found with careful examination of the face, muzzle, or pinnae. Clinical signs are usually evident within several hours of the bite.

✓ Dogs and cats present with acute, progressive, flaccid quadriparesis and may appear mildly sedated. Limb spinal reflexes are absent, and reduced nociception often occurs. Some tail movement may be preserved. Reduced palpebral reflexes, reduced facial sensation, and dysphagia are often seen. A characteristic feature of coral and tiger snake envenomation is hemolysis and hemoglobinuria. Ventricular tachycardia may also occur.

✓ Changes on the EMG are similar to those of tick paralysis. Coral snake antivenin is available and may help to reduce the severity of clinical signs if given promptly. The dose of antivenin is controversial and is usually given empirically (one to four vials slowly IV). **Antivenin is expensive and may cause anaphylaxis. Thus, a skin test of 1:10 dilution, 0.2 ml intradermally may be considered before IV administration. Not all animals need antivenin to survive.**

♥ Therapy mainly involves providing supportive care as described in Table 9-2 and allowing time for the toxin to exit the body. Animals that have progressive respiratory muscle paresis may require assisted ventilation. A CBC and urinalysis should be monitored for hemolysis. Fluid therapy at 2 to 3 times maintenance levels should be administered if hemolysis occurs to protect the kidneys. Blood gases should be monitored for hypoxia and increased pCO_2 or decreased pO_2 should be corrected. The overall prognosis depends on the size of the snake and amount of venom received. **With supportive care, the prognosis for recovery from paralysis is often excellent and many animals make a complete recovery in 7 to 10 days.**

Myasthenia Gravis

✓ Generalized myasthenia gravis may cause acute quadriparesis in dogs and cats. The quadriparesis may worsen with exercise. The diagnosis and treatment of myasthenia gravis are discussed in Section 11.

Botulism

✓ Ingestion of toxin from the organism *Clostridium botulinum* is a rare cause of flaccid quadriparesis or quadriplegia in dogs. Cases documented in dogs have been associated with type C toxin. Naturally occurring botulism has not been documented in cats. The most common source of infection is probably through ingestion of carrion, although clostridial infections may play a role. The toxin interferes with the release of acetylcholine from the endplates of motor neurons, resulting in failure of neuromuscular transmission.

✓ Acute, progressive quadriparesis develops over a 12–24 hour period and varies in severity, depending on the amount of toxin ingested. All spinal reflexes of the limbs are depressed or absent, and muscle tone is reduced. Facial paralysis, dysphonia, dysphagia, and megaesophagus from cranial nerve involvement are often seen. Constipation and urine retention have also been documented. As the toxin only affects the motor endplates, sensation remains intact.

✓ The EMG changes are similar to those of tick paralysis and coral snake envenomation. The toxin can be identified in the serum, feces, vomitus, or carrion by a mouse neutralization test, although this must be done early in the disease process to be useful. Although a Type C antitoxin is available, to be effective it must be administered before entry of the toxin into the nerve endings, and most cases already have neurologic signs on presentation.

✓ Paresis then paralysis of intercostal and diaphragmatic muscles can occur, so respiration should be monitored to detect hypoventilation and hypoxia. Blood gas determinations should be evaluated if possible to detect increased pCO_2 and decreased pO_2. Oxygen therapy or assisted ventilation may be necessary for a few days in some cases. The required nursing care and physical therapy are outlined in Table 9-2. Stool softeners, suction of the oropharynx, and administration of artificial tears for corneal protection may be needed. Antibiotic therapy is usually not indicated unless concurrent infection is present, because ingestion of the preformed toxin, rather than infection with the organism, causes the neurologic impairment in dogs. Many affected dogs recover fully within 2 to 3 weeks.

💣※ Aminoglycoside and ampicillin administration should be avoided, as these antibiotics can worsen neuromuscular weakness.

Acute Polyneuropathies

✓ Other acute polyneuropathies can cause acute quadriparesis or quadriplegia but are probably rare compared with acute polyradiculoneuritis. These diseases have many underlying causes and usually present with a chronic, progressive, or waxing and waning course and are discussed in Section 10.

Aminoglycoside Intoxication

✓ Aminoglycoside antibiotics (gentamicin, amikacin, kanamycin, and others) can cause or exacerbate blockade of the neuromuscular junction. This leads to acute, flaccid quadri-paresis. In animals with neuromuscular disease, these antibiotics can worsen the paresis. Discontinuation of the drug results in reversal of the paresis in most cases.

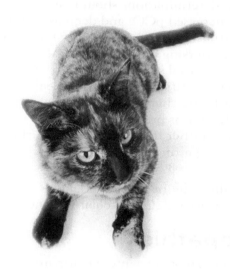

Chronic Quadriparesis

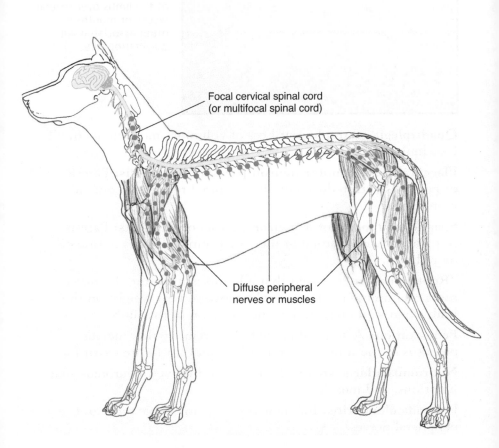

Focal cervical spinal cord
(or multifocal spinal cord)

Diffuse peripheral
nerves or muscles

Definitions

Chronic quadriparesis: Quadriparesis that progresses over 1 week to several months.

Quadriparesis (tetraparesis): Weakness (paresis) in all four limbs, which can be mild (ambulatory), moderate (nonambulatory, sternal recumbency), or severe (nonambulatory, lateral recumbency), but some voluntary limb movement is retained (Figure 10-1); most ambulatory animals with quadriparesis also show ataxia and conscious proprioceptive deficits.

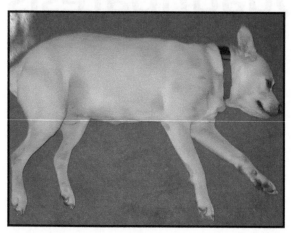

Figure 10-1 Progressive quadriparesis with depressed spinal reflexes of the limbs over several weeks or months is often associated with polyneuropathy.

Quadriplegia (tetraplegia): Loss of voluntary movements in all four limbs.

Flaccid or lower motor neuron paresis or paralysis: Paresis or paralysis with reduced or absent spinal reflexes in one or more limbs.

Spastic or upper motor neuron paresis or paralysis: Paresis or paralysis with normal or increased spinal reflexes in one or more limbs.

"Root signature": A sign that a lesion is irritating the nerve roots to a limb; manifests as reluctance to bear weight on the limb when standing and lameness or pain of the limb.

Fenestration: A surgical procedure to remove the nucleus pulposus of the intervertebral disk to prevent future extrusions.

Neuromuscular system: The peripheral nerves, neuromuscular junctions, and muscles.

Polyradiculoneuritis: Inflammation of many nerve roots and peripheral nerves.

Decubital ulcer: A deep wound with sloughing skin and muscle; occurs over bony prominences due to constant pressure from lying in one position too long; the bone is often exposed.

Meningomyelitis: Inflammation of the meninges and spinal cord.

Myelitis: Inflammation of the spinal cord.

Lesion Localization

✓ The location of lesions that cause chronic quadriparesis are shown in Figure 10-2. These lesions usually occur in the:

- Focal cervical and cranial thoracic spinal cord (C1-T2)

- Multifocal cervical, thoracic, and lumbar spinal cord (C1- L7)

- Diffuse neuromuscular system (peripheral nerves, neuromuscular juctions or muscles)

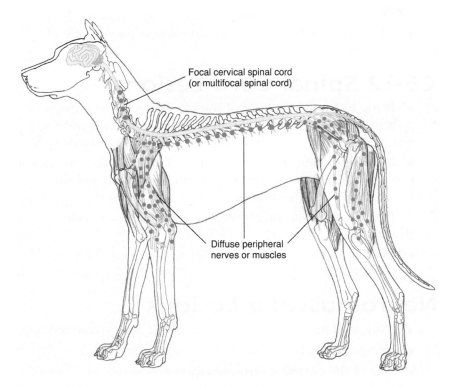

Figure 10-2 Chronic progressive quadriparesis can be associated with a focal cervical lesion, a multifocal spinal cord lesion, or a generalized neuromuscular lesion (dots indicate lesion localization).

Differentiation of Spinal Cord and Neuromuscular Lesions

✓ An algorithm on how to differentiate spinal cord from neuromuscular lesions is shown in Section 9, Figure 9-3.

C1-C5 Spinal Cord Lesions

✓ If crossed extensor reflexes are present in the thoracic limbs and the pelvic limb spinal reflexes are normal or hyperactive, then the lesion is localized to C1-C5.

✓ If the spinal reflexes of all four limbs are normal or if thoracic limb spinal reflexes are normal and pelvic limb spinal reflexes are hyperactive, the lesion could be at either C1-C5 or C6-T2.

✓ May have unilateral Horner's syndrome on the side of the lesion.

C6-T2 Spinal Cord Lesions

✓ If the lesion affects most of the C6-T2 region, the flexor reflexes of the thoracic limbs are reduced or absent, and the spinal reflexes in the pelvic limbs are normal or exaggerated.

✓ If the lesion affects only part of the C6-T2 region, the flexor reflexes of the thoracic limbs may still be normal, and this lesion cannot be distinguished from a C1-C5 lesion.

✓ May have unilateral Horner's syndrome on the side of the lesion.

✓ May be loss of cutaneous trunci response on the side of the lesion.

Neuromuscular Lesions

✓ Decreased or absent thoracic and pelvic limb spinal reflexes.

✓ Decreased or absent muscle tone in all four limbs.

✓ Loss of the cutaneous trunci response.

Differential Diagnosis

Spinal Cord Disorders

✓ Degenerative intervertebral disk disease—common in dogs, rare in cats

✓ Caudal cervical spondylomyelopathy—common in large-breed dogs

✓ Meningomyelitis—common in dogs, occasional in cats

✓ Diskospondylitis—common in dogs, rare in cats

✓ Neoplasia—occasional in dogs and cats

✓ Lysosomal storage disorders—rare in dogs and cats

✓ Spinal cord cysts and syringomyelia—rare in dogs and cats

✓ Leukoencephalomyelopathy—rare in dogs

Neuromuscular Disorders

✓ Hypothyroid neuromyopathy—occasional in dogs

✓ Chronic idiopathic polyneuropathy—occasional in dogs, rare in cats

✓ Protozoal polyradiculoneuritis—occasional in dogs, rare in cats

✓ Polymyopathies—occasional in dogs and cats

✓ Myasthenia gravis—occasional in dogs and cats

✓ Diabetic polyneuropathy—rare in dogs and occasional in cats

✓ Insulinoma polyneuropathy—rare in dogs

✓ Paraneoplastic polyneuropathy—rare in dogs and cats

✓ Toxic polyneuropathy—rare in dogs and cats

✓ Congenital or hereditary polyneuropathies—rare in dogs and cats

Diagnostic Evaluation

Important Historical Questions

- Onset, progression, and duration of signs?
- Behavior changes or seizures?
- Anorexia, depression, or other signs of illness?
- Neck pain?
- Voice change?
- Past or present history of neoplasia?

- Exposure to toxins?
- Current or recent medications and response to therapy?
- Raw meat diet (toxoplasmosis)?

Physical and Neurologic Examinations

✓ Examine the ocular fundus for chorioretinitis.

✓ Examine for evidence of other systemic disease or neoplasia.

✓ Differentiate spinal cord from neuromuscular lesions.

✓ Check if Horner's syndrome is present (suggests a C1–T2 spinal cord disorder).

✓ Determine if one or more cranial nerves are affected (indicates neuromuscular disorders).

✓ Determine if pain is a feature of the disease process.

Applicable Diagnostic Tests

✓ A complete blood count (CBC), serum chemistry profile, and urinalysis are performed to detect systemic illness and as part of the preanesthetic evaluation.

✓ Thoracic and abdominal radiographs and abdominal ultrasonography are indicated if neoplasia is suspected or abnormalities are found on the physical examination.

✓ Serum creatine kinase (CK) and serum acetylcholine receptor antibody levels are evaluated if polymyopathy or myasthenia gravis is suspected.

✓ The following are tests that are performed under general anesthesia, as well as their potential findings:

- Cerebrospinal fluid (CSF) analysis may show leukocytosis with or without elevated protein in cases of meningomyelitis and some neoplastic processes or, in chronic intervertebral disk disease, myelitis, neoplasia, cysts, and spinal cord compression elevated protein only.

- Routine vertebral column radiographs may show calcified cervical intervertebral disks, diskospondylitis, spondylosis deformans, and vertebral neoplasia.

- A myelogram with dynamic views is useful to evaluate the instability and ligamentous hypertrophy associated with caudal cervical spondylomyelopathy.

- A myelogram may also demonstrate spinal cord compression in animals with intervertebral disk disease, cysts or neoplasia;

primary spinal cord neoplasia may cause the spinal cord to appear swollen on the myelogram.

- Computed tomography (CT) and magnetic resonance imaging (MRI) can be useful to evaluate intervertebral disk disease, diskospondylitis, spinal cord neoplasia and cysts, and syringomyelia.

- Electromyography (EMG), including needle EMG, motor nerve-conduction velocity, repetitive nerve stimulation, and F-waves, are evaluated to determine if a diffuse neuromuscular disease is present and if the lesion is affecting the nerve roots, peripheral nerves, neuromuscular junction, and/or muscle.

- Muscle and nerve biopsies may be performed if peripheral nerve or muscle disease is suspected.

✓ Serum and CSF immunoassays for infectious diseases are indicated if CSF analysis shows evidence of inflammation.

Spinal Cord Disorders

Degenerative Intervertebral Disk Disease

✓ Hansen Type II intervertebral disk disease (IVDD) is associated with fibroid degeneration and slow protrusion of the anulus fibrosus into the vertebral canal, causing chronic progressive quadriparesis (Section 7, Figure 7-5). Type II IVDD is more common in older, nonchondrodystrophic dogs of any size or breed but can also be seen in chondrodystrophic breeds, such as dachshunds and Pekingese. On occasion, Hansen Type I IVDD (Section 7, Figure 7-4) can cause slow extrusion of the nucleus pulposus, producing quadriparesis that progresses over several weeks. Cervical disk disease is rare in cats. Mildly affected dogs may have a stiff, short-strided gait and may have neck pain. Quadriparesis may be mild or progress to a nonambulatory condition. Limb spinal reflexes are usually normal or hyperactive.

✓ Since Type II IVDD rarely causes disk calcification or a narrowed disk space, routine radiographs are usually normal. CSF analysis should be performed before myelography to rule out meningomyelitis; such analysis often shows elevated protein levels. Spinal cord compression is usually obvious on the myelogram with or without CT (Figure 10-3). CT and MRI can be noninvasive ways to evaluate disk degeneration and spinal cord compression (Section 7, Figures 7-8, 7-9, and 7-10).

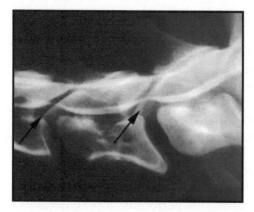

Figure 10-3 A lateral myelogram of a 7-year-old Doberman pinscher with chronic progressive quadriparesis from Type II intervertebral disk protrusion at two sites, C5-6 and C6-7 (arrows).

✔ Many dogs may respond temporarily to medical management (Section 9, Table 9-1). Acupuncture treatments may also help relieve the pain and quadriparesis. Lifestyle changes should be recommended as outlined in Section 7, Table 7-4. **Surgery is often required for dogs that worsen when medication is discontinued or those that are nonambulatory.** Chronic compression can lead to spinal cord atrophy from disruption of the normal blood flow, which can reduce the effectiveness of surgery. A ventral slot surgical technique is most commonly performed (Section 7, Figure 7-11). The prognosis for return to normal function with surgery is usually good, but in large-breed dogs recovery may involve 4 to 8 weeks of intensive nursing care (see Section 9, Table 9-2).

✔ As discussed in Section 9, pneumonia can be a fatal complication, so dogs are turned and respiration and body temperature are monitored. Turning reduces the chances of decubital ulcers. The dog must be kept on a clean, padded surface. Dermatitis can occur secondary to irritation from urine and contamination from feces, so cleanliness is essential. The bladder should be expressed so excessive distention does not damage the bladder wall. Most dogs will defecate reflexively, but an enema or stool softener may be needed if they become constipated.

✔ Prophylactic fenestration of other cervical disks at the time of surgery is usually performed in small breed dogs and may help to prevent further recurrence of the disease at another site.

Caudal Cervical Spondylomyelopathy

✔ Caudal cervical spondylomyelopathy (CCSM) is seen most commonly in Great Danes and Doberman pinschers but can occur in any large-breed dog. Because ataxia of all four limbs is often the initial sign, CCSM has been referred to as wobbler's syndrome. On close examination, quadriparesis or paraparesis with conscious proprioceptive deficits is usually also present. Spinal cord decompression and stabilization are usually undertaken when affected dogs are ataxic, before quadriparesis becomes severe. Diagnosis and therapy of CCSM are presented in Section 8.

Meningomyelitis

✓ The same inflammatory diseases of the brain discussed in Section 2 can affect the spinal cord. Meningomyelitis or myelitis can cause chronic quadriparesis with or without cervical pain. The diagnosis is suspected by finding leukocytic pleocytosis and elevated protein levels on CSF analysis. CSF from the lumbar subarachnoid space may have a higher leukocyte count and protein content than that of the cerebellomedullary cistern due to the caudal flow of CSF. An inflammatory focus may be visible on MRI. Serum and CSF immunoassays for specific organisms may be performed. Diagnosis and treatment of infections and other inflammatory disorders are discussed in Section 2, Tables 2-8, 2-9, 2-10, and 2-11)

Diskospondylitis

✓ Diskospondylitis can cause spinal cord compression due to inflammation and swelling of the intervertebral disk and surrounding tissues. This pathologic process causes progressive quadriparesis, but most dogs are evaluated for severe neck pain. Diagnosis and treatment of diskospondylitis are discussed in Section 7.

Neoplasia

✓ Osteochondromatosis, also known as multiple cartilaginous exostoses, is proliferation of benign masses of cartilage and bone at metaphyseal growth plates, which often occurs at multiple sites in young animals. Cervical vertebral osteochondromas can compress the spinal cord and cause chronic progressive quadriparesis and neck pain. Ostechondromas can also produce chronic paraparesis and are discussed in Section 13.

✓ Primary or metastatic neoplasia of the vertebrae can produce chronic progressive quadriparesis from spinal cord compression. Osteosarcoma, chondrosarcoma, fibrosarcoma, hemangiosarcoma, multiple myeloma, and metastatic prostatic or mammary adenocarcinomas are the most common types of vertebral neoplasia. Bony proliferation or lysis is usually visible on routine radiographs of the vertebral column and can be further visualized with CT (see Section

7, Figures 7-18 and 7-19). Pain is a primary feature of vertebral neoplasia. Spinal cord compression or expansion secondary to neoplasia can be seen on a myelogram with or without CT (Figure 10-4). Neoplasia may be extradural (in the epidural space), intradural-extramedullary (between the spinal cord and dura) (Figure 10-5), or intramedullary (within the spinal cord).

✓ Most spinal cord tumors are best evaluated with MRI. An elevated protein level without leukocytic pleocytosis is most frequently seen on CSF analysis. Occasionally, mild pleocytosis occurs. Atypical lymphocytes may also occasionally be found in the CSF in animals with spinal lymphoma, but other tumor cells are rare. In some cases, fluoroscopy-guided needle aspiration of the spinal mass may enable collection of tissue for cytologic examination and identification of the neoplasm. The most common types of spinal cord tumors are listed in Table 10-1.

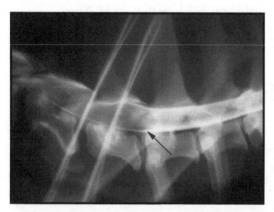

Figure 10-4 Lateral myelogram of a 7-year-old Dalmatian with chronic progressive quadriparesis and a nerve sheath tumor that has compressed the spinal cord at C7 (arrow).

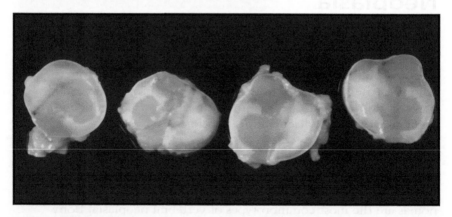

Figure 10-5 Transverse sections of the spinal cord of the dog in Figure 10-4 obtained at recropsy showing growth of the nerve sheath tumor into the spinal cord on cross-section.

Table 10-1
Common Tumors of the Spinal Cord

Extradural (often painful)

- Vertebral neoplasia (primary and metastatic)
- Lymphosarcoma

Intradural extramedullary (often painful)

- Meningioma
- Neurofibroma
- Neurofibrosarcoma
- Schwannoma

Metastatic intramedullary (often nonpainful)

- Hemangiosarcoma
- Mammary gland adenocarcinoma
- Lymphosarcoma

Primary intramedullary (often nonpainful)

- Ependymoma
- Astrocytoma
- Ependymoma

✋ Meningiomas and peripheral nerve sheath neoplasms are the most common spinal cord tumors in dogs. Gliomas and ependymomas are the most frequent primary intramedullary spinal cord tumors. Neoplasia, which metastasizes to the spinal canal or spinal cord, includes hemangiosarcoma, adenocarconomas from mammary and prostate glands and lymphoma. Lymphoma is the most common spinal tumor of cats. Progressive painful paraparesis is the most common clinical sign in cats, as there is a predilection for the lymphoma to be localized in the thoracic and lumbar vertebral canal (see Section 13).

♥ The appropriate therapy for spinal neoplasia depends on tumor location, size, and histologic type. **The immediate goal of therapy is to relieve the deleterious effects of spinal cord compression, which is achieved with corticosteroids and possibly decompressive surgery.** Pain is controlled as described in Section 7, Table 7-2. Prednisone 0.25–1 mg/kg PO every 12 hours may improve quadriparesis, but the disorder returns when prednisone is reduced or discontinued. If an extradural or intradural-extramedullary neoplasm is suspected, exploratory dorsal laminectomy or hemilaminectomy is performed to remove as much of the tumor as possible and to collect tissue samples for histologic identification of the tumor type.

✓ Postoperative radiation therapy may reduce or delay re-growth of neoplastic tissue in some dogs and cats with meningiomas. In some cases of lymphoma, multiple myeloma, and other neoplasms, chemotherapeutic and radiation protocols are available. Dogs and cats with spinal neoplasia generally have a poor long-term prognosis, but in some cases clinical signs can be alleviated for a year or more.

Lysosomal Storage Disorders

✓ Lysosomal storage disorders result from congenital absence or inactivity of a specific lysosomal enzyme. The substrate normally metabolized by that enzyme accumulates within cells causing cell dysfunction and death. Clinical signs vary depending on the type of enzyme deficiency. The types of lysosomal storage disorders that cause progressive quadriparesis are listed in Section 2, Table 2-15.

Spinal Cord Cysts and Syringomyelia

✓ Depending on their location, epidermoid dermoid and arachnoid cysts may compress the spinal cord and cause progressive quadriparesis or paraparesis in dogs and cats. Diagnosis and treatment of spinal cord cysts are discussed in Section 13.

✓ Syringomyelia can cause progressive quadripanesis and is discussed in Section 9.

Leukoencephalomyelopathy

✓ Progressive ataxia and quadriparesis, associated with areas of demyelination in the spinal cord, brainstem, and cerebellum, are seen in adult Rottweilers. This condition is known as leukoencephalomyelopathy. CSF analysis, EMG, radiographs, and myelography are normal. MRI may show lesions within the spinal cord white matter. There is no treatment. Quadriparesis progresses over 6 to 12 months until the dog is recumbent. The diagnosis is usually confirmed on necropsy. An inherited cause is suspected.

Neuromuscular Disorders

Hypothyroid Neuromyopathy

✋ Hypothyroid neuromyopathy can cause progressive quadriparesis, muscle atrophy, and depressed spinal reflexes in dogs.

Systemic signs of hypothyroidism, such as obesity and alopecia, may not be evident. Other neurologic signs include head tilt, facial paralysis, laryngeal paresis, and megaesophagus (Section 6). Microcytic anemia and elevated cholesterol may be found on the CBC and chemistry profile, respectively. Fibrillation potentials and positive sharp waves in limb and paravertebral muscles, slow nerve-conduction velocities, and decreased amplitudes of evoked muscle action potentials support the presence of polyneuropathy on EMG. The diagnosis is best confirmed by demonstration of a decreased serum total thyroxine (T4) or free T4 in conjunction with an elevated serum thyroid-stimulating hormone level. Neurogenic atrophy is seen on histologic examination of muscle, and demyelination and axonal degeneration are seen on nerve biopsies. **Levothyroxine sodium (Soloxine, Daniels Pharmaceuticals) 0.02 mg/kg PO every 12 hours is administered,** and after 4 weeks the serum T4 level is rechecked, and the dosage is adjusted until results are within the high normal range. Neurologic signs usually respond to treatment within 3 months.

Chronic Idiopathic Polyneuropathy

✓ Chronic idiopathic polyneuropathy primarily affects adult dogs and rarely cats. Clinical signs of flaccid paraparesis that progress to flaccid quadriparesis may develop over several months to years and can be characterized by periodic remissions and recurrences. Cranial nerve deficits are occasionally seen (Section 6). Sensory nerve involvement can result in ataxia (Section 8), reduced or absent conscious proprioception, and a reduced response to noxious stimuli. Abnormalities on the EMG—diffuse fibrillation potentials, positive sharp waves, complex repetitive discharges, slowed motor nerve conduction velocities, and F-wave disturbances—support the diagnosis of polyneuropathy. Denervation atrophy of the muscle and inflammation, segmental demyelination, or axonal loss of nerves can be seen on histologic examination of biopsy specimens.

♥ **Some animals may benefit from prednisone 0.25–1 mg/kg PO every 12 hours.** If improvement occurs, then alternate-day prednisone 0.25–1 mg/kg PO may be useful as a long-term therapy to prevent relapses. **If there is no response to prednisone alone, another immunosuppressant drug may be added, such as cyclophosphamide or azathioprine.** The prednisone dose is reduced to 0.5 mg/kg PO every 12 hours, and cyclophosphamide (Cytoxan, Bristol Myers Squibb) 1–2 mg/kg PO is administered once daily for 4 days, discontinued for 3 days, and then given again for 4 days in a repeating cycle then discontinued when remission is achieved or after 4 months of therapy, or if hemorrhagic cystitis occurs. Although it may take longer to become effective, azathioprine (Imuran, Glaxo Wellcome) 2 mg/kg/day PO, given until improvement is seen and then reduced to every other day indefinitely, is another alternative for dogs. Hemograms and platelet numbers should be closely monitored. Hepatoxicity can occur with azathioprine, so serum chemistry profiles and bile acids should be monitored. In some cases, there is no response to any therapy and the prognosis is grave.

Protozoal Polyradiculoneuritis/Polymyositis

✓ Protozoal polyradiculoneuritis due to either *Neospora caninum* or *Toxoplasma gondii* may occur in dogs and cats, particularly young or immunosuppressed animals. Puppies usually have accompanying myositis and are presented with progressive paraparesis and pelvic limb extension (Section 13). The infection may also cause meningoencephalomyelitis (Section 2). The EMG abnormalities of diffuse fibrillation potentials, positive sharp waves, complex repetitive discharges, slowed motor nerve-conduction velocities, and F-wave disturbances support the diagnosis of polyneuropathy. CSF abnormalities include mixed-cell leukocytic pleocytosis and elevated protein, but the CSF can also be normal. Serum and CSF immunoassays for *N. caninum* or *T. gondii* may support the diagnosis if high IgM or rising IgG levels are noted. Diagnosis is confirmed by observing organisms on histologic examination of a muscle biopsy.

♥ **Toxoplasmosis and neosporosis can be treated for 2 to 4 weeks with oral trimethoprim-sulfadiazine 15 to 30 mg/kg every 12 hours or ormetoprim-sulfadimethoxine (Primor, Pfizer) 15 mg/kg every 12 hours. Clindamycin (Antirobe, Pfizer) 5–10 mg/kg every 12 hours in dogs and cats may be added. Pyrimethamine (Daraprim, Glaxo Wellcome) 0.5–1.0 mg/kg once daily for 3 days then reduced to 0.25 mg/kg once daily for 14 days in dogs and cats may also be used.** Bone marrow suppression has been reported with the use of pyrimethamine in small animals necessitating CBC monitoring. The prognosis is guarded, especially if there is severe accompanying muscle damage or contractures.

Polymyopathies

✋ Chronic progressive quadriparesis may be associated with chronic polymyositis or other polymyopathies. The spinal reflexes are often preserved, and polymyopathies may be difficult to differentiate from spinal cord diseases on the neurologic examination. Distinguishing features may be conscious proprioceptive deficits with some spinal cord lesions, and generalized muscle pain or atrophy with some polymyopathies. If the spinal reflexes are depressed, polymyopathy may be difficult to distinguish from polyneuropathy. Some endocrine disorders, such as hypothyroidism, can cause polymyopathy concurrent with polyneuropathy. Serum CK levels may be elevated or normal. Fibrillation potentials, positive sharp waves, and complex repetitive discharges (bizarre high-frequency discharges) on the EMG indicate neuromuscular disease. Histologic examination of a muscle biopsy specimen confirms polymyopathy and may give insight into the cause. The differential diagnosis, diagnosis, and treatment of polymyopathies are discussed in Section 11.

Myasthenia Gravis

✓ Dogs and cats with myasthenia gravis can present with chronic progressive quadriparesis, but episodic or exercise-induced paraparesis and quadriparesis are more common. Spinal reflexes and conscious proprioception are usually normal. Myasthenia gravis is discussed in Section 11.

Diabetic Polyneuropathy

🐾 Clinical and subclinical polyneuropathy occurs in dogs and especially in cats with diabetes mellitus. The causes and mechanisms of peripheral nerve degeneration remain controversial and are probably multifactorial. Pathologic findings include active axonal degeneration and regeneration and demyelination and remyelination. Progressive paraparesis and quadriparesis with proprioceptive deficits, muscle atrophy, and depressed spinal reflexes may be seen. Cats often assume a plantigrade posture in the pelvic limbs. Animals may have hyperesthesia. Diagnosis of diabetes mellitus is based on the finding of persistent hyperglycemia with glycosuria. EMG abnormalities consisting of diffuse fibrillation potentials, positive sharp waves, complex repetitive discharges, slowed motor nerve conduction velocities, or abnormal F-waves support the diagnosis of polyneuropathy.

♥ **Partial or full recovery can occur within 6 to 12 months through adequate control of diabetes with insulin therapy.** Some cats may remain hyperesthetic and resist being handled. **Antioxidant therapy with oral vitamin E 10 to 25 IU/kg once daily and vitamin C 15 mg/kg may protect the peripheral nerves from further damage** and slow disease progression. **N-acetylcysteine 25 mg/kg PO every 8 hours daily for 2 weeks then reduced to every other day is another effective antioxidant therapy.** Vitamin C may cause diarrhea, so a lower dose may be used initially and slowly increased. High doses of vitamin E may affect blood coagulation and should be used cautiously in animals with coagulopathies.

Insulinoma Polyneuropathy

✓ A common cause of hypoglycemia in middle-aged and older dogs is insulinoma (Section 2). German shepherds, Irish setters, and boxers seem to be predisposed to this type of tumor. Hypoglycemia or a paraneoplastic process secondary to insulinoma may be responsible for polyneuropathy, but the pathophysiologic process is not well understood. Clinical signs include paraparesis that progresses to quadriparesis with depressed or absent spinal reflexes. EMG may show fibrillation potentials and positive sharp waves in all muscles, slow nerve-conduction velocities, and decreased amplitudes of evoked muscle action potentials; these findings support the presence of polyneuropathy. Neurogenic atrophy is seen on histologic examination of muscle biopsies. Loss of axons and myelin may be found on histologic examination of nerve biopsies. Diagnosis and treatment of insulinomas are discussed in Section 2. Neuropathy often improves once the primary tumor is removed.

Paraneoplastic Polyneuropathy

✓ Neoplasms other than insulinomas can cause a variety of systemic abnormalities remote from the site of tumor invasion. Collectively, these are called paraneoplastic disorders. Dogs presenting with a chronic progressive polyneuropathy should be evaluated for a neoplastic process. As with insulinomas, if the underlying tumor is successfully treated, polyneuropathy may resolve.

Toxic Polyneuropathy

✓ Whenever polyneuropathy of unknown cause is found, toxic polyneuropathy should be considered. Many types of neuromuscular intoxication cause acute weakness, which worsens with exercise. These are discussed in Section 11. Chemicals documented to produce chronic polyneuropathies in animals are presented in Table 10-2, but ingestion of these chemicals is rare in dogs and cats. Degeneration of intramuscular nerve endings is found on histologic examination of a muscle biopsy. These neuropathies are known as distal axonopathies, or dying-back neuropathies, and are associated with abnormal axonal transport. Organophosphate and carbamate intoxication may produce neuromuscular weakness and tremors in dogs and cats without signs of salivation, diarrhea, or miosis. These intoxications are discussed in Sections 4 and 11. Dogs appear to be relatively resistant to delayed organophosphate intoxication.

✓ Polyneuropathy may occur in dogs receiving vincristine sulfate (Oncovin, Lilly). The neuropathy usually improves after the drug is discontinued. As chemotherapeutic treatment of various tumors becomes more commonplace, toxic polyneuropathies are likely to be recognized more frequently. When in doubt about whether a substance has caused intoxication, contact the ASPCA National Animal Poison Control Center (888-426-4435) or another poison control center.

Table 10-2
Chemicals That Cause Polyneuropathies

HEAVY METALS

Lead, mercury, thallium, copper, zinc, and antimony

INDUSTRIAL COMPOUNDS

Trichlorethylene, N-hexane, acrylamide, malathion, carbon disulfide, methyl bromide, lindane, carbon tetrachloride, gasoline, methyl butyl ketone, zinc pyridinethione

DRUGS

Clioquinol, diphenylhydantoin, disulfiram, isoniazid, nitrofurantoin, thalidomide, vincristine, vinblastine, ampicillin, erythromycin, and tetracycline

Congenital or Hereditary Polyneuropathies

✓ Congenital and hereditary polyneuropathies are progressive, breed-specific diseases that affect young cats and dogs. Affected animals may initially appear paraparetic, but quadriparesis with generalized muscle atrophy eventually becomes apparent. There is no treatment. Some polyneuropathies progress rapidly, and affected animals are often euthanized. Others polyneuropathies slowly progress over years or stabilize so affected animals may have a reasonable quality of life. Diagnosis is based on the breed, history, and clinical signs and findings on the EMG and histologic examination of a nerve or muscle biopsy. The breeds affected and key features of specific congenital or hereditary polyneuropathies are outlined in Table 10-3.

Table 10-3

Congenital or Hereditary Polyneuropathies That Cause Quadriparesis

Disease	Breeds Known To Be Affected	Key Features
Chronic spinal muscular atrophy (motor neuronopathies)	Swedish laplands, Brittany spaniels, English pointers, German shepherds, Rottweilers, Cairn terriers, salukis, griffon briquet vendeens	Progressive degeneration of motor neurons in spinal cord and nuclei of brainstem; progressive denervation of muscle fibers results in weakness and severe muscle atrophy by 2-4 months of age; dogs with chronic forms may live several years
Progressive axonopathy	Boxers	Primary axonal disease with secondary demyelination; initial pelvic limb ataxia at 2 to 3 months of age progressing to thoracic limbs; disease may stabilize by 1-2 years of age
Giant axonal neuropathy	German shepherds	Autosomal recessive trait; axons of central and peripheral nervous systems affected; both sensory and motor fibers affected; clinical signs begin at 14 to 16 months of age and slowly progress over years
Hypertrophic neuropathy	Tibetan mastiffs	Autosomal recessive trait; primarily demyelination of peripheral nerves; generalized weakness begins at 2 to 3 months of age and quadriplegia occurs within a few weeks
Globoid cell leukodystrophy (Krabbe's disease)	Cairn terrier, West Highland White terrier, cats	Autosomal recessive lysosomal storage disease that results in progressive degeneration of white matter of the central and peripheral nerves from 3-6 months of age (see Section 2, Table 2-15)
Distal polyneuropathy	Rottweilers	Axonal necrosis and demyelination in dogs 1-4 years of age affecting sensory and motor nerves

Hypomyelinating neuropathy	Golden retrievers	Hypomyelination of peripheral nerves, pelvic limb ataxia at 7 weeks of age progressing to crouched stance, mild pelvic limb atrophy, and weakness; may improve with age but will probably never be normal
Sensory and motor polyneuropathy	Alaskan malamutes	Paraparesis progressing to quadriparesis; coughing and regurgitation usually beginning by 1 year of age; megaesophagus may be seen; axonal degeneration present; may stabilize then deteriorate
Distal polyneuropathy (axonopathy)	Birman cats	Progressive paraparesis due to reduced numbers of myelinated axons in central and peripheral nervous systems
Hyperoxaluria	Domestic shorthaired cats	Hereditary defect causing deposition of oxalate crystals in the kidneys and renal failure at 5-9 months of age; L-glycerate found in urine; progressive quadriparesis with swollen axons distended with neurofilaments in the dorsal root ganglia, ventral nerve roots, and intramuscular nerves
Hyperchylomicronemia	Cats	Inherited lipoprotein lipase deficiency; peripheral nerves are compressed by lipid granulomas

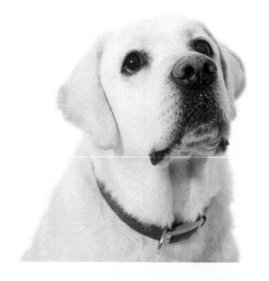

Episodic and Exercise-induced Weakness

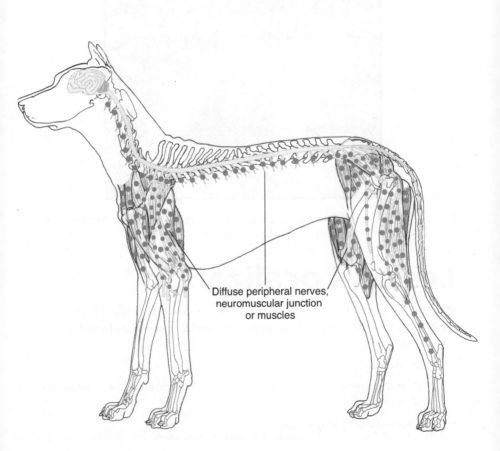

Diffuse peripheral nerves, neuromuscular junction or muscles

Definitions

Episodic or exercise-induced weakness: weakness of the pelvic limbs or all four limbs and neck that occurs periodically and/or worsens with exercise (Figure 11-1); there is no evidence that consciousness is impaired during the episode.

Neuromuscular disorder: disease of the peripheral nerves (lower motor neurons), neuromuscular junctions, or muscles.

Neuromuscular junction: The terminal part of the peripheral nerve and the acetylcholine receptor (AchR) on the skeletal muscle cell membrane.

Myotonia: Tonic spasms of muscles with delayed relaxation.

Cataplexy: sudden loss of muscle tone associated with narcolepsy (see Section 16).

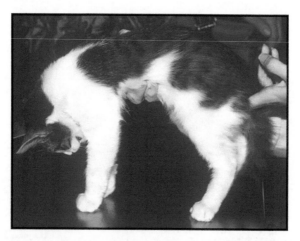

Figure 11-1 A cat with generalized weakness and ventral neck flexion from hypokalemia. (Courtesy of Dr. Michael Schaer.)

Lesion Localization

✓ The following types of lesions, the locations of which are shown in Figure 11-2, cause episodic and exercise-induced weakness:

- Systemic

- Neuromuscular (peripheral nerves, neuromuscular junctions and muscles)

- Brainstem (cataplexy)

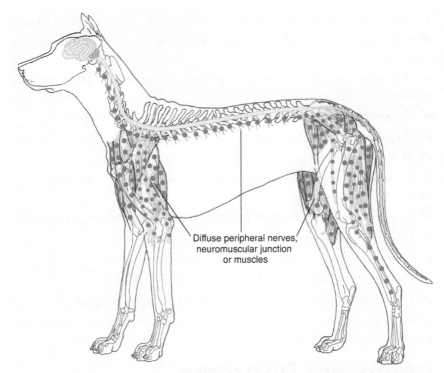

Figure 11-2 Exercise-induced weakness is often associated with a generalized neuromuscular lesion (dots indicate lesion localization; dots are on nerve roots diffusely not on the spinal cord itself).

Differential Diagnosis

Systemic Disorders

✓ Cardiopulmonary disease—common in dogs and cats

✓ Anemia—common in dogs and cats

✓ Renal failure—common in dogs and cats

✓ Hypoadrenocorticism—common in dogs

✓ Hypoglycemia—common in dogs, occasional in cats

Neuromuscular Disorders

✓ Iatrogenic corticosteroid polymyopathy—common in dogs, occasional in cats

✓ Polymyositis—occasional in dogs and cats

✓ Myasthenia gravis—occasional in dogs and cats

✓ Hypokalemic polymyopathy—occasional in cats, rare in dogs

✓ Subacute organophosphate intoxication—occasional in dogs and cats

✓ Hyperadrenocorticism polymyopathy—occasional in dogs and rare in cats

✓ Hypoadrenocorticism polymyopathy—occasional in dogs

✓ Hypothyroid neuromyopathy—occasional in dogs

✓ Hyperthyroid neuromyopathy—occasional in cats

✓ Episodic intermittent collapse of Labrador retrievers—rare breed-specific

✓ Congenital and inherited polymyopathy—rare in dogs and cats

✓ Lipid storage myopathy—rare in dogs and cats

✓ Mitochondrial myopathy—rare in dogs and cats

✓ Nutritional polymyopathy—rare in dogs and cats

✓ Paraneoplastic polymyopathy—rare in dogs and cats

✓ Polyneuropathies—usually cause acute or chronic quadriparesis (see Sections 9 and 10)

Brainstem Disorders

✓ Cataplexy—rare in dogs and cats

Differential Diagnosis of Ventral Neck Flexion in Cats

✓ Hypokalemic polymyopathy—occasional

✓ Subacute organophosphate intoxication—occasional

✓ Myasthenia gravis—occasional

✓ Hyperthyroid neuromyopathy—occasional

✓ Polymyositis—occasional

✓ Thiamine deficiency—rare

Diagnostic Evaluation

Important Historical Questions

- Does the problem worsen with exercise, or do episodes of collapse occur spontaneously?
- Is the problem associated with the environmental temperature?
- Frequency of occurrence?
- Onset, progression, and duration of signs?
- Regurgitation or vomiting?
- Coughing, increased respiration, or dyspnea?
- Polyuria or polydipsia?
- Anorexia or polyphagia?
- Depression or other signs of illness?
- Diet?
- Exposure to toxins?
- Problems in littermates or other relatives?
- Muscle or other pain?
- Past or present neoplasia?
- Recent or current use of corticosteroids, over-the counter drugs, herbal preparations, nutriceuticals, or other medications?

Physical Examination

✓ Examine the mucous membranes for pallor or cyanosis.

✓ Evaluate the strength of the pulse.

✓ Auscultate the heart to detect cardiac murmurs or arrhythmias and evidence of abnormal lung sounds.

✓ Examine the skin for hair loss or dermatitis, which might be associated with dermatomyositis, hypothyroidism, or hyperadrenocorticism.

✓ Monitor for fever, which may be present with systemic disease or during an episode in exercise-intolerant Labrador retrievers.

✓ Examine for other evidence of systemic disease or neoplasia.

✓ Determine if muscle atrophy, pain, or cramping is present.

Neurologic Examination

The neurologic examination can be normal between episodes or may have one or more of the following signs:

✓ Paraparesis or quadriparesis, which worsens with exercise.

✓ Ventroflexion of the neck or inability to lift the head due to neck weakness; this is common in cats with neuromuscular disorders.

✓ Muscle cramping or pain.

✓ Sustained muscle contraction; this is seen as a dimple when the muscle is tapped with the percussion hammer in myotonic myopathies.

✓ Moderate to severe muscle atrophy in all limbs.

✓ Reduced muscle tone in all four limbs.

✓ Normal-to-decreased spinal reflexes in the thoracic and pelvic limbs.

✓ If there is a concurrent neuropathy, conscious proprioceptive deficits may be present in the pelvic limbs or all four limbs.

Applicable Diagnostic Tests

✓ A complete blood count (CBC), serum chemistry profile, and urinalysis can be useful to detect anemia, hypokalemia, hypoglycemia, renal or bladder disease, and other systemic disorders and as part of the preanesthetic evaluation.

✓ Serum creatine kinase (CK) levels may be elevated in some cases of polymyopathy.

✓ Serum antinuclear antibody (ANA) may be positive in some animals with immune-mediated polymyositis.

✓ Serum acetylcholine receptor (AchR) antibody levels are usually elevated in cases of myasthenia gravis.

✓ Serum cholinesterase levels are usually reduced in animals with organophosphate intoxication.

✓ Thoracic and abdominal radiographs and abdominal ultrasonography are indicated if neoplasia is suspected or if abnormalities are found on the physical examination. Megaesophagus and aspiration pneumonia may be seen.

✓ Electrocardiography (ECG) and echocardiography may be abnormal in cardiac diseases.

✓ A tensilon test (IV edrophonium chloride) usually results in a temporary return to normal exercise tolerance in cases of myasthenia gravis with exercise intolerance; cases with mild weakness from other causes can also appear stronger.

✓ An adrenocorticotropic (ACTH)-stimulation test often shows reduced serum cortisol in cases of hypoadrenocorticism and increased serum cortisol in cases of hyperadrenocorticism; a dexamethasone-suppression test often shows increased cortisol levels in cases of hyperadrenocorticism; a urine cortisol-creatinine ratio is often elevated in hyperadrenocorticism; serum endogenous ACTH levels can be normal or elevated with pituitary-dependent hyperadrenocorticism and low or undetectable with adrenal tumors.

✓ Serum total thyroxine (T4) or free T4 may be low, and serum thyroid-stimulating hormone (TSH) may be elevated in cases of hypothyroidism. Serum T4 and free T4 will be elevated in cases of hyperthyroidism.

✓ Some polymyopathies may have elevated pre- and post-exercise serum lactate and pyruvate levels.

✓ Urine organic acids and amino acids may be helpful in characterizing metabolic myopathies.

✓ The following is a list of tests for which anesthesia is required and their potential findings:

- Electromyography (EMG), including needle EMG, motor nerve-conduction velocity, repetitive nerve stimulation, and F-wave evaluation is performed to determine if diffuse neuromuscular disease is present and if the lesion affects the peripheral nerves, neuromuscular junction, or muscle.

- A muscle biopsy is performed to diagnose and classify muscle disease.

- A nerve biopsy is obtained if neuropathy is suspected.

Systemic Disorders

♥ Cardiopulmonary disorders may result in exercise-induced weakness and collapse. Careful examination, including auscultation, ECG, echocardiography, and thoracic radiographs may be indicated to evaluate the heart and lungs. A Holter or cardiac event monitor may be useful to record the ECG during an episode of collapse to ensure that cardiac arrhythmia is not the inciting cause. Animals with collapse from laryngeal paralysis usually have stridor (Section 6). A routine CBC and serum chemistry profile will detect anemia, renal failure, electrolyte abnormalities, and hypoglycemia, which may be causing episodic or exercise-induced weakness. Abdominal radiography and ultrasonography may be helpful to further characterize these diseases. An ACTH stimulation test, dexamethasone-suppression test, urine cortisol-creatinine ratio, and serum endogenous ACTH should be considered in suspected cases of hypoadrenocorticism and hyperadrenocorticism.

Neuromuscular Disorders

Iatrogenic Corticosteroid Myopathy

♥ Dogs treated with long-term corticosteroid therapy for a variety of chronic diseases commonly develop a myopathy characterized by potentially profound weakness and muscle atrophy. Classic signs of hyperadrenocorticism, such as thinning of the hair coat and skin and a pendulous abdomen, often accompany the myopathy. Dogs that have had fewer than 4 weeks of corticosteroid administration rarely develop a clinically significant disorder. Myopathy is more common after administration of the fluorinated corticosteroids, such as triamcinolone, betamethasone, and dexamethasone.

✓ The EMG may be normal, but the diagnosis is usually made on histologic examination of a muscle biopsy. The treatment of choice is to reduce or discontinue the corticosteroids. Improvement usually follows but can take many weeks to months. Because of the catabolic effect of corticosteroids, optimizing nutritional status is important. Protein supplementation is recommended. Inactivity worsens myopathy, and exercise may prevent the development of weakness. Physical therapy, such as swimming, whirlpool therapy, and massage, may be useful to prevent and treat muscle weakness and wasting in patients receiving corticosteroids.

Polymyositis

♥ Polymyositis, a generalized inflammatory process of the muscles, may be inherited or acquired. The acquired form is associated with immune-mediated, infectious, paraneoplastic, or idiopathic processes in dogs and cats. An autosomal dominant inherited dermatomyositis in collies and Shetland sheepdogs begins with facial dermatitis and masticatory muscle atrophy at approximately 8 to 10 weeks of age. This disorder can progress to signs of generalized polymyositis. Immune-mediated polymyositis may be associated with systemic lupus erythematosus, polyarthritis, lymphocytic thyroiditis, and other known immune-mediated disorders. Infections with *Toxoplasma gondii* and *Neospora caninum* can occasionally cause polymyositis in dogs and cats. An underlying neoplastic process elsewhere in the body can also cause polymyositis. Idiopathic polymyositis could be immune-mediated. Any age, breed, or sex of dog or cat may develop polymyositis.

✓ Clinical findings include acute or chronic exercise intolerance and muscle weakness, which can be continuous or episodic. Anorexia, dysphagia, weight loss, and pyrexia may also occur. Some dogs present with recurrent bouts of aspiration pneumonia secondary to dysphagia and megaesophagus (Figure 11-3). A stiff, stilted gait and muscle pain and atrophy are often present.

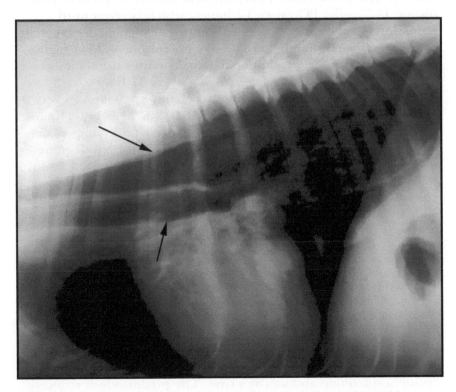

Figure 11-3 Megaesophagus (arrows) is a common finding in dogs with weakness that worsens on exercise due to polymyositis or myasthenia gravis.

✋ The CBC may be normal or show leukocytosis. Serum CK is often elevated. Areas of positive sharp waves, fibrillation potentials, and complex repetitive discharges can be seen on EMG examination, but the EMG may also be normal. Serum immunoassays for *N. caninum* or *T. gondii* may support an infectious cause. An ANA test may be positive, which supports an immune-mediated process, but the test is often normal in cases suspected to have immune-mediated polymyositis. Histologic evidence of muscle inflammation is found on examination of a muscle biopsy. Organisms associated with toxoplasmosis or neosporosis are occasionally found within muscle biopsy samples. A thorough evaluation for concurrent neoplasia should be performed, including thoracic and abdominal radiographs and abdominal ultrasonography.

♥ Any underlying disease process, such as neoplasia or infection, must be treated. The treatment of toxoplasmosis and neosporosis is outlined in Section 2, Table 2-11. **Animals with suspected cases of immune-mediated polymyositis usually respond to prednisone 1–2 mg/kg PO every 12 hours, which is given until remission is achieved. The dosage can then be gradually tapered over several weeks, and alternate-day prednisone 0.25–1 mg/kg PO can be given for an additional 1 to 2 months.** Oral famotidine (Pepcid AC, Merck) 0.5–1 mg/kg every 12 hours, cimetidine (Tagamet, SmithKline Beecham) 5–10 mg/kg every 8 hours, or misoprostol (Cytotec, Searle) 1–3 µg/kg every 8 hours may be given to reduce the chance of gastrointestinal upset or ulcers when the dose of corticosteroid therapy is high. If signs recur when prednisone is discontinued, therapy is started again to obtain remission, and then alternate-day prednisone therapy is given indefinitely. Serum CK should be monitored during and after therapy on a monthly basis. If the levels are elevated, prednisone is re-instated or the dose is increased.

> **Warning:** Prednisone therapy often causes polyuria/polydipsia, polyphagia, and panting. Give extra water but feed the normal amount. Long-term corticosteriod therapy can cause gastrointestinal ulcers, hepatopathy, and myopathy.

✔ If the animal does not respond to prednisone alone, another immunosuppressant drug may be added. Options include oral cyclophosphamide and azathioprine. The prednisone is reduced to 0.5 mg/kg every 12 hours, and oral cyclophosphamide

(Cytoxan, Bristol Myers Squibb) 1 to 2 mg/kg PO is administered once daily for 4 days, discontinued for 3 days, then given for 4 days in a repeating cycle and discontinued when remission is achieved, after 4 months of therapy, or if hemorrhagic cystitis occurs. Although it may take longer to become effective, another alternative for dogs is azathioprine (Imuran, Glaxo Wellcome) 2 mg/kg/day PO given until improvement is seen and then reduced to every other day indefinitely. Hemograms and platelet numbers should be closely monitored. Because hepatoxicity can occur with azathioprine, serum chemistry profiles and bile acids should also be monitored. Most animals respond well to therapy, but chronic immunosuppression may be necessary as recurrence is common. Megaesophagus with aspiration pneumonia can complicate the treatment. If an underlying neoplastic process is detected and corrected, polymyositis should resolve. Routine vaccination can cause a relapse of immune-mediated polymyositis.

Myasthenia Gravis

♥ Myasthenia gravis commonly presents as episodic or exercise-induced weakness due to impaired transmission of acetylcholine (ACh) at the neuromuscular junctions of skeletal muscles. Other clinical presentations of myasthenia gravis include dysphagia, laryngeal paresis, regurgitation (Section 6), paraparesis, and quadriparesis. Myasthenia gravis may be congenital or acquired and associated with an immune-mediated or paraneoplastic process. Congenital myasthenia gravis occurs in Jack Russell terriers, smooth fox terriers, Samoyeds, and various breeds of cats. Acquired myasthenia gravis may occur in some cats 2 to 4 months following initiation of methimazole (Tapazole, Jones Medical Industries) therapy for hyperthyroidism. Weakness resolves after the drug is discontinued.

✓ In immune-mediated myasthenia gravis, antibodies are formed against the ACh receptor of skeletal muscles, and these antibodies interfere with normal muscle contraction. Affected animals progressively develop a shortened stride with exercise, which eventually becomes total fatigue and inability to walk. Strength returns with brief rest, and they are again able to ambulate for short distances. The palpebral reflex becomes fatigued with repeated testing, and sometimes facial nerve paresis is present. Despite profound weakness, conscious proprioception and spinal reflexes are usually normal. Megaesophagus and dysphagia are common in dogs and can result in excessive salivation, regurgitation, aspiration pneumonia, and death.

✓ Intravenous administration of the short-acting anti-cholinesterase edrophonium chloride (Tensilon, ICN) 1 to 5 mg in dogs and 0.2 to 1 mg in cats may dramatically improve strength during an episode of collapse. If higher doses are given, a cholinergic crisis of bradycardia, profuse salivation, dyspnea, cyanosis, and limb tremors may result, and this can be reversed with atropine 0.05 mg/kg IV. Improvement with edrophonium chloride does not necessarily rule myasthenia gravis in or out, as other causes of weakness, like polymyositis, commonly improve with edrophonium chloride. A definitive diagnosis can be made with serologic testing documenting elevated AchR antibodies. As some cases may be falsely seronegative, re-testing is important in all weak animals suspected to have myasthenia gravis. The severity of clinical signs may not correspond with the degree of elevation of ACh receptor antibody titers.

✓ Megaesophagus and aspiration pneumonia may be seen on thoracic radiographs (Figure 11-3). In paraneoplastic myasthenia gravis, thymoma may be seen as a cranial mediastinal mass on thoracic radiographs. A thorough physical and radiographic workup, including abdominal ultrasonography should be performed to search for neoplasia. Some dogs with myasthenia gravis have concurrent hypothyroidism, and weakness does not improve until both disorders are treated. In hypothyroidism, serum total T4 or free T4 levels are usually reduced and TSH levels are usually elevated. Myasthenia gravis and polymyositis may also occur together, and serum CK levels may be elevated. EMG is often normal except for a decremental evoked muscle response on repetitive nerve stimulation of 5/second.

♥ **Initial therapy usually consists of pyridostigmine bromide (Mestinon, ICN) 0.5–3 mg/kg PO every 8 to 12 hours with food.** A liquid formulation of pyridostigmine bromide is recommended so that the dose can be easily adjusted to the level needed to control clinical signs. With high doses, weakness may occur as a result of a cholinergic crisis; thus, a low dose of pyridostigmine is initially given then slowly increased until weakness resolves. Famotidine (Pepcid AC, Merck) 0.5–1 mg/kg every 12 hours PO may reduce the nausea and gastrointestinal irritation from the pyridostigmine bromide.

♥ **Concurrent hypothyroidism is treated with levothyroxine sodium (Soloxine, Daniels) 0.02 mg/kg PO every 12 hours.** After 4 weeks of therapy, a serum total T4 is obtained and the dosage adjusted until the total serum T4 is maintained within the normal range. **Surgical removal of the thymoma or other**

neoplasm is necessary to achieve remission in cases of paraneo-plastic myasthenia gravis. Concurrent immune-mediated polymyositis must also be treated as described above to resolve the weakness.

♥ If response to the pyridostigmine bromide is limited and aspiration pneumonia is not present, prednisone 0.25–1 mg/kg PO every 12 hours may be given. In a few cases, weakness may worsen temporarily when prednisone therapy is intiated. Prolonged prednisone therapy is avoided because iatrogenic corticosteroid-induced myopathy may cause further weakness. If clinical signs improve, alternate-day prednisone therapy at the lowest effective dose is administered. If there is no response to prednisone alone, azathioprine (Imuran, Glaxo Smith Kline) 2 mg/kg PO once daily may be given until improvement is seen as described above for polymyositis. Aspiration pneumonia must be treated aggressively with antibiotics as it can be life-threatening. Aminoglycoside antibiotics, ampicillin, and other drugs that might further reduce neuromuscular transmission are avoided.

✓ Most dogs have megaesophagus and to avoid regurgitation should be fed small amounts of moist food made into small balls two or three times daily from an elevated surface. The dog is then held vertically (i.e., with the front feet on a chair and the back feet on the floor) for 10 to 15 minutes after eating to assist the movement of food into the stomach. Small amounts of water are offered often, and the dog must drink with the head elevated. When regurgitation is severe, gastrostomy tube feeding may be necessary to maintain nutrition, ensure the administration of pyridostigmine therapy, and avoid aspiration pneumonia.

✓ Serial monitoring of AchR antibody levels on a bimonthly then monthly basis can help track the disease progress. The prognosis varies. Most animals respond well to therapy, others have no response, and still others have recurrent bouts of aspiration pneumonia that necessitate intensive therapy. Animals that have little response to routine therapy should have serial evaluations for an underlying neoplastic process. Spontaneous remission can occur within 3 to 12 months in animals with immune-mediated myasthenia gravis. As clinical signs improve, pyridostigmine bromide doses are reduced and therapy is discontinued when remission occurs. Although megaesophagus can be permanent, regurgitation improves with remission. Recurrences can be seen. Routine vaccination may cause a relapse of immune-mediated myasthenia gravis.

Hypokalemic Polymyopathy

♥ Hypokalemia in cats may cause acute onset of generalized weakness, persistent ventral flexion of the neck, and occasionally muscle pain (Figure 11-1). Conscious proprioception and spinal reflexes are normal. These signs are rare in dogs. The serum potassium level is often 1.5–3.5 mEq/L (normal, 4–5 mEq/L). Serum CK is often 500 to 10,000 U/L (normal, 250 U/L). Chronic renal failure with a loss of potassium in the urine is a common cause of hypokalemia in cats, and serum blood urea nitrogen (BUN) and creatinine levels are elevated. Animals consuming diets containing less than 0.6% potassium or acidifying high-protein diets may develop hypokalemic polymyopathy. Other conditions that may result in hypokalemia include hyperthyroidism, diuretic therapy, anorexia, chronic vomiting or diarrhea, and hepatic disease. A suspected inherited hypokalemia may occur in Burmese cats from 2 to 6 months of age.

✓ EMG may be normal or have areas of positive waves and fibrillation potentials. Histologic examination of muscle biopsies may be normal or show muscle fiber necrosis with little or no evidence of inflammation.

♥ **Potassium gluconate (Tumil K, Daniels) 2–4 mEq PO every 12 hours may be used in all animals.** The dosage is adjusted until serum potassium levels are normal. In cats with renal dysfunction, oral supplementation must be continued, but in others a diet with greater than 0.6% potassium is enough. Severely hypokalemic cats may die of respiratory paralysis and can be cautiously treated with potassium chloride 0.2–0.4 mEq/kg/hour IV diluted in intravenous fluids with constant cardiac monitoring and evaluation of serum potassium every 4 hours until the potassium level reaches 3.5 mEq/L. Ventilatory support may be necessary.

✓ Serum CK and potassium levels may be monitored, and both should return to normal as the cat clinically improves. Serum BUN and creatinine levels often return to normal as potassium levels return to normal in cats with renal disease. Regular monitoring of serum potassium levels is important for long-term management. The prognosis for resolution of weakness is good.

Subacute Organophosphate Intoxication

♥ A common cause of persistent ventral flexion of the neck and exercise-induced weakness in cats and generalized weakness in both dogs and cats is subacute organophosphate intoxication.

Chlorpyrofos is a typical organophosphate that causes subacute organophosphate intoxication 7 to 10 days after exposure. The acute signs of miosis, salivation, and tremors are often absent in these cases. Nonpainful neuromuscular weakness with ventral flexion of the neck may be the only presenting sign in cats. Conscious proprioception and spinal reflexes are normal. A history of toxic exposure and a low serum cholinesterase level support the diagnosis. Cats with serum cholinesterase levels below 500 IU (normal, 900 to 1200 IU) have neurologic signs. **Administration of diphenhydramine (Benadryl, Parke-Davis) 4 mg/kg PO every 8 hours may significantly improve the weakness.** Most cats return to normal in 3 to 6 weeks. Cholinesterase levels may be monitored and will increase slowly as the clinical signs improve.

Other Intoxications

✓ Some drugs and chemicals are toxic to the neuromuscular system and cause acute weakness. The possibility of exposure to prescription and over-the-counter medications and toxic chemicals and plants should be discussed with the owner. When in doubt about whether a substance can cause intoxication, the ASPCA National Animal Poison Control Center (888-426-4435), or any other poison control center can be consulted.

Hyperadrenocorticism (Cushing's Myopathy)

♥ The prevalence of subclinical myopathy in hyperadrenocorticism (Cushing's disease) in dogs may be high. A distinct myopathy has not been reported in cats with hyperadrenocorticism, but muscle wasting can be a prominent finding. Clinical manifestations are similar to those of exogenous corticosteroid myopathy with muscle atrophy and weakness. Unilateral or bilateral pelvic limb stiffness from muscle fibrosis may occur initially, and the thoracic limbs may become involved over time. Severe pelvic limb rigidity with myotonia can occur in some dogs with chronic myopathy. Serum CK may be elevated in some dogs. Trains of positive waves and complex repetitive discharges may be observed on EMG. Histologic examination of a muscle biopsy shows muscle fiber necrosis and fibrosis. **If clinical signs are mild, some dogs improve over a period of several months if the disease is effectively treated.** Improvement in motor function appears to be inversely related to the duration of disease prior to therapy, and some deficits often persist.

Hypoadrenocorticism

✓ Muscle weakness and exercise intolerance occur frequently in association with hypoadrenocorticism (Addison's disease) in dogs. Adrenal insufficiency impairs muscle carbohydrate metabolism, water and electrolyte balance, muscle blood flow, and adrenergic sensitivity, all of which are factors that contribute to the myopathy associated with Addison's disease. Weakness is usually generalized and may involve the pharyngeal or esophageal musculature as well. Serum CK, EMG, and muscle biopsy may be normal. Correction of the electrolyte imbalance and glucocorticoid deficiency usually eliminates the clinical weakness.

Hypothyroid Neuromyopathy

✓ Hypothyroidism can cause muscle weakness due to neuromyopathy in dogs. The classic clinical signs of hypothyroidism, including lethargy, weight gain, seborrhea, and hair loss are not always obvious. Clinical signs suggestive of neuromuscular dysfunction in hypothyroid dogs include weakness, stiffness, muscle pain, reluctance to move, and muscle wasting. If both peripheral nerves and muscles are affected, then conscious proprioceptive deficits, depressed spinal reflexes, and cranial nerve deficits may be found. Microcytic anemia and elevated cholesterol may be found on the CBC and chemistry profile, respectively. Serum CK levels can be elevated but may also be normal. The diagnosis is confirmed when serum total T4 and free T4 levels are reduced and serum TSH levels are elevated. Muscle biopsy sections show atrophy of the type II muscle fibers. **Levothyroxine sodium (Soloxine, Daniels Pharmaceuticals) 0.02 mg/kg PO every 12 hours is given. After 4 weeks of therapy, serum T4 levels are rechecked and the dosage is adjusted until T4 levels are maintained within the normal range.** Weakness usually responds to treatment within 3 months.

Hyperthyroid Neuromyopathy

✓ A few cats with hyperthyroidism may be weak and an even fewer will have ventral flexion of the neck. Owners will report a decreased ability to jump and fatigue associated with physical exertion such that cats may lie down or rest when moving from one place to another. Serum total T4 levels are usually elevated. **Treatment of hyperthyroidism in cats may involve administration of radioactive iodine, oral methimazole (Tapazole, Lilly), or thyroidectomy.** There are risks and benefits associated with each type of therapy, which are beyond the scope of this book. The weakness resolves once a euthyroid state is achieved. Acquired myasthenia gravis may occur in some cats 2 to 4 months after initiation of methimazole therapy. The weakness resolves and AchR antibodies return to the normal range after therapy is discontinued.

Exercise-induced Collapse of Labrador Retrievers

✓ Young Labrador retrievers between 7 months and 2 years of age may present with weakness and collapse during exercise. Weakness begins in the pelvic limbs but can progress to total collapse followed by a period of confusion. The body temperature is often severely elevated (up to 41.6° C [107° F]), and severe alkalosis is present on blood gas analysis immediately following exercise. Most mildly affected dogs return to normal within 20 minutes. All remaining clinicopathologic and electrodiagnostic tests and histologic examination of muscle biopsies are normal. An inherited metabolic myopathy associated with insulin and glucose uptake in the muscle is suspected. There is no specific therapy available; however, empiric treatment for metabolic myopathies can be tried. Such therapy **consists of carnitine 50 mg/kg PO every 12 hours, co-enzyme Q 100 mg PO once daily, and riboflavin 100 once daily PO.** Any store carrying nutritional supplements will have these products.

♥ Lifestyle changes are essential to avoid hyperthermic brain damage or death. Exercise during high ambient temperatures, excitement, and continuous intense exercise are avoided. Hunting dogs may be less affected during cold weather. The clinical signs do not progress with age and can usually be managed with lifestyle changes.

Congenital and Inherited Myopathies

There are many breed-specific generalized muscle disorders in dogs and cats. In many of these disorders, finding characteristic muscle changes on histologic examination of muscle biopsies provides the definitive diagnosis. There are no specific treatments. The clinical course of these disorders varies—some animals become stable and can maintain a good quality of life, while others deteriorate with severe muscle atrophy and fibrosis and death. Table 11-1 outlines the diseases, affected breeds, and a few key features of each disorder.

Table 11-1
Congenital and Inherited Myopathies

Disease	Breeds Known To Be Affected	Key Features
Muscular dystrophy	Golden retrievers, Irish terriers, Samoyeds, miniature schnauzers, Belgian shepherds, Rottweilers, German shorthaired pointers, Pembroke Welsh corgis, Japanese spitz	Often X-linked inherited disease but has been described in females as well as males; progressive weakness, stiff gait, and muscle atrophy from 2-3 months of age
Feline muscular dystrophy	Domestic shorthaired cats, Devon Rex, European shorthaired	Hypertrophic form of the X-linked disease; progressive muscle hypertrophy and stiffness from 3 months of age
Glycogenosis type II (Pompe's disease)	Lapland dogs	Glycogen storage disease due to α-1,4-glucosidase (acid maltase) deficiency; gradual progressive generalized weakness occurring after 6 months of age; regurgitation from megaesophagus; accumulation of glycogen in skeletal muscles
Glycogenosis type III (Cori's disease)	German shepherds, Akitas	Defect of the glycogen debranching enzyme amylo-1,6-glucosidase (glycogenosis type III), similar to Cori's disease in humans; muscle weakness is evident by 2 months of age; accumulation of glycogen in skeletal muscles
Glycogenosis type IV	Norwegian Forest cats	Deficiency of the glycogen-branching enzyme; clinical signs include generalized muscle tremors and weakness progressing to quadriplegia apparent at about 5 months of age; accumulation of glycogen in skeletal muscles

Glycogenosis type VII	English springer spaniels, American cocker spaniels	Autosomal recessive form of phosphofructokinase deficiency; usually have compensated hemolytic anemia, intravascular hemolysis, and hemoglobinuria without overt muscle weakness but myopathy can be present
Distal myopathy	Rottweilers	Familial; progressive distal limb weakness from 6-8 weeks of age
Labrador retriever myopathy	Labrador retrievers	Autosomal recessive disease. Weakness and marked deficiency of skeletal muscle mass with progressive exercise intolerance from 3 months of age; stabilizes at 6-12 months of age
Myotonic myopathy	Chow chows, Staffordshire terriers, Great Danes, Rhodesian ridgebacks, West Highland White terriers, miniature schnauzers; domestic shorthaired cats	Persistent active muscle contraction after voluntary movement from 6-8 weeks of age; dimpling of the muscle seen on percussion; may be acceptable pets
Nemaline rod myopathy	Domestic shorthaired cats; border collies, silky terriers	Weakness progressing to tremors at 6 months of age in cats and from 3 months of age in dogs
Central core myopathy	Great Danes	Inherited; progressive muscle wasting and exercise intolerance with collapse exacerbated by excitement from 6 months of age
Hypertonic myopathy	Cavalier King Charles spaniels	Episodic exercise- and excitement-induced muscle cramping that causes collapse from 3 months of age; can usually be acceptable pets
Devon Rex myopathy	Devon Rex cats	Autosomal recessive; generalized limb weakness, ventral flexion of the neck, megaesophagus from 1-6 months of age

Lipid Storage Myopathy

✓ A biochemical defect within the muscle can lead to excessive storage of lipid. The clinical presentation varies and includes muscle atrophy, weakness, and in some cases dramatic muscle pain. Serum CK and EMG may be normal. Excessive lipid deposition is observed on histologic examination of a muscle biopsy specimen using special staining techniques. Further investigations, including evaluation of urinary organic acids; plasma amino acid concentrations; and quantification of total, free, and esterified carnitine in plasma, urine, and muscle can be performed to try to determine specific metabolic abnormalities.

♥ **Treatment with carnitine 50 mg/kg PO every 12 hours, coenzyme Q 100 mg PO once daily, and riboflavin 100 mg/day PO can result in an improvement of clinical signs in 4 to 6 weeks.** Any store that sells nutritional supplements will carry these products.

Mitochondrial Myopathies

✓ Inherited enzymatic defects within the mitochondrial electron-transport chain can lead to polymyopathy. Clumber and Sussex spaniels, Old English sheepdogs, boxers, and Jack Russell terriers have been affected. Clinical signs associated with mitochondrial myopathies include exercise-induced weakness, cramping with minimal exercise, chronic progressive quadriparesis, and muscle atrophy. Resting and post-exercise plasma lactate and pyruvate concentrations are elevated. Massive proliferation of abnormal mitochondria is seen on histologic examination of a muscle biopsy specimen with special staining techniques. The aggregates of abnormal mitochondria stain red with the Gomori-modified trichrome stain in frozen biopsy sections, creating the pathologic representation of ragged-red muscle fibers.

♥ **Treatment as described above for lipid storage myopathies may be tried, but mitochondrial myopathies may rapidly progress and are often fatal.**

Nutritional Polymyopathies

✓ Diets low in vitamin E and selenium can cause a nutritional polymyopathy referred to as white muscle disease. This condition is rarely seen now that diets with adequate vitamin E and selenium are routinely fed. Serum CK is elevated, and necrosis is found on histologic examination of a muscle biopsy specimen. If muscle damage is not severe, correcting the diet improves the myopathy and weakness.

Paraneoplastic Polymyopathy

✓ In confirmed cases of polymyositis of unknown origin, the possibility of an underlying neoplastic disorder should be considered. A thorough examination for neoplasia should be done whenever neuromyopathy of unknown origin is diagnosed. The myopathy often improves with treatment of the neoplastic process

Thiamine Deficiency

✓ Because of routine feeding of well-balanced pet foods, thiamine (vitamin B1) deficiency rarely occurs. Thiamine deficiency may initially manifest as ventral neck flexion in cats, but it rapidly progresses to cause dementia, stupor, or seizures. This disorder is discussed in Section 2.

Brainstem Disorders

Cataplexy

Cataplexy is sudden loss of muscle tone with excitement or exercise and is associated with narcolepsy. The weakness may only involve the pelvic limbs, and the animal may not fall asleep. A discussion of the diagnosis and treatment of narcolepsy and cataplexy is found in Section 16.

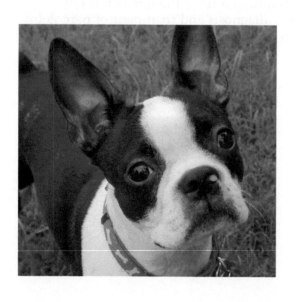

Section 12

Acute Paraparesis or Paraplegia

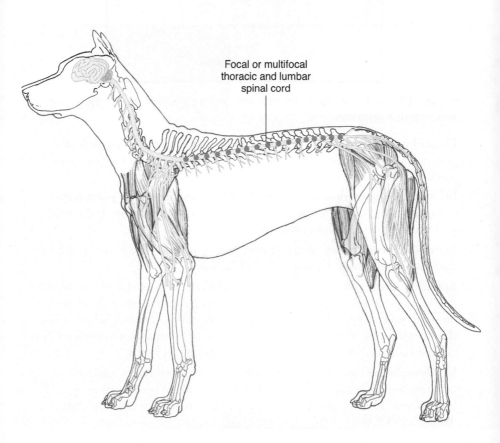

Focal or multifocal
thoracic and lumbar
spinal cord

Definitions

Acute paraparesis or paraplegia: neurologic signs occur immediately or within 72 hours.

Paraparesis: weakness and reduced voluntary movement of the pelvic limbs.

Paraplegia: loss of voluntary movement of the pelvic limbs (Figure 12-1).

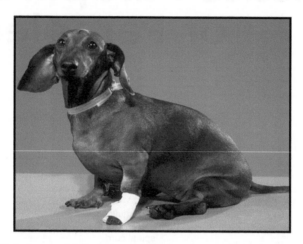

Figure 12-1 A 4-year-old dachshund with acute paraplegia from a Type I intervertebral disk extrusion.

Flaccid or lower motor neuron (LMN) paraparesis or paraplegia: paraparesis or paraplegia with reduced or absent spinal reflexes and muscle tone in the pelvic limbs.

Spastic or upper motor neuron (UMN) paraparesis or paraplegia: paraparesis or paraplegia with normal or exaggerated spinal reflexes and muscle tone in the pelvic limbs.

Schiff-Sherrington syndrome: extensor rigidity of the thoracic limbs and paraplegia from an acute T3-L3 lesion.

Spinal walking: alternating flexion and extension of the pelvic limbs due to hyperactive reflexes beginning 1 to 2 months after development of severe T3-L3 lesions; using functional paravertebral muscles, the animal may stand and appear to be taking steps; is involuntary but can be confused with recovery of voluntary movement.

Myelomalacia: necrosis and hemorrhage of the spinal cord; can progressively ascend and descend from the site of an injury over a 72-hour period after acute spinal cord trauma and intervertebral disk disease (IVDD).

Fenestration: a surgical procedure to remove the nucleus pulposus of the intervertebral disk to prevent future extrusions.

Neuromuscular disorder: disease of the peripheral nerves (LMN), neuromuscular junctions, and muscles.

Decubital ulcer: a deep wound with sloughing skin and muscle; occurs over bony prominences due to constant pressure from lying in one position too long; the bone is often exposed.

Lesion Localization

✓ The location of lesions that cause acute paraparesis or paraplegia are shown in Figure 12-2. These lesions are usually found in the:

- Neuromuscular system—bilateral lumbosacral nerves and muscles of the pelvic limbs
- T3-L3 spinal cord segments
- L4-S2 spinal cord segments or nerve roots

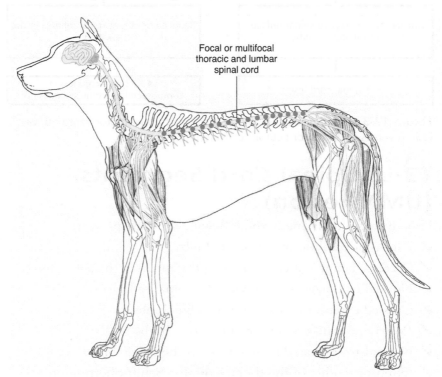

Focal or multifocal
thoracic and lumbar
spinal cord

Figure 12-2 Acute paraparesis or paraplegia is associated with a lesion in the spinal cord or nerves below T3 (dots indicate lesion localization).

Differentiation of Upper Motor Neuron and Lower Motor Neuron Lesions

Figure 12-3 is an algorithm showing differentiation of lesions of the upper versus the lower motor neurons.

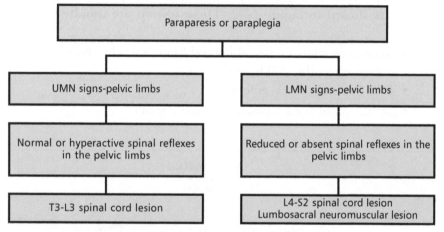

Figure 12-3 Algorithm showing differentiation of upper motor neuron (UMN) lesions versus lower motor neuron (LMN) lesions.

T3-L3 Spinal Cord Segments (UMN Lesion)

Usually, more than one of the following signs are present:

✓ Paresis or paralysis of the pelvic limbs

✓ Decreased or absent conscious proprioception in the pelvic limbs

✓ Normal or exaggerated pelvic limb spinal reflexes

✓ Crossed extensor reflexes in the pelvic limbs

✓ Positive Babinski's sign in the pelvic limbs

✓ Normal-to-increased muscle tone in the pelvic limbs

✓ Extensor rigidity of the thoracic limbs (Schiff-Sherrington syndrome)

✓ Normal or spastic anal reflex

✓ Bladder difficult to express initially then within 10 days reflex urination may begin with frequent spastic expulsion of small amounts of urine

✓ Reduced or absent cutaneous trunci response at the site of the lesion and caudally

✓ Reduced or absent superficial pain sensation at the site of the lesion and caudally

✓ Pain at the site of the lesion

L4-S2 Spinal Cord Segments or Nerve Roots (LMN lesion) and Lumbosacral Neuromuscular Lesions

One or more of the following signs are usually present:

✓ Paresis or paralysis of the pelvic limbs

✓ Decreased or absent conscious proprioception in the pelvic limbs

✓ Decreased or absent patellar reflex (L4-5)

✓ Decreased or absent cranial tibial, gastrocnemius, sciatic, and flexor reflexes (L6-S2)

✓ Decreased or absent anal reflex (S1-3)

✓ Constant or frequent dribbling of urine from a distended bladder that is easy to express (S1-3) in dogs; may be difficult to express in cats

✓ Decreased or absent muscle tone in the pelvic limbs

✓ Pain at the site of the lesion

✓ Cutaneous trunci response is usually normal

Differential Diagnosis

✓ Aortic thromboembolism—common in cats, rare in dogs

✓ Degenerative intervertebral disc disease (IVDD)—common in dogs, rare in cats

✓ Spinal cord trauma—common in dogs and cats

✓ Fibrocartilaginous embolism—common in dogs, rare in cats

✓ Meningomyelitis—occasional in dogs and cats

✓ Neoplasia—occasional in dogs and cats

Diagnostic Evaluation

Important Historical Questions

- Acute onset over 24 to 72 hours?
- Progressive or nonprogressive?
- Possibility of recent trauma? (If so, obtain vertebral radiographs before proceeding further.)
- Is the animal in pain?
- Difficulty jumping or going up or down stairs?
- Have there been past episodes of paraparesis?
- Past or present neoplasia?
- Is urinary or fecal incontinence present?
- Can the animal urinate voluntarily?
- Any difficulty breathing, depression, anorexia, or other signs of systemic illness?
- Any recent or current medication?
- Effectiveness of attempted therapies?

Physical and Neurologic Examinations

✓ Auscultate the chest for evidence of cardiopulmonary disease and other systemic disease

✓ Examine hind limb pulses and perfusion

✓ Localize the lesion to either T3-L3, L4-S2, or lumbosacral neuromuscular

✓ Determine the severity of signs—ataxia, paresis, paralysis, loss of deep pain (Table 12-1)

✓ Determine if painful and location

✓ If urinary incontinence is present, determine whether the bladder is easy or difficult to express

Applicable Diagnostic Tests

✓ A complete blood count, serum chemistry profile, and urinalysis are performed to detect systemic illness and as part of the preanesthetic evaluation.

✓ Thoracic and abdominal radiographs and abdominal ultrasonography are indicated if neoplasia is suspected or abnormalities are found on the physical examination.

Table 12-1
Severity of Acute Thoracolumbar Spinal Cord Lesions*

- Paraparesis with UMN signs

- Paraparesis with LMN signs

- Paraplegia with UMN signs

- Paraplegia with LMN signs

- Paraplegia with UMN signs and loss of deep pain

- Paraplegia with LMN signs and loss of deep pain

- Paraplegia with LMN signs and loss of deep pain and the cutaneous trunci response above L4 (could be an ascending and descending lesion, such as myelomalacia from trauma)

*In order of best to worst prognosis.

✓ Thoracic radiographs show cardiac enlargement with or without pulmonary edema in cats with cardiomyopathy.

✓ A Doppler-flow sensing device placed on the dorsomedial aspect of the metatarsals can be used to evaluate blood flow in distal pelvic limbs.

✓ Ultrasonography of the distal aorta and illiac arteries may often demonstrate a thrombus and obstruction of blood flow.

✓ Electrocardiogram and echocardiography can be useful to evaluate cardiomyopathy.

✓ Coagulation tests, such as activated clotting time (ACT), prothrombin time (PT), and partial thromboplastin time (PPT) may be indicated for animals with thromboembolism and no evidence of cardiac disease.

✓ The following tests are done under anesthesia; potential findings are also noted.

- Cerebrospinal fluid (CSF) analysis may show leukocytosis with or without elevated protein levels in animals with acute IVDD, meningitis, and some neoplastic processes; or elevated protein alone may be noted in IVDD, trauma, and neoplasia.

- Routine vertebral column radiographs can detect vertebral fractures and luxations, calcified intervertebral disks, narrowed intervertebral disk spaces, and vertebral neoplasia.

- Myelography is useful to detect spinal cord compression from IVDD or neoplasia or spinal cord expansion from neoplasia or edema secondary to fibrocartilaginous embolism.

- Computed tomography (CT) and magnetic resonance imaging (MRI) can be useful to evaluate IVDD, fibrocartilaginous embolism, and an inflammatory focus or neoplasm of the spinal cord.

- Surgical exploration of the spinal canal can enable removal or biopsy of masses for histologic examination.

✓ Serum and CSF immunoassays for infections diseases are indicated if CSF analysis shows evidence of inflammation.

Neuromuscular Disorders

Aortic Thromboembolism

♥ Thromboembolism of the aorta or iliac arteries (saddle thrombus) occurs commonly in cats and rarely in dogs. In cats, it is often associated with hypertrophic cardiomyopathy. A large thromboembolus can lodge in the caudal aorta or the iliac arteries and cause pelvic limb pain, symmetric or asymmetric paraparesis, or paraplegia from ischemia of the peripheral nerves and muscles. Femoral pulses are often absent, and reduced blood flow to the pelvic limbs is often found using a Doppler-flow sensing device placed on the dorsomedial metatarsal region. The footpads may be cyanotic, and distal limbs usually feel cool. The pelvic limb muscles, particularly the gastrocnemius muscles, are often firm and painful. Spinal reflexes and deep pain are usually absent. Affected cats often have a murmur or gallop rhythm on auscultation of the heart.

✓ Cardiac enlargement and pulmonary edema may be seen on thoracic radiographs. Echocardiography usually shows evidence of cardiac disease, and thrombi may be visualized in the left atrium. Ultrasonography of the distal aorta and iliac arteries may allow visualization of the thrombus. Coagulation tests, such as ACT, PT, and PPT may be indicated for animals with no evidence of cardiac disease.

✓ Therapy involves addressing the underlying disease process and trying to prevent further nerve and muscle damage. Aspirin, warfarin, and heparin have been used to reduce the chances of further thromboembolism, but therapy must be closely monitored to reduce the possibility of undesirable side effects. Streptokinase and tissue-type plasminogen activator have been given to try to reduce the size of the thrombus but have had variable results, and cause hemorrhage and other adverse effects. Pain is controlled as outlined in Section 7, Table 7-2. **Treatment protocols are complex and change constantly. Consultation with a specialist is recommended.** Some cats can re-canalize the thrombus and regain some pelvic limb function. The long-term prognosis is often poor because of the severity of the underlying disease process and the likelihood of recurrence.

Spinal Cord Disorders

Degenerative Intervertebral Disk Disease

♥ Hansen Type I IVDD is the most common cause of acute paraparesis and paraplegia of dogs. As discussed in Section 7, in Type I IVDD, the nucleus pulposus ruptures through the anulus fibrosus, causing contusion and compression of the spinal cord (Section 7, Figure 7-4). A disk rarely extrudes into the spinal canal between T2-T10 because of the presence of the conjugal (intercapital) ligament, which traverses the space between the ribs immediately dorsal to the disk. Because the size of the lumbar vertebral canal is small compared with that of the spinal cord, there is little room for extruded disk material without significant spinal cord compression. In addition, because the spinal cord is shorter than the vertebral column in dogs and spinal cord segments L4-Cd5 are located within the L4-L7 vertebral canal, several spinal cord segments and nerve roots can be compressed by a single disk (Section 1, Figure 1-2). The mobility of the thoracolumbar junction results in a high incidence of IVDD in this region. Jumping off the couch or similar sharp moves of the vertebral column can cause the disk to extrude with a force that can render the dog paralyzed for life. As a result, thoracolumbar disk extrusion causes more extensive spinal cord injury than cervical disk extrusion (Section 9).

♥ Dachshunds, Pekingese, Lhasa apsos, beagles, cocker spaniels, Shih Tzus, and many other small-breed dogs and some large-breed dogs are at risk for acute paraparesis and paraplegia from acute Type I IVDD. The incidence in Dachshunds exceeds that of other dogs. Acute IVDD is rare in cats unless it is associated with trauma. Severity of the spinal cord injury can be evaluated as outlined in Table 12-1. The extruded disk is usually on the side of the most affected pelvic limb if asymmetric paresis is present. If paraplegia with or without deep pain is found, there is some hope for return of function, but emergency medical and surgical therapy are essential to ensure the best possible outcome. **If dogs are presented within 24 hours of the onset of paraplegia, IV methylprednisolone sodium succinate (MPSS) is immediately administered as outlined in Table 12-2, and referral to a specialist for emergency surgical decompression is recommended.**

Table 12-2
Methylprednisolone therapy for acute paraplegia

Acute paraplegia presented within 8 hours of onset:
- **Methylprednisolone sodium succinate (MPSS) 30 mg/kg IV**.
(Refer immediately for emergency surgical decompression if the animal is stable.)

- Two hours after the initial dose, MPSS 15 mg/kg IV is given and repeated every 6 hours for 24-48 hours if voluntary movement is still absent.

- **To prevent gastrointestinal complications,** give IV famotidine (Pepcid AC) 0.5-1 mg/kg every 12-24 hours or cimetidine (Tagamet) 5-10 mg/kg every 8 hours.

Acute paraplegia between 8 hours and 24 hours of onset:
- MPSS 15 mg/kg IV every 6 hours for 24 hours. (Refer for emergency surgical decompression after the first dose if the animal is stable.)

Warnings

- **Do not use MPSS** at higher doses, in ambulatory animals, or if the patient presents more than 24 hours after the onset of injury, as the pathologic condition may be worsened.

- **Stop treatment if melena or vomiting occurs**

✓ If the dog can still move voluntarily, then high-dose MPSS IV is not necessary. Aside from the immediate spinal cord tissue damage done by the extruded disk material, secondary neurotoxic processes result in the formation of oxygen containing free radicals and a cycle of progressive spinal cord destruction that continues over 24 to 48 hours. The antioxidant and other neuroprotective properties of MPSS have been shown to reduce spinal cord destruction if a specific dose range is administered IV within 8 hours of an induced spinal cord injury in experimental laboratory animals. These doses and time intervals have been extrapolated for use in dogs.

✓ Although dogs usually lose the cutaneous trunci response before the deep pain response, sometimes the opposite occurs, and this may indicate that spinal cord damage is most significant deep in the white matter. Many of these dogs can still recover adequate function. A few dogs with severe spinal cord injury can develop ascending myelomalacia and die from respiratory paralysis regardless of therapy. Most of these dogs have paraplegia, loss of pelvic limb and anal reflexes, loss of deep pain, and a progressive ascending loss of the cutaneous trunci response on serial neurologic examinations.

✓ It is common to see multiple calcified disks on plain radiographs especially in chondrodystrophic breeds of dogs. A narrowed disk space and calcified material in the spinal canal may also be present (Figure 12-4), but the lesions obvious on routine radiography may not be associated with the current problem. CSF analysis should always be performed first to rule-out meningomyelitis, although a mild increase in the number of leukocytes may occur in cases of acute disk extrusion.

✓ Diagnostic imaging is used to determine the diagnosis and the site of spinal cord compression prior to surgery. Deviation of the contrast columns or diffuse spinal cord swelling with thinning or absence of contrast media over one or more vertebrae can be observed on a myelogram (Figure 12-5). CT after the myelogram can further delineate the extent of a compressive lesion. CT in chondrodys-trophic breeds and MRI if available are preferred to avoid the deleterious effects of myelography (see Section 7, Figures 7-8, 7-9, 7-10, and Section 9, Figures 9-5, and 9-6). CT and MRI are extremely useful for identifying lateral disk extrusion as well as the extent of any associated extradural and subarachnoid hemorrhage.

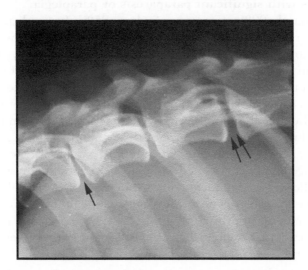

Figure 12-4 Routine lateral radiograph showing a narrowed intervertebral disk space (arrow) and calcified disk in the intervertebral foramen at T11-T12 and a calcified nucleus pulposus at T13-L1 (double arrows) in a 4-year-old dachshund with acute paraplegia.

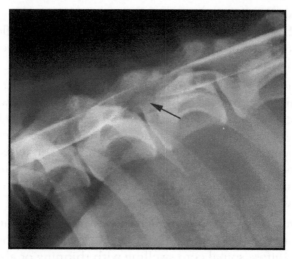

Figure 12-5 A lateral myelogram of the dog in Figure 12-4 showing the spinal cord compression at T11-T12 (arrow) from a Type I intervertebral disk extrusion.

♥ **Decompressive surgery for acute paraplegia from disk extrusion is most effective within 24 hours of the onset of signs, and emergency referral is important. Surgery is recommended for most dogs with significant paraparesis or paraplegia.** Approximately 90% of paraparetic dogs, 85% of paraplegic dogs with response to deep pain, and 50% of paraplegic dogs with no response to deep pain recover with surgery. Some dogs with paraparesis can recover without surgery, but the likelihood of recovery is reduced the longer surgery is postponed. In addition, recovery times with surgical intervention are usually much shorter than with medical therapy alone, and prophylactic fenestration can be performed to prevent recurrence of thoracolumbar disk extrusion in the future. Medical management of mildly paraparetic dogs that are not having surgery is outlined in Table 12-3. The same protocol can be followed in paraplegic dogs when the expense makes surgery prohibitive for some owners. Physical therapy and nursing care should be given as outlined in Table 12-4, but strict rest is essential, so whirlpool baths, swimming, sling walks, and other exercise are avoided for 4 weeks.

Table 12-3
Medical Management of Paraparetic Dogs Not Having Surgery

• **Strict crate confinement** for 4 weeks (activity is limited to short leash walks with a harness for urinating and defecating). No walking around the house. If possible, the animal is gently carried.

• **Oral prednisone 0.25–1 mg/kg every 12 hours with tapered doses over 7-14 days** is given to reduce spinal cord swelling from compression. If the animal improves then relapses as the dose is reduced, increase prednisone dose again and recommend surgery.

• **Famotidine** (Pepcid AC, Merck) **0.5–1 mg/kg PO every 12-24 hours, cimetidine** (Tagamet, SmithKline Beecham) **5–10 mg/kg PO every 12 hours, or misoprostol** (Cytotec, Searyl) **1–3 μg/kg PO every 8 hours** or another gastrointestinal (GI) protectant drug must be given to reduce GI ulceration when the prednisone dose is high.

• **Oral diazepam 0.5–2 mg/kg every 6-8 hours as needed (not to exceed 10 mg every 6 hours)** may help relieve painful muscle spasms.

• **If pain is severe, see Section 7, Table 7-2.**

Table 12-4
Nursing Care and Physical Therapy for Paraplegic Dogs

• Keep on a clean, padded surface and turn to the opposite side every 6 hours to avoid decubital ulcers.

• Monitor for fever twice daily for 1 week after surgery.

• Express bladder every 6-8 hours if unable to urinate, and monitor the urine for blood.

• Assist in defecation if needed.

• Keep skin dry and free of urine and feces (apply water-repellent ointment to perineal and caudal abdominal areas).

• Feed a well-balanced diet, and have water readily available.

• Ensure strict rest for 4 weeks if surgery is not performed.

• Massage and perform passive range-of-motion exercise of the pelvic limbs for 15 minutes 3-4 times a day until able to walk.

• Whirlpool baths and swimming can begin 5-7 days after surgery but should not be done for 4 weeks if surgery is not performed or for 6 weeks if a vertebral fracture has been repaired.

• Assist attempts to stand and support weight 3-4 times a day.

• Sling walks can begin when some movement returns but not for 4 weeks if surgery is not performed or for 6 weeks if a vertebral fracture has been repaired.

♥ The goal of surgery is to decompress the spinal cord and remove extruded disk material. The type of surgery performed is usually determined by the location of the extruded disk. Hemilaminectomy is performed for T10-L4 extrusions (Figure 12-6); dorsal laminectomy is performed for extrusions caudal to L4 because the ilia prevent a dorsolateral approach (Figure 12-7).

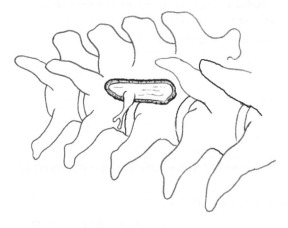

Figure 12-6 (above)
The hemilaminectomy surgical technique. Removal of the dorsolateral vertebral lamina to expose the spinal cord and interverbral disc space on one side.

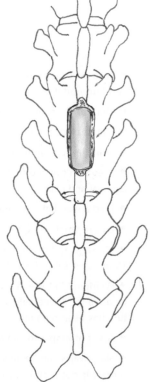

Figure 12-7 (right)
The dorsal laminectomy surgical technique. Removal of the dorsal vertebral lamina to expose the top of the spinal cord.

✓ If the animals' response to deep pain is absent, durotomy may be performed to visualize the spinal cord parenchyma and assess the prognosis. Liquefaction of the cord indicates myelomalacia, which carries a poor prognosis. Following decompressive surgery, prophylactic fenestration of the T11-12 to L3-4 disks may be performed in small chondrodystrophic dogs to prevent future extrusion of other disks. Only prophylactic fenestration of obviously degenerate disks is performed in larger dogs because vertebral instability can result and cause future problems.

♥ Postoperative pain is controlled as outlined in Section 7, Table 7-2. **Oral prednisone 0.25 mg/kg every 12 hours for 3 days then tapered over 7 to 14 days may be given after surgery. Famotidine (Pepcid AC, Merck) 0.5–1mg/kg PO every 12 to 24 hours, cimetidine (Tagamet, SmithKline Beecham) 5–10 mg/kg PO every 12 hours, or misoprostol (Cytotec) 1 to 3 µg/kg PO every 8 hours or another gastrointestinal protectant is given to reduce upset or ulceration from the prednisone. Oral muscle relaxants, like diazepam 0.5–2 mg/kg every 6 to 8 hours as needed (not to exceed 10 mg every 6 hours) may help relieve painful muscle spasms and also make the bladder easier to express.**

♥ Paraplegic dogs are easier to care for than quadriplegic dogs. Decubital ulcers, urine contact dermatitis, and bladder infections are the biggest complications. Postoperative nursing care and physical therapy are outlined in Table 12-4. The bladder may have to be expressed for up to 10 days after surgery, but with T3-L3 lesions, reflex or voluntary urination usually begins shortly after that time. The bladder may have to be expressed for a longer period in patients with L6-S2 lesions. As voluntary limb movement appears, control of urination often returns. If the response to deep pain testing is absent for more than a month, paraplegic dogs are unlikely to recover function. Voluntary movement, which indicates improvement of function, must be distinguished from spinal walking, which occurs 1 to 2 months after injury. Deep pain is usually absent in dogs that are spinal walking. Most dogs have an excellent prognosis and continue to improve for 6 to 12 months following surgery. Dogs with paraplegia often enjoy exercise in a wheeled cart placed under their pelvic limbs. Several carts are commercially available for paraplegic dogs of all sizes and can be found on the Internet. Dogs with permanent paralysis must be monitored and treated for cystitis but can live otherwise active lives. Lifestyle changes as outlined in Table 12-5 are recommended.

Table 12-5
Advice to Dog Owners: Strategies to Reduce the Chances or Effects of Future Intervertebral Disk Disease

Do's

- Reduce weight if obese.

- Feed a well-balanced diet.

- Provide daily antioxidant supplementation of vitamin E 10-25 IU/kg and vitamin C 15 mg/kg.

- Use a harness instead of a collar.

- Can go for daily walks on a leash (after recovery).

- Can do obedience training (no jumping).

Don'ts

- No jumping on and off furniture, running down stairs, sitting up to beg, or dancing on the hind legs.

- No playing frisbee or "tug of war," chasing balls, shaking toys, or participating in other activities that cause quick, sharp turns of the neck or back.

- No rough play with other dogs.

- No agility training that necessitates jumping or climbing.

- No jogging and "road work" behind a vehicle.

Spinal Cord Trauma

♥ Acute spinal cord trauma most commonly results from fractures, subluxation, or luxation of the vertebrae. The diagnosis of trauma is often apparent from the history and physical examination. Life-threatening problems, such as shock and hemorrhage, are treated, and a thorough physical examination is performed to identify the extent of nonneural injuries. Diaphragm or urinary bladder rupture is common in traumatized, paraplegic dogs. Assessment of voluntary movement, pelvic limb spinal reflexes, and cutaneous trunci and deep pain responses is carefully performed to avoid moving the vertebral column. Pain medication is administered as soon as possible. Ideally, the patient should be rigidly immobilized on a radiolucent board, which prevents further damage from excessive movement while allowing radiographs to be taken with minimal manipulation. Intravenous methylprednisolone sodium succinate is administered as soon as possible to paraplegic dogs and cats as outlined in Table 12-2.

✔ When the animal is sedated or anesthetized, the stabilizing effect of paravertebral muscle tone is lost, and vertebral instability can cause further spinal cord damage. Two radiographic views are imperative to assess the degree of instability at the site of a fracture or subluxation. Additional imaging is important, even if a lesion has been detected on routine radiography, to determine the extent of the lesion, identify additional spinal cord injuries remote from the obvious lesion, and to plan surgical intervention. The degree of spinal cord compression and edema can be visualized on myelography, CT, or MRI (Figure 12-8). CT may be useful to detect small fractures not visible on routine radiographs.

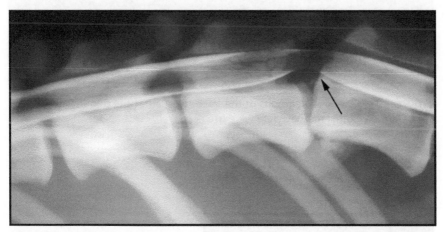

Figure 12-8 Lateral myelogram of a 1-year-old mixed-breed dog that had been paraplegic with deep pain for 1 month; note the spinal cord compression from a fracture subluxation of L1-2 (arrow); surgical decompression and stabilization were performed (Figures 12-9 and 12-10), and the dog became ambulatory in the pelvic limbs in 3 months.

♥ **If significant hemorrhage, bone fragments, or other space-occupying lesions are found within the spinal canal, hemilaminectomy or dorsal laminectomy and decompression of the spinal cord may be necessary (Figures 12-6 and 12-7). Visible vertebral fractures or subluxation should be surgically stabilized.** Steinmann pins or orthopedic screws and polymethyl methacrylate are typically used to stabilize the vertebrae (Figures 12-9 and 12-10). If hemorrhage but no spinal cord compression is present, recovery from spinal trauma can be achieved through the medical approach outlined in Table 12-3. Placement of a brace or cast to stabilize the spine should be considered, which helps to minimize movement and provides some support. Adequate analgesia should be provided at all times as outlined in Section 7, Table 7-2.

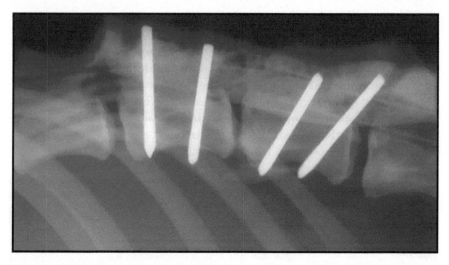

Figure 12-9 Lateral radiographs of the fracture repair of the dog in Figure 12-8; pins and polymethyl methacrylate were used.

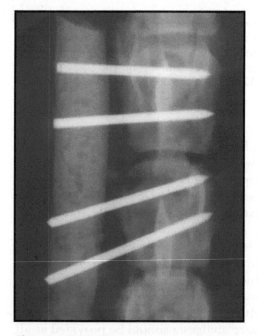

Figure 12-10 A ventrodorsal radiograph of the fracture repair of dog in Figure 12-8; pins and polymethyl methacrylate were used.

✓ Postoperative nursing care and physical therapy are outlined in Table 12-4. The prognosis for recovery for paraparetic and paraplegic dogs that respond to deep pain is good in most cases. Improvement often continues for 9 to 12 months. The prognosis for animals with paraplegia and no deep pain response as a result of injury is often worse than that for IVDD because of the degree of traumatic forces upon the spinal cord. As discussed for IVDD, if there is no response to deep pain for more than a month, paraplegic dogs are unlikely to recover function. Voluntary movement, which indicates improvement of function, must be distinguished from spinal walking, which occurs 1 to 2 months after injury. Animals with permanent paraplegia may adapt to a cart as suggested for IVDD. Spinal fractures that occur spontaneously or with minimal trauma should be evaluated for the presence of an underlying neoplasm (pathologic fractures).

Fibrocartilaginous Embolism

🖐 A common cause of asymmetric paraparesis or paraplegia in large dogs is spinal cord infarction from fibrocartilaginous emboli (FCE). Small dogs and cats are affected less frequently. Clinical signs develop acutely and progress rapidly (within 1 to 2 hours) to unilateral or bilateral paraplegia (Figure 12-11). The diagnosis and treatment of FCE are presented in Section 9. Infarction of T3-L3 has a good prognosis for recovery. If unilateral infarction

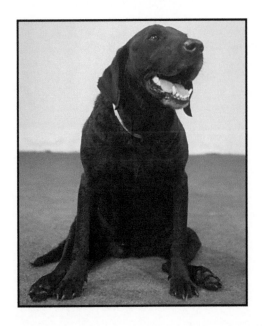

Figure 12-11
A 5-year-old Labrador retriever with acute paraplegia from a fibrocartilaginous embolism.

of L4-S2 occurs with absent spinal reflexes in one pelvic limb, recovery is possible but slow. If bilateral infarction of L4-S2 occurs and no pelvic limb spinal reflexes or response to deep pain are present, the prognosis for complete recovery can be poor. Even if some limb function recovers, the ability to voluntarily urinate can remain permanently impaired.

Meningomyelitis

✓ Inflammation of the spinal cord due to canine distemper virus, toxoplasmosis, neosporosis, rickettsia, fungi, bacteria, and immune-mediated dysfunction rarely cause acute onset of paraplegia. Such inflammatory processes are more commonly associated with diseases that have a chronic, progressive course. Diagnosis and treatment of inflammation of the nervous system are discussed in Section 2.

Neoplasia

✓ Spinal cord neoplasia rarely presents as acute paraplegia unless a pathologic vertebral fracture or spinal cord hemorrhage or infarction has occurred. Spinal cord neoplasia is discussed in Section 10.

Section 13

Chronic Paraparesis

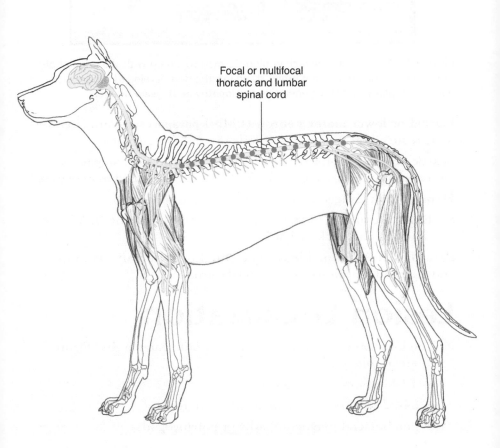

Focal or multifocal
thoracic and lumbar
spinal cord

Definitions

Chronic paraparesis: Neurologic signs that progress over a week to several months.

Paraparesis: Weakness and reduced voluntary movement of the pelvic limbs.

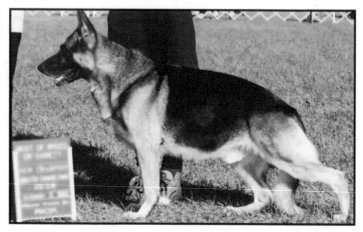

Figure 13-1 A Best-in-Breed champion German shepherd with the angulation of the pelvic limbs that is the breed standard; the dog developed progressive pelvic limb paresis from degenerative myelopathy at 10 years of age.

Flaccid or lower motor neuron (LMN) paraparesis: Paraparesis with reduced or absent spinal reflexes and muscle tone.

Spastic or upper motor neuron (UMN) paraparesis: Paraparesis with normal or exaggerated spinal reflexes and increased muscle tone.

Hyperpathia: Exaggerated response to painful stimuli.

Scoliosis: Deviation of the vertebral column resulting in a curvature of the neck or back.

Paresthesia: Abnormal burning or tingling; often affects limbs and feet and manifests as self-mutilation.

Lesion Localization

✓ The location of lesions that cause chronic paraparesis (Figure 13-2) are as follows:

- T3-L3 spinal cord segments
- L4-S2 spinal cord segments or nerve roots
- Lumbosacral polyneuropathy or polymyopathy

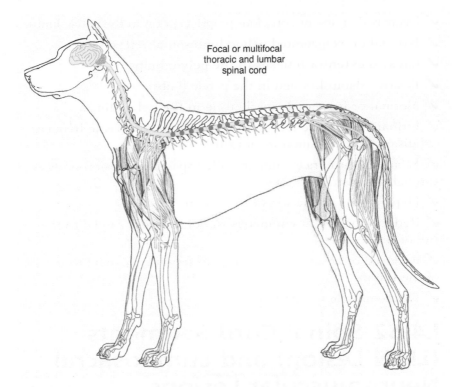

Figure 13-2 Chronic paraparesis is usually associated with a lesion in the spinal cord below T3 (dots indicate lesion localization).

Differentiation of Upper Motor Neuron and Lower Motor Neuron Lesions

Differentiating the type of motor neuron lesions that cause chronic paraparesis is shown in Section 12, Figure 12-3.

T3-L3 Spinal Cord Segments (UMN Lesion)

Animals with these lesions usually have more than one of the following signs:

✓ Paresis or paralysis of the pelvic limbs

✓ Decreased or absent conscious proprioception in the pelvic limbs

✓ Normal or exaggerated pelvic limb spinal reflexes

✓ Crossed extensor reflexes in the pelvic limbs

✓ Positive Babinski's sign in the pelvic limbs

✓ Normal or increased muscle tone in the pelvic limbs

✓ Urinary incontinence—reflex urinations, or spastic frequent expulsion of small amounts of urine

✓ Fecal incontinence—uncontrolled spastic expulsion of feces through a constricted anus

✓ Hyperpathia at the site of the lesion

✓ Reduced or absent cutaneous trunci response caudal to the site of the lesion

✓ Reduced or absent superficial pain sensation caudal to the site of the lesion

✓ Disuse muscle atrophy

L4-S2 Spinal Cord Segments (LMN Lesion) and Lumbosacral Neuromuscular Lesions

Usually more than one of the following signs occur:

✓ Paresis or paralysis of the pelvic limbs

✓ Decreased or absent conscious proprioception in the pelvic limbs

✓ Decreased or absent patellar reflex (L4-5); increased if the lesion is caudal to L5

✓ Decreased or absent cranial tibial, gastrocnemius, sciatic, and flexor reflexes (L6-S2)

✓ Decreased or absent muscle tone in the pelvic limbs

✓ Decreased or absent anal reflex (S1-3)

✓ Constant or frequent dribbling of urine from a distended bladder that is easy to express (S1-3) in dogs; may be difficult to express in cats

✓ Fecal incontinence—uncontrolled defecation through a dilated anus

✓ Usually normal cutaneous trunci response

✓ Hyperpathia at the site of the lesion

✓ Neurogenic muscle atrophy

Differential Diagnosis

✓ Degenerative intervertebral disk disease (IVDD)—common in dogs, occasional in geriatric cats

✓ Degenerative myelopathy—common in German shepherds, occasional other dogs

✓ Lumbosacral degeneration—common in large-breed dogs

✓ Meningomyelitis—common in dogs and cats

✓ Diskospondylitis—common in dogs, rare in cats

✓ Hemivertebrae and other vertebral malformations—occasional in dogs, rare in cats

✓ Neoplasia—occasional in dogs and cats

✓ Spinal cord cysts—rare in dogs and cats

✓ Lysosomal storage disorders—rare in dogs and cats

✓ Polyradiculoneuritis/myositis—rare in dogs

✓ Other polyneuropathies or polymyopathies—rare in dogs and cats

Diagnostic Evaluation

Important Historical Questions

• Onset, course and duration of signs—progression over weeks or months?

• Is the animal in pain?

• Difficulty rising in the pelvic limbs?

• Difficulty going up stairs or jumping onto furniture or into the car?

• Have there been previous episodes of paraparesis?

• Change in tail carriage?

• Past or present neoplasia?

• Is urinary or fecal incontinence present?

• Can the animal urinate voluntarily?

• Any signs of systemic illness?

• Any recent or current medications?

• Is the dog doing agility training or other work involving climbing or jumping?

• Effectiveness of attempted therapies?

Physical and Neurologic Examinations

✓ Localize the lesion to T3-L3 or L4-S2 (includes neuromuscular lesions).

✓ Determine the severity of signs; in order of progressive severity: ataxia, paraparesis, paraplegia with deep pain response, paraplegia with no deep pain response (Section 12, Table 12-1). Most animals are presented at the paraparesis stage as this progresses over a week or more.

✓ Evaluate the thoracic limbs carefully as a cervical or diffuse neuromuscular lesion can appear to only affect the pelvic limbs.

✓ Determine the source of pain, if any.

✓ If urinary incontinence is present, determine whether the bladder is easy or difficult to express.

Applicable Diagnostic Tests

✓ A complete blood count (CBC), serum chemistry profile, and urinalysis are performed to detect systemic illness and as part of the preanesthetic evaluation.

✓ Thoracic and abdominal radiographs and abdominal ultrasonography are indicated if neoplasia is suspected or abnormalities are found on the physical examination.

✓ Tests for which the animal must be anesthetized as well as their potential findings are as follows:

- Cerebrospinal fluid (CSF) analysis may show leukocytic pleocytosis with or without elevated protein levels in cases of meningomyelitis; lumbar CSF may have more significant abnormalities than does cerebellomedullary CSF.

- CSF analysis may show elevated protein in IVDD, degenerative myelopathy, spinal cord neoplasia, and some lysosomal storage disorders. Lumbar CSF may show the greatest changes.

- CSF cholinesterase levels are elevated in German shepherd degenerative myelopathy.

- Electromyography (EMG) may show positive sharp waves and fibrillation potentials in the paravertebral, limb, or tail muscles in the area of a focal lesion; EMG may detect multifocal lesions or a generalized neuromuscular disorder.

- Spinal cord evoked potentials may be abnormal.

- Routine vertebral column radiographs often show calcified intervertebral disks, diskospondylitis, and vertebral malformations or neoplasia; spondylosis deformans and dural ossification are usually incidental findings in older animals.

- Myelography is useful to detect spinal cord compression from IVDD, neoplasia, vertebral abnormalities, and cysts or to demonstrate spinal cord expansion from neoplasia.

- Computed tomography (CT) and magnetic resonance imaging (MRI) can be useful to evaluate IVDD, diskospondylitis, vertebral and spinal cord neoplasia, vertebral anomalies, cysts, and lumbosacral degeneration.

- Surgical exploration of the spinal canal can enable removal or biopsy of masses for histologic examination.

- Muscle and nerve biopsy is obtained if a neuromuscular lesion is suspected.

✓ Serum and CSF titers for organisms or cultures are obtained if meningomyelitis is suspected.

✓ Urine and blood cultures are obtained if diskospondylitis is suspected.

Spinal Cord Disorders

Degenerative Intervertebral Disk Disease

♥ The most common cause of chronic progressive paraparesis in dogs is Hansen Type II IVDD. Middle-aged or older nonchondrodystrophic, large-breed dogs, like German shepherds and Labrador retrievers, are most commonly affected, although any breed of dog and geriatric cats may be affected. As discussed in Section 7, the anulus fibrosus slowly protrudes into the spinal canal with Type II IVDD and compresses the spinal cord (Section 7, Figure 7-5). In some instances, spinal cord compression is partially or solely related to hypertrophy of the dorsal anulus fibrosus and the dorsal longitudinal ligament. Chronic Type II IVDD often occurs at the more mobile points of the vertebral column, such as the thoracolumbar and the lumbosacral regions. Type II IVDD rarely occurs between T1-T10 because the conjugal (intercapital) ligament between the rib heads reinforces the region immediately dorsal to the disk.

✓ Initial clinical signs may be weakness on rising, reluctance to jump into the car or onto the furniture, and difficulty climbing stairs. Although acute exacerbations are possible, clinical signs usually reflect a chronic, progressive, focal spinal cord lesion and include asymmetric or symmetric pelvic limb ataxia, paraparesis, conscious proprioceptive deficits (Figure 13-3), and focal hyperpathia. In some animals, no evidence of hyperpathia can be found, so it can be difficult to differentiate Type II IVDD from degenerative myelopathy on initial clinical evaluation. Fecal and urinary incontinence may also be present.

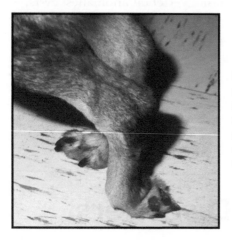

Figure 13-3 Loss of conscious proprioception helps differentiate orthopedic and spinal cord disease in dogs with mild paraparesis; conscious proprioception is reduced or absent in spinal cord disease and usually normal in orthopedic disease.

🖐 Elevated protein levels with normal leukocyte counts and cytologic findings are common on lumbar CSF analysis. Positive sharp waves and fibrillation potentials may be found in affected paravertebral, limb, and tail musculature on EMG and can help determine whether more than one site is involved. Routine radiographs may show spondylosis deformans and bony proliferation of the dorsal articular facets, or they may be normal. Dural ossification may be an incidental radiographic finding. Calcification of the nucleus pulposus and narrowed disk spaces are rarely seen on routine radiographs of animals with Type II IVDD, and myelography, CT, or MRI is necessary to document spinal cord compression. Severe compression may be found in animals with only mild to moderate paraparesis, as the spinal cord can adjust to slow rates of compression and neurologic signs may develop only after it can no longer compensate. Myelography is the most efficient technique to outline multiple thoracolumbar and cervical lesions. Paraparesis may be worse (usually transiently) following myelography so MRI is preferred if the lesion can be well localized. **The treatment of Type II IVDD can be medical, surgical, or both and depends on the factors outlined in Table 13-1.**

Table 13-1
Factors Affecting Treatment Choices
in Dogs with Type II
Intervertebral Disk Disease

- Condition of the animal
- Duration and severity of the paraparesis
- Presence of multifocal lesions
- Suspicion of concurrent degenerative myelopathy
- Economic situation of the client.

♥ If an elderly animal is in good physical condition, has no concurrent significant medical problems, and has only a single disk protrusion, surgical intervention should not be excluded on the basis of age alone. Animals with paraparesis from a single lesion that has progressed over a few weeks tend to do better with surgery than those with signs that have been progressing for several months or longer. Surgery may not be beneficial for long-term compression, as spinal cord atrophy is often irreversible. If an animal with a focal disk protrusion responds well to prednisone therapy, then decompressive surgery may be more likely to be effective. **Medical management of Type II IVDD is outlined in Table 13-2.** The use of carprofen (Rimadyl, Pfizer), etodolac (Etogesic, Fort Dodge), buffered aspirin, or other nonsteroidal anti-inflammatory drugs (NSAIDs) should be discontinued during prednisone therapy. Unfortunately, when prednisone is discontinued, clinical signs often return, as spinal cord compression is still present. Rest is not essential as in Type I IVDD because exercise does not worsen the protrusion, and moderate exercise, such as walking or swimming, is important in elderly animals. If possible, surgical decompression of the spinal cord offers a better long-term solution than does prednisone therapy. Referral for alternative therapies, such as acupuncture, herbs, massage, and other forms of physical therapy, should also be considered. However, prednisone may have to be discontinued as it may inhibit their effectiveness.

✔ As discussed in Section 12, the type of surgery is usually determined by the location of the protrusion. **Hemilaminectomy is usually performed for protrusions between vertebrae T10-L4, and dorsal laminectomy is done for protrusions caudal to L4** (Section 12, Figures 12-6 and 12-7). A Type II disk can be very firm and may have to be excised with a scalpel. Surgery for chronic Type II IVDD often requires more manipulation of the meninges and spinal cord than is needed in acute Type I disk extrusions. As a result, paresis is often more severe after surgery. However, this is usually a temporary setback and the long-term prognosis is very good to excellent in most cases. The postoperative nursing care and physical therapy are similar to that described in Section 12 for acute paraplegia and are outlined in Table 13-3.

Table 13-2
Medical Management of Type II Thoracolumbar Intervertebral Disk Disease

- Permit moderate exercise, such as walking and swimming.

- Avoid jumping, going up and down stairs, or rough play.

- Administer prednisone 0.25-1 mg/kg PO every 12 hours with tapered doses over 30 days. If improvement is noted but relapse occurs when the dose is reduced, increase the dose again and recommend surgery. If surgery is not an option, continue with the lowest dose of prednisone that will control the signs (preferably alternate-day therapy).

- Oral famotidine (Pepcid AC, Merck) 0.5-1 mg/kg every 12-24 hours, cimetidine (Tagamet, SmithKline Beecham) 5-10 mg/kg every 12 hours, misoprostol (Cytotec, Searyl) 1-3 µg/kg every 8 hours or other GI protectant may be given to reduce gastrointestinal upset from the prednisone.

- Administer diazepam 0.5-2 mg/kg PO every 6-8 hours as needed (not to exceed 10 mg every 6 hours) if muscle spasms are present.

- Pain is unlikely to be severe, but if needed, conduct pain management as outlined in Chapter 7, Table 7-2.

Warning: Prednisone therapy often causes polyuria/polydipsia, polyphagia, and panting. Give extra water but feed a smaller amount of a high-quality, low-calorie diet because the dog will not be able to exercise as much as in the past. Long-term corticosteroid therapy can cause gastrointestinal ulcers, hepatopathy, and myopathy.

Warning: Never use carproden (Rimadyl), etodolac (Etogesic), buffered aspirin, or other non-steroidal antiinflammatory drugs in combination with prednisone or other corticosteroids as gastrointestinal ulcers and perforation can lead to death.

Table 13-3
Nursing Care and Physical Therapy for Paraparetic Dogs

- Keep on a clean, padded surface and turn to the opposite side every 6 hours to avoid decubital ulcers.

- Monitor for fever twice daily for 1 week after surgery.

- Express bladder every 6-8 hours if unable to urinate, and monitor the urine for blood.

- Use enemas or stool softeners to assist in defecation if needed.

- Keep skin dry and free of urine and feces (apply water-repellent ointment to perineal and caudal abdominal areas).

- Feed a well-balanced diet, and have water readily available.

- Massage and perform passive range-of-motion exercises of the pelvic limbs for 15 minutes 2-3 times a day.

- Assist attempts to stand and support weight 3-4 times a day; may use a hoist.

- Whirlpool baths and swimming can begin 5-7 days after surgery.

- Sling walks can begin when some movement returns.

Degenerative Myelopathy

✓ German shepherd degenerative myelopathy (GSDM) is seen in German shepherd dogs between 5 and 14 years of age (Figure 13-1). Similar degenerative myelopathies (DMs) occur in boxers, Pembroke Welsh corgis, Belgian tervurens, Old English sheepdogs, Rhodesian ridgebacks, Weimaraners, Great Pyrenees mountain dogs, and other large-breed dogs within the same age range. However, fewer data are available in these dogs, so it is difficult to determine whether the pathophysiologic process is the same as that of GSDM. DM has also been reported in cats. The exact cause of GSDM is unknown, but an immune-mediated disease process is suspected.

♥ Nonpainful pelvic limb ataxia and paresis are seen. These signs progress over several months and may have a waxing and waning course. Weakness evident on rising may be the first indication of a problem. As many German shepherds and other large breeds commonly develop osteoarthritis of the hips and stifles and spondylosis deformans, difficulty rising may be attributed to discomfort associated with these disorders. If reduced or absent conscious proprioception is found in one or both pelvic limbs, then a neurologic disorder is likely (Figure 13-3). As DM progresses, ataxia and paraparesis are obvious, and pelvic limb spinal reflexes are normal or hyperactive, indicating a spinal cord lesion between T3-L3. Patellar reflexes may become depressed or absent due to degeneration of axons in the dorsal root later in the disease process. Affected dogs finally become unable to rise or walk with the pelvic limbs and develop urinary and fecal incontinence. Severe paraparesis typically develops within 3 to 6 months after identification of GSDM. The thoracic limbs can become progressively involved, leading to quadriparesis within 9-12 months and finally the animal succumbs from respiratory paralysis. Few patients with GSDM survive beyond 18 months without treatment.

Since German shepherds and other large-breed dogs also commonly develop Type II IVDD and lumbosacral degeneration, DM must be differentiated from these and other spinal cord disorders. Some German shepherds may have GSDM concurrently with other spinal cord disorders. Radiographs of the vertebral column may be normal or show concurrent spondylosis deformans. Myelography is unremarkable in DM. However, affected dogs may be more paretic (usually transiently) after myelography, and MRI may be preferred to rule out Type II IVDD and other causes of paraparesis. Spinal cord evoked potentials can confirm spinal cord dysfunction. Diagnosis of DM is suspected after ruling out other causes of chronic progressive paraparesis. The clinical criteria for the diagnosis of GSDM are outlined in Table 13-4. Other animals with DM may have similar findings. A definitive diagnosis of DM can only be achieved with histologic examination of the spinal cord obtained at necropsy.

Table 13-4
Diagnostic Criteria for German Shepherd Degenerative Myelopathy

- Signalment: German shepherd or German shepherd mixed-breed dogs 5 years of age or older

- History: Chronic, progressive, non-painful paraparesis of several months duration

- Neurologic examination: Symmetric or asymmetric paraparesis; conscious proprioceptive deficits; normal, hyperactive, or depressed patellar reflexes; all other spinal reflexes normal or hyperactive

- EMG: Normal

- Spinal cord evoked testing: Slowed spinal cord conduction

- Lumbar CSF analysis: Normal cytologic characteristics with elevated protein levels

- Lumbar CSF cholinesterase levels: Elevated

- Neuroimaging (routine radiography, myelography, CT, routine MRI): No lesions affecting the spinal cord to account for clinical signs

♥ Elevated CSF cholinesterase, interleukin 6, and ubiquitin concentrations suggest the presence of inflammation in GSDM. The clinical stage and severity of GSDM correlate with depressed lymphocyte blastogenesis to plant mitogens, resulting from the genesis of circulating suppressor cells. Some dogs with GSDM also exhibit antigen-binding cells specific to canine myelin basic protein. Increased circulating immune-complexes in the serum and CSF are similar to other inflammatory diseases and are not specific to GSDM. **The treatment of GSDM is directed at controlling the inflammatory processes associated with the underlying immune disorder and is outlined in Table 13-5.** This treatment may also be helpful in other dogs with DM.

Table 13-5
Treatment of German Shepherd Degenerative Myelopathy

- **Oral epsilon aminocaproic acid** (Amicar) 500 mg every 8 hours
- **Oral N-Acetylcysteine** 25 mg/kg every 8 hours daily for 2 weeks then reduced to every other day
- **Oral vitamin E** 1000–2000 IU once or twice daily
- **Oral vitamin C** 250–500 mg once or twice daily
- **Regular walking or swimming**
- **High-quality, balanced diet**
- Referral to a holistic veterinarian who can provide supportive treatment with acupuncture, herbs, dietary supplements, homeopathy, and/or massage

♥ Circulating immune complexes damage endothelial cells in the blood vessels of the spinal cord and cause deposition of fibrin in the perivascular spaces. Fibrin degradation attracts inflammatory cells into the lesions, causing further tissue damage. Epsilon aminocaproic acid (EACA) is an antifibrinolytic agent that reduces the inflammation associated with fibrin degradation. EACA causes gastric irritation and should be given with food to prevent nausea and vomiting.

♥ The inflammatory cells release prostaglandins and cytokines, which ultimately lead to the formation of oxygen-containing free radicals that further damage the tissues. N-Acetylcysteine (NAC) is a potent antioxidant that prevents free radical-induced tissue destruction. NAC comes as a 20% solution and must be diluted with chicken broth (or other compatible water substitute) to 5% and given with food to prevent nausea and vomiting. Some compounding pharmacies may be able to formulate medications at a reduced cost. Therapeutic doses of oral vitamin E and vitamin C can also be given to reduce tissue damage from oxygen containing free radicals. As high doses of vitamin C may induce diarrhea, low doses are initially given then increased if tolerated. High doses of vitamin E may inhibit coagulation and should be avoided in animals with coagulopathies. Treatment with EACA, NAC, and vitamins E and C is aimed at slowing the progression of GSDM or achieving remission. Almost all GSDM patients show some short-term benefit from EACA and antioxidant therapy. Remission has been seen in cases treated early in the course of disease. Dogs with GSDM may live long enough to develop other age-related problems. Periodic assessments of their general health are important.

♥ Diet may have a powerful influence on the development of chronic degenerative diseases and should be closely monitored. Complementary therapies may prolong life and increase its quality. Many dogs with DM develop severe paraparesis and incontinence despite all treatment attempts. A cart can be used to support the pelvic limbs for walks, but the disease process will eventually affect the thoracic limbs. Owners usually decide on euthanasia prior to this stage when quality of life becomes poor.

✓ On necropsy, widespread demyelination and loss of axons are found, especially in the thoracolumbar spinal cord (Figure 13-4). Nearly all funiculi are vacuolated. Similar lesions are occasionally seen scattered throughout the white matter of the brain. Many patients have evidence of plasma cell infiltrates in the kidneys or throughout the gastrointestinal tract, providing a hint to the underlying immune disorder that causes GSDM. Immunoglobulins and complement are found in the spinal cord lesions of dogs with this disorder.

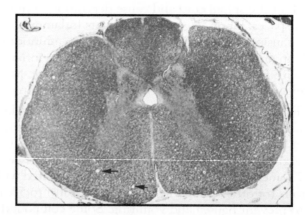

Figure 13-4 Transverse histologic section showing loss of axons and myelin leaving holes in the white matter of the spinal cord (arrows) of a German shepherd with degenerative myelopathy.

Lumbosacral Degeneration

✓ Pain associated with lumbosacral degeneration (LSD) may cause difficulty in rising, jumping into the car or onto furniture, and going up stairs. On occasion, compression of L7-S1 nerve roots may result in paraparesis with atrophy of the semimembranosis, semitendinosis, gastrocnemius, and cranial tibial muscles. **Dogs with LSD initially have lumbosacral pain, and diagnosis and treatment are discussed in Section 7.** Later in the course of the disease the nerve roots to the bladder, anus, and tail are primarily affected (Section 15).

Meningomyelitis

✓ Meningomyelitis and myelitis can cause chronic progressive paraparesis and are associated with infectious organisms as well as an unknown inflammatory process. Myelitis associated with the canine distemper virus can cause paraparesis that progresses to paraplegia within a few weeks, and the thoracic limbs may be normal or only mildly paretic. Meningomyelitis and myelitis often cause acute and chronic quadriparesis (see Sections 9 and 10). The diagnosis, treatment, and prognosis of central nervous system inflammation are discussed in Section 2, Tables 2-8 to 2-11.

Diskospondylitis

✓ Back pain is the most common initial clinical sign of thoracolumbar diskospondylitis, and difficulty rising in the pelvic limbs is often associated with pain rather than paresis. If diskospondylitis is left untreated, progressive ataxia and paraparesis can result from spinal cord compression due to inflammation and swelling of the intervertebral disk and surrounding tissues. **Diagnosis, treatment, and prognosis of diskospondylitis are discussed in Section 7.**

Hemivertebra and Other Vertebral Malformations

✓ Vertebral malformations are seen most commonly in the thoracic vertebral column of brachycephalic dogs, such as Boston terriers, pugs, and English and French bulldogs. Such malformations include hemivertebrae (Figure 13-5), butterfly vertebra, transitional vertebrae, and block vertebrae. Although usually an incidental radiographic finding, these malformations occasionally cause scoliosis and compression of the spinal cord. Ataxia and paraparesis may worsen as the animal grows as a result of increasing compression or tethering (stretching from tying down of the cauda equina) of the spinal cord. The lesion may not necessarily cause pain. Although vertebral malformation is obvious on routine radiographs, spinal cord compression is visualized with myelography and CT or MRI (Figure 13-6). **Decompression of the spinal cord can be attempted but may worsen the paraparesis or paraplegia.** Some animals with chronic compression have concurrent syringomyelia, hydromyelia, or spinal cord atrophy, which complicates therapy and recovery.

✓ Spina bifida or incomplete fusion of the dorsal spinous process may be found on routine radiography and CT. Myelography or MRI may demonstrate a meningeal sac (meningocele) protruding through the dorsal opening in the vertebra. Progressive paraparesis can result. Spina bifida is most common in the sacral region (Section 15) but occurs in the thoracic area as well.

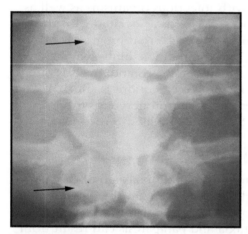

Figure 13-5
Ventrodorsal radiograph of hemivertebrae (arrows).

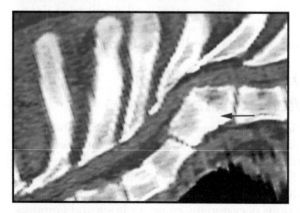

Figure 13-6
Reconstructed sagittal CT image of the spinal column of the dog in Figure 13-5 showing the hemivertebrae and spinal cord compression at the arrow.

Neoplasia

✓ Vertebral osteochondromas are benign, proliferative masses of cartilage and bone that occur at metaphyseal growth plates. Osteochondromas of the thoracolumbar vertebrae may compress the spinal cord and cause progressive paraparesis in young, growing animals. Occurrence at multiple skeletal sites is referred to as multiple cartilaginous exostoses. Pain can often be localized to the site of the lesion. Radiodense circular lesions protruding from the vertebra into the spinal canal may be seen on routine vertebral column radiographs. Myelography and MRI document spinal cord compression. CT with or without myelography can be useful to show the extent of the osteochondroma.

♥ Growth of the osteochondroma may stop when the animal reaches skeletal maturity. Those without spinal cord compression may not require therapeutic intervention. **However, for paraparetic animals with significant spinal cord compression from osteochondroma, decompressive laminectomy with removal of the mass results in improvement of the paraparesis and recovery within a few months.** Histologic examination of the mass is important to confirm the diagnosis and to differentiate osteochondroma from a malignant neoplasm. Malignant transformation of osteochondromas is rare but has been reported in dogs. Osteochondromas may be an inherited disorder in dogs.

✓ Chronic progressive paraparesis may be associated with a vertebral or extradural, intradural, or intramedullary spinal cord tumor. Tumors of the vertebrae and those that affect the meninges and nerve roots cause pain and are described in Section 7. Lymphoma commonly causes painful progressive paraparesis in cats. Neoplastic lymphocytes may be found on analysis of lumbar CSF. Myelography and MRI demonstrate spinal cord compression and aspiration of the mass can be attempted for cytologic evaluation.

♥ **Surgical resection of the mass followed by chemotherapy or radiation therapy may improve paresis and prolong the survival time of both dogs and cats with spinal cord neoplasia.** Diagnosis and treatment of spinal cord tumors are discussed in Section 10.

Spinal Cord Cysts

✓ Epidermoid, dermoid, and arachnoid cysts may compress the spinal cord and cause progressive paraparesis or quadriparesis, depending on their location, in dogs and cats. During fetal development, adjacent skin-determining ectoderm and mesoderm remain attached to the neural tube and become enclosed in the meninges, brain, or spinal cord as they form. Epidermoid cysts are lined with squamous cell epithelium, contain keratin and a few inflammatory cells, and are usually intramedullary (located within the spinal cord). Dermoid cysts have a more complex wall and are filled with sebaceous glands, sweat glands, and hair follicles. A dermoid cyst may have a draining tract that communicates with the skin; such cysts are called a dermoid sinus. Although dermoid cysts are common in Rhodesian ridgebacks, they rarely cause spinal cord compression and paraparesis. Arachnoid cysts usually form in the meninges on the dorsal midline and can cause intradural-extramedullary compression of the spinal cord; they may also be an incidental finding. Arachnoid cysts are filled with CSF. Spinal dysraphia (incomplete closure of the neural tube) may accompany arachnoid cysts, as a congenital defect. Clinical signs may occur in adult dogs, indicating that the cysts may enlarge over time.

✓ Cysts may be visible on myelography, and CT following myelography may further delineate the degree of spinal cord compression. MRI is superior to visualize the extent of the cyst and associated spinal dysraphia.

♥ **Decompressive surgery through dorsal laminectomy (see Section 12, Figure 12-7) and removal of an arachnoid cyst may result in complete recovery.** Epidermoid cysts may be more difficult to completely remove, and although they may improve, neurologic signs may recur.

Lysosomal Storage Disorders

✓ Lysosomal storage disorders result from congenital absence or inactivity of a specific lysosomal enzyme. The substrate normally metabolized by that enzyme accumulates within cells, ultimately causing their death. The clinical signs vary with different enzyme deficiencies. The types of lysosomal storage disorders that cause progressive paraparesis are listed in Section 2, Table 2-15. There is no treatment.

Neuromuscular Disorders

Polyradiculoneuritis/Myositis

✓ Puppies as young as 4 weeks of age may develop progressive asymmetric or symmetric paraparesis and a "bunny-hopping" gait from *Toxoplasma gondii* and *Neospora caninum* infections of the lumbosacral nerve roots and muscles (polyradiculomyositis).

Although affected limbs have no spinal reflexes, they are stiff because of muscle fibrosis and tendon contracture. Diffuse fibrillation potentials and trains of positive sharp waves are found in the lumbar paravertebral and pelvic limb musculature. CSF analysis may show leukocytic pleocytosis and/or an elevated protein level. The diagnosis is suspected from the history and clinical findings, but serum and CSF immunoassays and histologic examination of a muscle biopsy can confirm the diagnosis. Serum titers for *T. gondii* and *N. caninum* may be elevated. A polymerase chain reaction test for the organisms may be more sensitive if available. Organisms are occasionally found within muscle biopsy sections.

✓ Early treatment with trimethoprim-sulfadiazine 15–30 mg/kg PO every 12 hours or ormetoprim-sulfadimethoxine (Primor, Pfizer) 15 mg/kg PO every 12 hours and clindamycin (Antirobe, Pfizer) 5–10 mg/kg PO every 12 hours may result in some improvement. Pyrimethamine (Daraprim, Glaxo Wellcome) 0.5–1.0 mg/kg PO once daily for 3 days then reduced to 0.25 mg/kg once daily for 14 days may be added to trimethoprim-sulfadiazine or ormetoprim-sulfadimethoxine therapy. Pyrimethamine may cause bone marrow suppression in small animals so blood counts must be carefully monitored. Improvement with early treatment may be seen, but recovery is often incomplete.

Other Polyneuropathies and Polymopathies

Some polyneuropathies and polymyopathies may initially appear to affect only the pelvic limbs and cause chronic progressive paraparesis with little thoracic limb paresis. The patellar reflex may be the only spinal reflex that is depressed or absent on the neurologic examination. Conscious proprioceptive deficits in the pelvic limbs and loss of the cutaneous trunci response often occur in animals with polyneuropathy. However, conscious proprioception and spinal reflexes are often normal in animals with polymyopathies. Positive waves and fibrillation potentials may be found in all paravertebral and pelvic and thoracic limb musculature on EMG. The diagnosis is confirmed by histologic examination of a nerve or muscle biopsy. Chronic progressive polyneuropathies are discussed in Section 10, because they eventually produce quadriparesis, and polymyopathies in Section 11, because they are often associated with episodic or exercise-induced weakness.

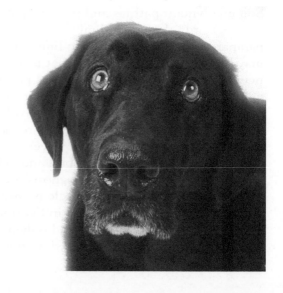

Section 14

Monoparesis or Monoplegia

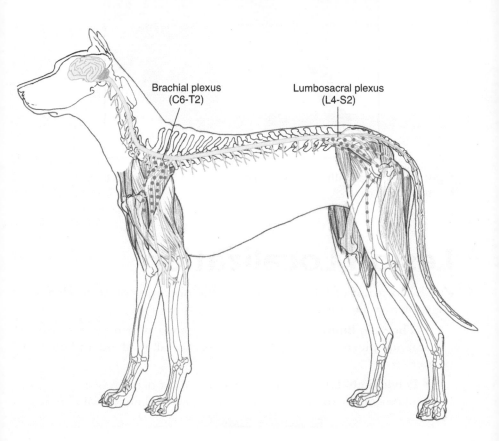

Brachial plexus
(C6-T2)

Lumbosacral plexus
(L4-S2)

Definitions

Monoparesis: Weakness of one thoracic or pelvic limb.

Monoplegia: Loss of voluntary movement of one thoracic or pelvic limb (Figure 14-1).

Nerve root avulsion: Tearing of the nerve roots from the spinal cord, as with brachial plexus avulsion.

Paresthesia: Abnormal burning or tingling; often affects limbs and feet and manifests as self-mutilation.

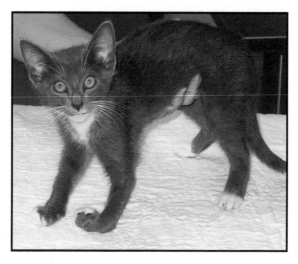

Figure 14-1 A cat with paralysis of the left thoracic limb from a traumatic brachial plexus injury.

Lesion Localization

✓ The location of lesions that cause monoparesis or monoplegia are shown in Figure 14-2. These locations are the:

- **Thoracic limb:** C6-T2 spinal cord segments or nerve roots; brachial plexus; or musculocutaneous, radial, median, and ulnar nerves

- **Pelvic limb:** L4-S2 spinal cord segments or nerve roots; lumbosacral plexus; or femoral, sciatic, peroneal and tibial nerves

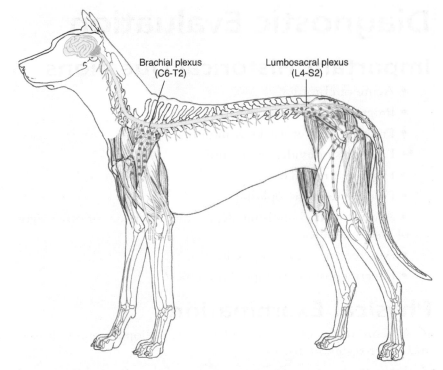

Figure 14-2 Monoparesis or monoplegia are most frequently caused by a lesion of the brachial plexus or lumbosacral plexus and their associated nerves (dots indicate lesion localization) and on rare occasions their associated spinal cord segments.

Differential Diagnosis

Acute Nonprogressive Monoparesis or Monoplegia

✓ Trauma—common in dogs and cats

✓ Fibrocartilagenous embolism—common in dogs, rare in cats

✓ Thromboembolism—occasional in cats, rare in dogs

Chronic Progressive Monoparesis or Monoplegia

✓ Degenerative intervertebral disk disease—occasional in dogs, rare in cats

✓ Neoplasia of nerve roots and peripheral nerves—occasional in dogs and rare in cats

Diagnostic Evaluation

Important Historical Questions

- Acute or chronic?
- Progressive or nonprogressive?
- Progression over weeks or months?
- Lameness or evidence of pain?
- History of trauma?
- Past or present neoplasia?
- Any difficulty breathing, depression, anorexia, or other signs of systemic illness?
- Any recent or current medication?
- Effectiveness of attempted therapies?

Physical Examination

✓ Auscultate the chest for evidence of cardiopulmonary disease and other systemic disease.

✓ Evaluate the pulse and temperature of the affected limb.

✓ Evaluate for orthopedic disease if lame.

✓ Examine for evidence of fractures or other traumatic lesions.

✓ Palpate the axillary or inguinal regions for pain.

Neurologic Examination

Deficits associated with specific nerves are outlined in Tables 14-1 and 14-2 and may include:

✓ Loss of voluntary flexion or extension of one or more joints

✓ Inability to support weight

✓ Loss of spinal reflexes of the limb

✓ Atrophy of specific muscles

✓ Loss of pain sensation in specific dermatomes

✓ Loss of conscious proprioception in the limb

✓ Neck, back or limb pain

Table 14-1
Thoracic Limb Peripheral Nerves and Associated Signs of Dysfunction

Nerve Affected	Spinal Cord Segments and Nerve Roots	Deficits	Will Limb Support Weight?	Reduced or Absent Spinal Reflexes	Major Muscles Atrophied	Loss of Pain Sensation
Suprascapular	C6-7	Loss of shoulder extension	Yes	None	Supraspinatus Infraspinatus	None
Axillary	C6-8	Loss of shoulder flexion	Yes	Flexor of shoulder	Deltoid	Dorsolateral surface shoulder to elbow
Musculocutaneous	C6-8	Loss of elbow flexion	Yes	Biceps and flexor of elbow	Biceps	Medial surface shoulder to elbow
Radial	C7-T2	Loss of elbow, carpus and digits extension	No	Triceps and extensor carpi radialis	Triceps, extensor carpi radialis, and digital extensors	Anterior surface of limb from elbow to toes
Median	C8-T2	Loss of carpus and digit flexion	Yes	Flexor of carpus	Superficial and deep digital flexors	Posterior surface of limb from elbow to toes
Ulnar	C8-T2	Loss of carpus and digit flexion	Yes	Flexor of carpus	Deep digital flexors	Fifth digit
Lateral thoracic	C8-T1	None	Yes	Loss of cutaneous trunci response	Not obvious, cutaneous trunci muscles	None
C6-T2 spinal cord or nerve roots* or brachial plexus	C6-T2	All or variation of the above signs	Yes or No	All, or variations of the above	All, or variations of the above	All, or variations of the above

*Horner's syndrome (ptosis, miosis, and enophthalmos) is often present if the lesion affects the C6-T2 spinal cord segments or nerve roots.

Table 14-2
Pelvic Limb Peripheral Nerves and Associated Signs of Dysfunction

Nerve Affected	Spinal Cord Segments And Nerve Roots	Deficits	Will Limb Support Weight?	Reduced Or Absent Spinal Reflexes	Major Muscles Atrophied	Loss of Pain Sensation
Obturator	L4-6	Loss of adduction of hip	Yes or No	None	Pectineus, Gracillus	None
Cranial and caudal gluteal	L6-S1	Reduced hip flexion	Yes	Reduced flexor of the hip	Gluteals	None
Femoral	L4-5	Loss of extension of the stifle	No	Patellar	Quadriceps	Medial surface of thigh and leg
Sciatic	L6-S2	Loss of extension of the hip, hock, tarsus, and digits and flexion of the stifle, hock, tarsus, and digits	Yes	Flexor, sciatic, cranial tibial and gastrocnemius	Biceps femoris Semimembranosis Semitendinosis Cranial tibial Gastrocnemius	Entire limb except medial surface of thigh and leg
Peroneal (Fibular)	L6-S2	Loss of extension of the hock, tarsus, and digits	Yes	Cranial tibial	Cranial tibial	Anterior surface of leg below the stifle
Tibial	L6-S2	Loss of flexion of the hock, tarsus, and digits	Yes	Flexor of hock and tarsus and gastrocnemius	Gastrocnemius	Posterior surface of leg below the stifle

Applicable Diagnostic Tests

✓ A complete blood count, serum chemistry profile, and urinalysis are performed to detect systemic illness and as part of the preanesthetic evaluation.

✓ Thoracic and abdominal radiographs and abdominal ultrasonography are indicated if neoplasia is suspected or if abnormalities are found on the physical examination.

✓ Thoracic radiographs show cardiac enlargement with or without pulmonary edema in cats with cardiomyopathy.

✓ A Doppler-flow sensing device placed on the dorsomedial region of the metatarsals or the palmer surface of the metacarpals can be used to evaluate blood flow in distal limbs.

✓ Electrocardiography and echocardiography can be useful to evaluate cardiomyopathy.

✓ Coagulation tests, such as activated clotting times (ACT), prothrombin time (PT), and partial thromboplastin time (PTT), may be indicated for animals with thromboembolism and no evidence of cardiac disease.

✓ The animal is anesthetized for the following tests; their potential findings are also noted:

- Electromyography (EMG) may show positive sharp waves and fibrillation potentials in the paravertebral and limb muscles associated with specific nerve involvement 7 to 10 days after onset of clinical signs.

- Nerve stimulation can be performed 72 hours after onset of clinical signs to determine nerve integrity.

- Routine radiographs may show calcified intervertebral disks, narrowed disk spaces, vertebral fractures or neoplasia.

- Myelography can be used to diagnose spinal cord compression from an intervertebral disk extrusion or protrusion or a nerve root tumor that may be growing through the intervertebral foramen into the spinal canal.

- Computed tomography (CT) and magnetic resonance imaging (MRI) can be useful to detect nerve root tumors, intervertebral disk disease, vertebral fractures, hemorrhage, or fibrocartilaginous embolism.

Disorders Causing Monoplegia or Monoparesis

Nerve Root, Plexus, or Nerve Trauma

♥ Trauma is the most common cause of acute monoparesis or monoplegia. Injury of the brachial plexus and subsequent paralysis of one thoracic limb is the most common type of trauma and is frequently seen after motor vehicle accidents (Figure 14-1). If the nerve roots of the brachial plexus are torn from the spinal cord (avulsion), Horner's syndrome of the eye, and loss of the cutaneous trunci reflex on the same side as the monoplegia are usually present (Section 6, Figure 6-8). In some cases of brachial plexus injury, the musculocutaneous nerve is spared and the limb is held flexed at the elbow. The type of nerve injuries and prognosis are outlined in Table 14-3.

Table 14-3
Types of Nerve Injury and Prognosis

- **Neurapraxia (axonapraxia):** Failure of nerve function in the absence of structural change due to blunt trauma, compression, or ischemia; **return to function normally ensues**.

- **Axonotmesis:** Disruption of the axon and myelin sheath with preservation of connective tissue fragments, resulting in degeneration of the axon distal to the injury site (Wallerian degeneration); regeneration of the axon is spontaneous and often of good quality.

- **Neurotmesis:** Partial or complete severance of a nerve, with disruption of the axon, its myelin sheath, and the connective tissue elements; **regeneration cannot occur unless the nerve segments are surgically reattached**.

✓ Most nerve injuries are caused by neurapraxia or neurapraxia and axonotmesis combined. Initially, all types of nerve injury can cause monoplegia with loss of superficial and deep pain sensations. If the deep pain response is present in all the digits, then the nerve is intact and chances for recovery are good. Since the prognosis varies with the nerve and type of injury, the EMG can be useful to determine which nerves have been injured and what type of injury has been sustained (Table 14-4).

Table 14-4
EMG Differentiation of Nerve Injuries

TYPE OF NERVE INJURY	EMG FIVE OR MORE DAYS AFTER INJURY	RESPONSE TO MOTOR NERVE STIMULATION
Neurapraxia	Normal	Normal
Axonotmesis	Positive sharp waves and fibrillation potentials in affected muscles	May have normal or slowed motor nerve conduction velocity
Neurotmesis	Positive sharp waves and fibrillation potentials in affected muscles	None

☡ The length of time for neurapraxia to resolve varies with the severity of the injury and may range from a few days to a few weeks. Although nerves with axonotmesis can regenerate, the distance between the site of the nerve injury and muscle must also be considered in the prognosis. Nerves grow approximately 2.5 cm/month, but after approximately 6 months neural sheath shrinkage and neurogenic muscle atrophy may inhibit further progress. Nerves injured greater than 15 cm proximal to the muscle may not be able to regenerate to the extent necessary to reach the muscle. If they do, their distal conduction times may be so slow that function is greatly impaired.

✓ If EMG is unavailable, serial neurologic examinations can be performed every month for the first 4 months. If monoplegia with absent superficial or deep pain response is still present 4 months after the injury, then recovery is unlikely.

♥ Routine radiographs, CT, or MRI may be useful to identify concurrent fractures or hemorrhage but can be normal. **Physical therapy is essential for recovery.** Tendon contracture can inhibit normal function even if the nerves regenerate. Manually flexing and extending affected joints and massaging all affected muscles for at least 15 minutes three times daily is recommended. If the limb drags on the ground, it should be placed in a sling tied around the animal's neck or covered with a protective boot to prevent injury. Splinting the limb may interfere with circulation and worsen the muscle damage.

✓ If brachial plexus avulsion has occurred, then recovery is unlikely (Figure 14-3). If the limb is placed in a sling, tendon contracture will occur within 3 to 6 months. The limb must be kept flexed so it does not drag on the ground and limb amputation can be avoided; however, some owners prefer limb amputation for esthetic reasons.

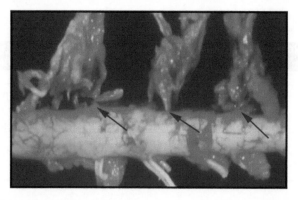

Figure 14-3 Necropsy specimen from a dog in which the brachial plexus has been torn from the spinal cord (arrows)

Fibrocartilaginous Embolism

✓ A small, unilateral infarction of the gray matter in the C6-T2 or L4-S2 spinal cord segments can cause paresis or paralysis of what appears to be just one limb. However, closer neurologic examination usually shows that the other limbs are affected to a lesser degree. The diagnosis and prognosis of fibrocartilaginous embolism of the spinal cord are discussed in Section 9.

Thromboembolism

✓ Thromboembolism of the aorta or iliac arteries (saddle thrombus) is common in cats but rare in dogs. This disorder typically causes acute paraplegia. Occasionally, one pelvic or thoracic limb may be affected. In cats, thromboembolism is often associated with hypertrophic cardiomyopathy. Coagulation tests, such as ACT, PT, and PTT, may be abnormal in other animals with thromboembolism. Tumor emboli can affect the blood supply to a limb and cause acute monoparesis or monoplegia. Diagnosis and treatment of thromboembolism are discussed in Section 12.

Degenerative Intervertebral Disk Disease

✓ Lameness of one limb that progresses over several days or weeks to monoparesis, decreased spinal reflexes, and muscle atrophy may be associated with lateralized Type I or Type II intervertebral disk extrusion or protrusion (Section 7, Figures 7-4 and 7-5). Neck or back pain is often associated with the limb dysfunction. The diagnosis is often best made with CT or MRI, as a myelogram may be normal. Surgical removal of the disk material is usually necessary, and the prognosis for recovery is excellent. Intervertebral disk disease is discussed further in Sections 7, 9, 10, 12, and 13.

Neoplasia

✓ Lameness of one limb that progresses over several weeks or months to paresis, reduction of spinal reflexes, and muscle atrophy may be associated with neoplasia of the nerve roots, plexus, or individual nerves. Pain is often detected on palpation of the neck, axilla, back, or inguinal regions, and paresis of other limbs often develops with time. Tumors of the peripheral nerve sheath (neurofibroma, schwannoma, neurofibrosarcoma) are the most common neoplasms identified. The diagnosis can be elusive until the tumor reaches a detectable size. The EMG can be useful to identify the presence of a nerve root or peripheral nerve disorder in animals with lameness and to determine which nerves are affected. Enlarged nerves may be visualized with MRI (Figure 14-4). Treatment of peripheral nerve sheath tumors entails removal of the tumor and nerve. However, if a plexus or many nerve roots are affected (Figure 14-5), then complete removal is often difficult and the tumor eventually grows into the spinal cord, causing quadriparesis or paraparesis (Section 10, Figures 10-4 and 10-5). Therefore, the prognosis for tumors of the plexus or nerve roots is guarded.

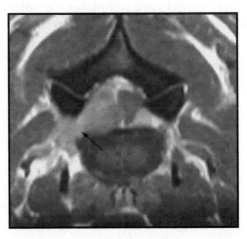

Figure 14-4 Transverse post-contrast T1-weighted MRI of a peripheral nerve sheath tumor that is growing through the intervertebral foramen and compressing the spinal cord (arrow).

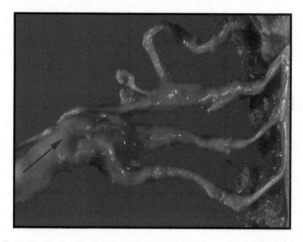

Figure 14-5 Necropsy specimen from a dog showing a peripheral nerve sheath tumor of the brachial plexus (arrows).

✓ Treatment is aimed at controlling the pain (Section 7, Table 7-2). Gabapentin (Neurontin, Parke-Davis) 6 to 15 mg/kg PO every 6 hours may be useful to reduce nerve pain; however, its expense limits its usefulness in veterinary medicine. Other new anticonvulsant drugs, like tiagabine, may be useful to control nerve pain in the future. Lymphosarcoma can infiltrate nerve roots, and other neoplastic processes may compress nerves and cause progressive paresis on one limb. Neoplasia of vertebrae can affect nerve roots and is discussed in Section 7. Other extradural and extramedullary spinal cord neoplams can affect nerve roots and cause monoparesis and are discussed in Section 10.

Section 15

Flaccid Tail, Anus, and Bladder

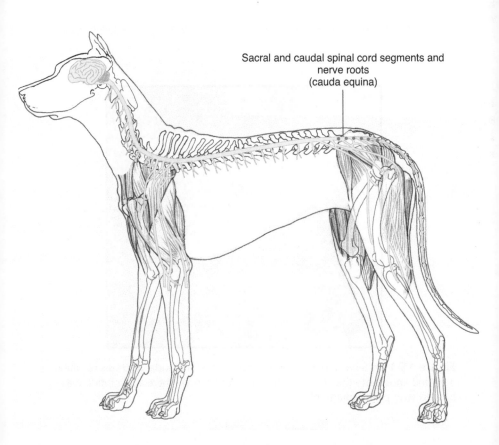

Sacral and caudal spinal cord segments and
nerve roots
(cauda equina)

Definitions

Cauda equina: The nerve roots L7-Cd5 that continue in the vertebral canal after the spinal cord has ended and before they exit after their respective vertebra; resembles a horse's tail.

Lower motor neuron (LMN) bladder: Reduced or absent tone in the detrusor and external sphincter muscles and loss of the micturition reflex.

Meningocele: A pouch of meninges and spinal fluid that herniates through a vertebral defect such as spina bifida.

Paresthesia: Abnormal burning or tingling; often affects limbs and feet and manifests as self-mutilation.

Spina bifida: Incomplete closure of the dorsal vertebral arches.

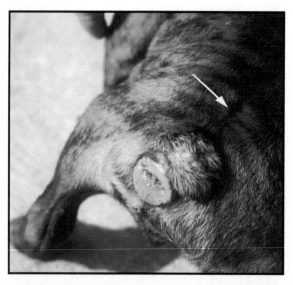

Figure 15-1 An 8-week-old bulldog puppy with sacrocaudal agenesis resulting in a dilated anus; note the abnormal hair growth (arrow) where spina bifida was located with plain radiographs.

Lesion Localization

✓ Lesions that can cause flaccid tail, anus, and bladder are located at S1-Cd5 spinal cord segments and nerve roots (Figure 15-2).

Differential Diagnosis

✓ Trauma—common in dogs and cats

✓ Lumbosacral degeneration—common in dogs

✓ Fibrocartilaginous embolism—common in dogs, rare in cats

✓ Diskospondylitis—common in dogs, rare in cats

✓ Sacrocaudal agenesis—common in Manx cats, occasional in dogs

✓ Abscess—occasional in dogs and cats

✓ Neoplasia—occasional in dogs and cats

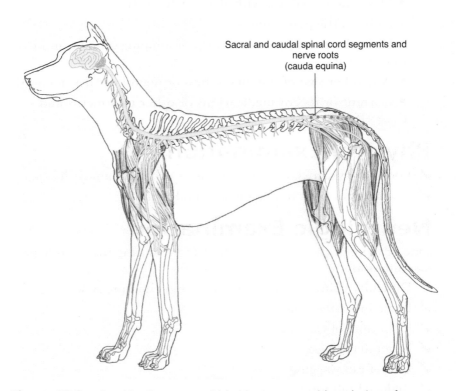

Sacral and caudal spinal cord segments and
nerve roots
(cauda equina)

Figure 15-2 A flaccid tail, anus, and bladder are caused by a lesion of the sacral and caudal spinal cord segments and nerve roots (dots indicate lesion localization).

Diagnostic Evaluation

Important Historical Questions

- Onset, course, and duration of signs?
- Painful or nonpainful?
- Is tail carriage normal?
- Does the tail wag?
- Is there straining to urinate or defecate?
- How frequent is bladder and/or bowel incontinence?
- Does the animal seem aware of the incontinence?
- Possibility of trauma? If so obtain lumbosacral radiographs.
- History of fighting or animal bites?
- Past or present neoplasia?
- Manx cat or bulldog with signs since birth?
- Lame in the pelvic limbs?
- Difficulty rising, going up stairs, or jumping onto furniture or into the car?
- Any other sign of systemic illness or neurologic dysfunction?
- Current or recent medications or other treatments and their effectiveness?

Physical Examination

✓ Look for evidence of bite wounds or other traumatic lesions.
✓ Evaluate for pain in the lumbosacral region.

Neurologic Examination

One or more of the following will be found during the neurologic examination:

✓ Difficulty rising in the pelvic limbs and climbing stairs
✓ Lame in a pelvic limb
✓ Uncurling of the tail
✓ Low tail carriage
✓ Loss of tail wagging
✓ Reduced tail tone
✓ Reduced or absent tail sensation
✓ Dilated anus

✓ Reduced or absent anal reflex

✓ Lack of anal sphincter contraction on rectal palpation

✓ Reduced or absent perineal sensation

✓ Pain on palpation of the dorsal lumbosacral vertebrae

✓ Pain on palpation of ventral surface of the lumbosacral vertebrae (per rectum)

✓ Large bladder that is easy to express in dogs but may be difficult to express in cats

✓ Loss of the micturition reflex

✓ Dribbling urine from the overflow of an engorged bladder

Applicable Diagnostic Tests

✓ A complete blood count, serum chemistry profile, and urinalysis can be useful to detect systemic illness and as part of the preanesthetic evaluation.

✓ Thoracic and abdominal radiographs and abdominal ultrasonography are indicated if neoplasia is suspected or abnormalities are found on the physical examination. Abdominal radiographs and ultrasonography may detect caudal sublumbar masses.

✓ The animal is anesthetized for the following tests; their potential results are also given:

> • An electromyogram (EMG) may show positive sharp waves and fibrillation potentials in the caudal gluteal, perineal, and tail muscles associated with specific nerve involvement 5 to 7 days after signs initially appear.

> • Nerve stimulation of the cauda equina can be performed, and evoked muscle potentials from the tail and anal sphincter are recorded to evaluate the integrity of the caudal and sacral nerve roots and nerves.

> • Routine lumbosacral radiographs can demonstrate sacrocaudal agenesis, spina bifida, spondylosis deformans, diskospondylitis, fractures or luxations, and vertebral neoplasia.

> • Lumbar cerebrospinal fluid (CSF) analysis may show neutrophilic pleocytosis in bacterial infections or elevated protein in compression lesions.

> • A myelogram may be useful to diagnose spinal cord compression from lumbosacral degeneration or a nerve root tumor, but contrast media may not descend caudally to outline the cauda equina. The extent of a meningocele may be determined with myelography.

- An epidurogram may be attempted to outline the cauda equina, but this test is often more difficult to interpret than other imaging studies and may be nondiagnostic.

- Computed tomography (CT) and magnetic resonance imaging (MRI) can be used to evaluate sacrocaudal agenesis, lumbosacral degeneration, diskospondylitis, abscesses, vertebral fractures, fibrocartilaginous embolism and neoplasia.

- Epidural needle aspirates may assist in diagnosing an abscess or epidural neoplasia, such as lymphosarcoma.

- Aspirates of the lumbosacral intervertebral disk space may be useful in the diagnosis of diskospondylitis.

✔ Urine and blood cultures and serum *Brucella canis* titers are obtained if diskospondylitis is found.

✔ Culture and sensitivity of needle aspirates or open biopsy samples should be performed if an abscess is identified.

Lumbosacral Disorders

Nerve Root Trauma

✔ Acute nerve root trauma most commonly results from fractures, luxations, or subluxation of the lumbosacral or sacral vertebrae. Such trauma is usually secondary to a motor vehicle accident. Fracture and/or luxation of the sacrocaudal junction may occur in animals that run when their tail is caught. Paralysis of the tail and urinary and fecal incontinence often result. While dogs have a flaccid urinary bladder that is easy to express, the bladder may be difficult to manually express in cats. Two radiographic views are imperative to assess the degree of displacement at the fracture site in most cases. CT can be useful to better visualize bone fragments in the spinal canal. Surgical decompression and stabilization may be required.

♥ Management consists of manual expression of the bladder and fecal evacuation if necessary. Low-dose propanolol 1.25 mg total dose PO every 8 to 12 hours may facilitate bladder expression in cats after several days of therapy. The prognosis is better if tail and perineal sensation is preserved. Sacrocaudal luxations (Figure 15-3) typically have a better prognosis for return of bowel and bladder function than do lumbosacral luxations. The tail may be permanently paralyzed and may eventually have to be amputated due to soiling or mutilation.

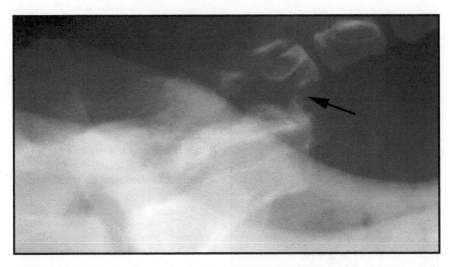

Figure 15-3 Lateral radiograph of a fracture-luxation of the caudal sacrum (arrow) causing a flaccid tail, dilated anus, and atonic bladder in a mixed-breed dog; the anal sphincter and bladder function returned over the following 3 months, but tail function did not.

Lumbosacral Degeneration

✓ Lumbosacral degeneration is common in large-breed dogs, and as discussed in Section 7, the pain associated with this disorder usually makes it difficult to rise, climb stairs, or jump onto furniture or into the car. Chronic joint instability and subluxation, proliferation of the surrounding ligaments and other soft tissues, and a Type II intervertebral disk protrusion (see Section 7, Figure 7-5) at L7-S1 produce a stenotic lumbosacral spinal canal.

✓ Affected dogs initially have low back pain (Section 7) and low tail carriage. As the disease progresses, paresis or paralysis of the tail and fecal or urinary incontinence may develop (Figure 15-4). Some dogs also bite the tail and leg and lick the genitals, which may be caused by paresthesia. Conscious proprioceptive deficits and pelvic limb paresis are rarely present. Lumbosacral radiographs and MRI often show profound changes if urinary and fecal incontinence is present (Figures 15-5 and 15-6). Surgical decompression of nerve roots if done early can result in significant improvement, but the chances for improvement decline once urinary or fecal incontinence develop. Further discussion of the diagnosis and treatment of lumbosacral degeneration is found in Section 7.

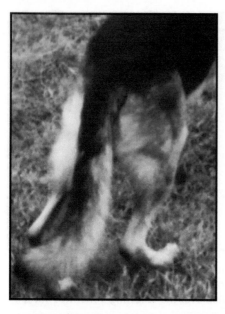

Figure 15-4
A flaccid tail and urinary and fecal
incontinence is associated with
advanced lumbosacral degeneration.

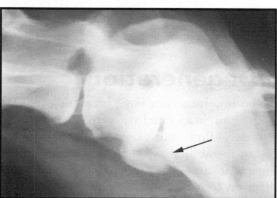

Figure 15-5
Lateral radiograph of
the spine of a dog
showing degenerative
changes in the L7-S1
vertebrae (arrows).

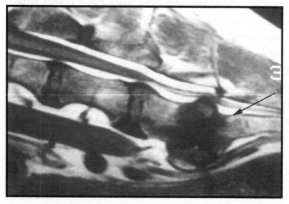

Figure 15-6
Sagittal T1-weighted MRI
of the dog in Figure 15-5
showing severe nerve
root compression over
L7-S1 resulting in fecal
and urinary incontinence
and tail paralysis.

Fibrocartilaginous Embolism

✓ Infarction of the sacrocaudal spinal cord from fibrocartilaginous emboli (FCE) can cause acute flaccid paralysis of the tail, anal sphincter, and bladder and occurs most commonly in large-breed dogs. If the infarction affects the L4-S2 spinal cord region, paraparesis or paraplegia will occur. Small dogs and cats are affected less frequently. **Diagnosis and treatment of FCE are presented in Section 9.** Although recovery is often possible, residual urinary and fecal incontinence may occur.

Diskospondylitis

✓Diskospondylitis is an infection of the vertebral endplates and intervertebral disk spaces. Vertebral osteomyelitis, or spondylitis, is an infectious process that affects the vertebral bodies. Diskospondylitis and spondylitis are usually caused by bacterial infection and are infrequently caused by a fungal infection such as aspergillosis,and migrations of foreign bodies (e.g. grass awns). Staphylococcal infections are most common and probably gain entrance by a hematogenous route. Pre-existing or concurrent skin, urinary tract, or cardiopulmonary infections are often present. Pain is located at the site of the affected vertebrae. Multiple vertebral sites may be involved, but the lumbosacral region is commonly affected (see Section 7, Figures 7-12, 7-13, and 7-14). If significant inflammation and compression of sacrocaudal nerve roots occurs, then a flaccid tail, anus, and bladder may result. **Diagnosis and treatment of diskospondylitis are discussed in Section 7.**

Sacrocaudal Agenesis

✓ Manx kittens and English bulldog puppies may present with fecal and urinary incontinence associated with a deformity of the sacrum and associated nerve roots. Spina bifida, or incomplete closure of the dorsal vertebral arches, is often present. The cauda equina is usually undeveloped and may be found within a meningocele. Innervation of the anus and bladder is reduced or absent. An abnormal hair pattern over the dorsal midline of the lumbosacral region and a palpable absence of the dorsal spinous process of the sacrum may be found on physical examination (Figure 15-1). There may be associated malformation of the lumbar spinal cord, so pelvic limb ataxia or paraparesis may also be present. The sacrocaudal agenesis can be seen on routine radiographs and CT or MRI.

There is no treatment to correct the malformation in most animals. Manual bladder expression and assistance to defecate must be performed. Chronic bladder infections must be treated with antibiotic therapy.

Bite Wound Abscess

✓ A flaccid tail, anus, and bladder may be associated with a focal bacterial epidural abscess of the nerve roots of the cauda equina secondary to a bite wound around the tailhead. Aspiration and culture of exudates from the epidural space confirm the diagnosis and assist in antibiotic selection. **Antibiotic therapy for bacterial infections is described with meningoencephalitis in Section 2, Table 2-11.** Antibiotics should be given for 4 to 6 weeks, and the prognosis for recovery can be good. Laminectomy for removal of debris is rarely necessary.

Neoplasia

✓ Neoplasia of the vertebrae, meninges, or nerve roots of the cauda equina can cause lumbosacral pain as well as flaccid tail, anus, and bladder. Lymphoma localized in the cauda equina is common in cats but only occurs occasionally in dogs. Bone and soft tissue changes can be best visualized with CT and MRI, respectively. Surgical removal, chemotherapy, and radiation therapy may improve the pain and prolong the survival time in both dogs and cats with neoplasia affecting the cauda equina. **Diagnosis and treatment of vertebral and spinal cord tumors are discussed in Sections 7 and 10; nerve root neoplasia is discussed in Section 14.**

Miscellaneous Neurologic Syndromes

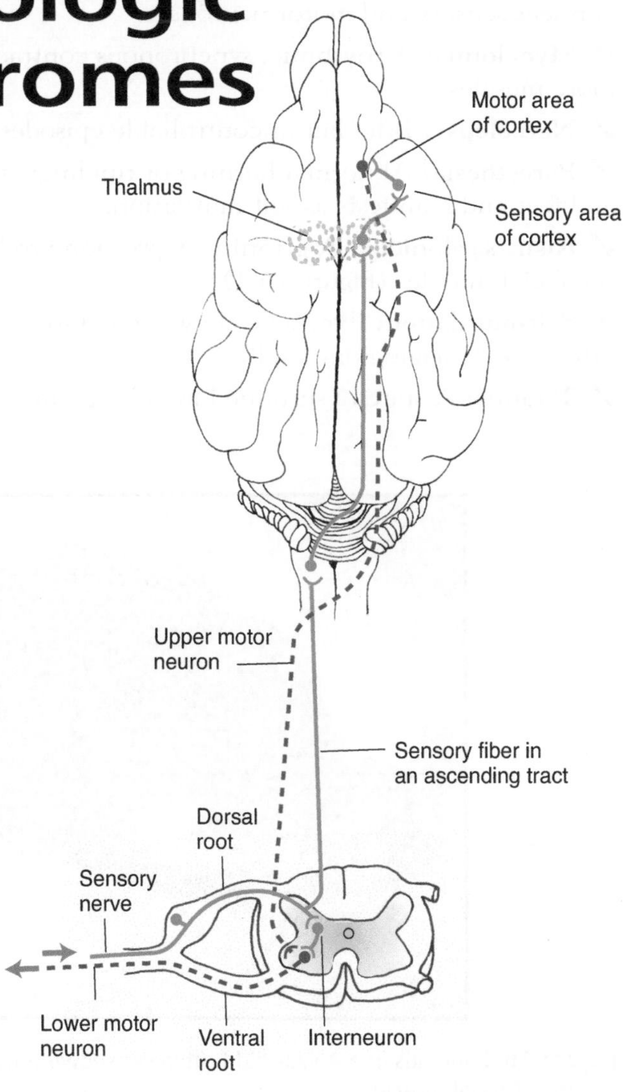

Motor area
of cortex

Thalmus

Sensory area
of cortex

Upper motor
neuron

Sensory fiber in
an ascending tract

Dorsal
root

Sensory
nerve

Lower motor
neuron

Ventral
root

Interneuron

Definitions

✓ **Cataplexy:** Abrupt attacks of weakness and loss of muscle tone triggered by emotional stimuli; a symptom of narcolepsy.

✓ **Episodic dyskinesia:** Involuntary, irregular contraction of trunk and limb muscles.

✓ **Hyperesthesia:** Increased sensitivity to stimulation resulting in a negative behavioral reaction.

✓ **Interneurons:** Neurons within the brain and spinal cord that connect sensory and motor neurons.

✓ **Myoclonus:** A rhythmic, synchronous contraction of one or more muscles.

✓ **Narcolepsy:** Brief but uncontrollable episodes of sleep.

✓ **Paresthesia:** Abnormal burning or tingling; often affects limbs and feet and manifests as self-mutilation.

✓ **Risus sardonicus:** A grinning expression produced by spasm of the facial muscles (Figure 16-1).

✓ **Self-mutilation:** Excessive chewing, licking, rubbing, or otherwise damaging one's self.

✓ **Tetanus:** A state of sustained muscle spasm.

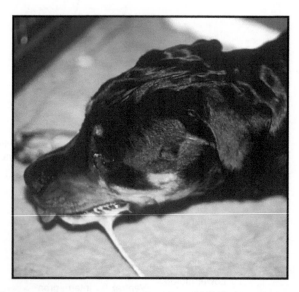

Figure 16-1 Tetanus in a 4-year-old Rottweiler showing the characteristic spasms of facial muscles.

Some distinct neurologic disorders in dogs and cats may be diagnosed on the basis of their characteristic clinical appearance. They include:

✓ **Tetanus**–rare in dogs and cats

✓ **Distemper myoclonus**–rare in dogs

✓ **Muscle cramping syndromes**–rare in dogs

✓ **Hyperesthesia and self-mutilation syndromes**–rare in dogs and cats

✓ **Dancing Doberman disease**–rare in Doberman pinschers

✓ **Narcolepsy**–rare in dogs

✓ **Rapid-eye-movement (REM) behavior disorder**–rare in dogs and cats

Lesion Localization

✓ **Tetanus:** Inhibitory interneurons of the brain stem and spinal cord

✓ **Distemper myoclonus:** Interneurons of the brainstem and spinal cord

✓ **Muscle cramping syndromes**

- Muscle
- Inhibitory interneurons of the brainstem and spinal cord
- Basal nuclei

✓ **Hyperesthesia and Self-Mutilation**

- Sensory peripheral nerves or sensory regions of the brainstem
- Muscle
- Anxiety disorder with associated neurochemical and neuro-hormonal imbalances

✓ **Dancing Doberman Disease**

- Gastrocnemius muscle

✓ **Narcolepsy:** Brainstem sleep centers

✓ **REM behavior disorder:** Brainstem sleep centers

Diagnostic Evaluation

✓ Because of the diversity of these disorders, the important historical questions, physical and neurologic examination findings, and possible diagnostic tests will be discussed with each disorder.

Miscellaneous Disorders

Tetanus

The bacteria *Clostridium tetani* usually gains entrance to the body through an external wound, although iatrogenic infection with improperly sterilized surgical instruments has been reported. The bacteria release a toxin that blocks inhibitory neurons in the brainstem and spinal cord, causing focal and generalized continuous muscle spasms. The characteristic contracture of facial muscles has been referred to as "risus sardonicus" (Figure 16-1). Masticatory and pharyngeal muscle spasms may lead to difficulty opening the mouth and dysphagia. Often, the ears are held erect and the nictitating membranes protrude or rhythmically contract. The limbs may be stiff as well and assume a saw horse stance. The diagnosis is based on the characteristic clinical appearance. Some dogs and particularly cats may develop focal tetanus, which causes stiffness or rigidity in one limb.

♥ Penicillin G procaine at 20,000–50,000 IU/kg IV is given every 4 hours to kill remaining bacteria. To control muscle spasms, methocarbamol (Robaxin, Robins) 55–220 mg/kg IV (not to exceed 330 mg/kg/day) may be given. One half the calculated dose is given rapidly, followed by slow administration after the animal relaxes. Diazepam 0.5 mg/kg not to exceed 10 mg every 4-6 hours IV, IM or rectally may be tried if methocarbamol does not control spasms. A diazepam constant rate infusion may be given as outlined in Section 3, Table 3-5. Stimulation by touch, light, and sound often induce muscle spasms and should be avoided. Intravenous tetanus antitoxin is given as soon as possible after diagnosis. A test dose of 0.1 to 0.2 ml SQ of equine origin tetanus antitoxin may be given, and if no adverse reaction occurs within 30 minutes, 100–1000 IU/kg/day IV is administered for dogs and cats. Intravenous fluids and supportive care are given until the effects of the toxin dissipate, which may be weeks. Muscle spasms associated with mastication, swallowing, and respiration can result in debilitation and necessitate intensive care. Dogs and cats that are focally affected often recover, but recovery may take weeks.

Canine Distemper Myoclonus

✓ A nonpainful, persistent, rhythmic contraction of a group of muscles, which continues even during sleep, may occur in dogs with an active or past infection with the canine distemper virus. The viral infection leads to a pacemaker-like electrical circuit in the spinal cord. Myoclonus or continuous rhythmic contractions of facial, masticatory, cervical, limbs, or other muscles can occur. Other signs of meningoencephalitis may be present (Section 2), or affected dogs may appear otherwise normal. Procainamide HCl (Pronestyl, Princeton) 6–8 mg/kg IV given over a 5-minute period (while monitoring the ECG) will minimize or eliminate the myoclonus. Procainamide (Procanbid, Monarch) 8–20 mg/kg PO every 12 hours may reduce myoclonus in mild cases but dogs should be closely monitored for adverse reactions. Although some animals can function well as pets, no treatment may be effective in severely affected animals and euthanasia may be required. Myoclonus can become less severe over a period of years after infection.

Muscle Cramping Syndromes

✓ Scottish terriers may develop a recessively inherited disorder characterized by muscle cramping with exercise, excitement, or cold, often before 6 months of age. Controlling environmental triggers and administering vitamin E 25 IU/kg/day PO may reduce or eliminate the muscle cramps. Diazepam 0.5 mg/kg PO every 8 hours may be used to control cramping if needed. Similar conditions have been reported in Dalmatians and Norwich terriers. Greyhounds may develop severe muscle cramping when racing after a prolonged period of rest that can lead to rhabdomyolysis and myoglobinuria. Episodic dyskinesia is associated with involuntary muscle contractions. Although rare, dyskinesia can be differentiated from seizures because there is no prodrome, autonomic signs, or postictal phase, and dyskinesia does not respond to anticonvulsant drugs. Excitement may initiate muscle cramping due to polymyopathy in Cavalier King Charles spaniels (Section 11). Myotonic myopathies may also cause muscle cramping and delayed relaxation after excitement (Section 11).

Hyperesthesia and Self-Mutilation

✓ Feline hyperesthesia syndrome is associated with twitching, rippling, or rolling of the skin along the thoracolumbar region. These signs are accompanied by vocalization, hysteria, and self-mutilation. Affected cats are hyperesthetic to light touching in the thoracolumbar region, and this may elicit the clinical signs. Paresthesias of unknown etiology are suspected to be the cause. Myopathy of the lumbar muscles has been documented in some cats, so electromyography and muscle biopsies of this region may be considered. Obsessive chin rubbing and tail chasing with or without mutilation are also observed in both dogs and cats. Sensory neuropathies, myopathies, hormonal imbalances, and psychological factors have all been suspected as the cause, but the exact mechanism is unknown. The best therapies appear to be those used to treat compulsive behavior disorders. Oral imiprimine (Tofranil, Novartis) 0.5–2 mg/kg every 8 to 12 hours in dogs or cats, clomipramine (Clomacalm, Pfizer) 1–3 mg/kg every 12 hours for dogs, fluoxetine (Prozac, Dista) 1 mg/kg every 24 hours in dogs, or buspirone (BuSpar, Bristol Myers Squibb) 2.5–15 mg every 8 to 12 hours in dogs or cats may be tried. Environmental changes, such as getting the pet a companion, increasing its exercise, or enriching the environment in other ways, may also alter the behavior. Behavior modification in conjunction with a pharmacologic therapy should be considered, although the response varies.

✓ Congenital sensory neuropathies that results in mutilation of the paws may occur in English setters, German shorthaired pointers, Dachshunds, and other dogs. There is no known effective treatment. Sensory neuropathies may be acquired secondary to neuronal damage from the canine distemper or herpes (pseudorabies) viruses, an extruded intervertebral disk, trauma, or neoplasia. Paresthesias are suspected to provoke licking and chewing of the affected area. Oral diphenylhydantoin (Dilantin, Parke-Davis) 25 to 30 mg/kg every 6 hours in dogs or gabapentin (Neurontin, Parke-Davis) 6 to 15 mg/kg every 6 hours in dogs may be tried to reduce the clinical signs associated with acquired sensory neuropathies. The expense of gabapentin may limit its use. Acupuncture may provide some relief from suspected paresthesias. Self-mutilation associated with intervertebral disk extrusion or protrusion, nerve injury, or neoplasia may improve over time or with correction of the underlying problem. If the underlying cause of acquired sensory neuropathy cannot be corrected, the prognosis is usually guarded.

Dancing Doberman Disease

✓ A breed-specific gastrocnemius myopathy occurs in Doberman pinschers from 1 to 10 years of age. Initially, one pelvic limb is affected and when the dog is standing still, the limb is held in flexion (Figure 16-2). The dog is not lame or paretic and usually has a normal gait. Over the ensuing months, the second pelvic limb may become affected, and when standing, the dog will alternately lift each pelvic limb in a dancing motion and then sit down. Positive sharp waves and fibrillation potentials are often found during electromyography of the gastrocnemius muscles. Myodegeneration is seen on histologic examination of the gastrocnemius muscle. There is no known treatment. No dogs have been known to spontaneously recover, but affected dogs can be acceptable pets.

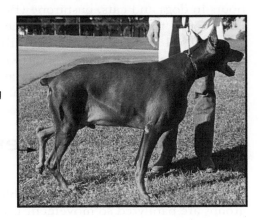

Figure 16-2 A 7-year-old male Doberman pinscher with dancing Doberman disease; note the flexion of the left pelvic limb at rest (arrow).

Narcolepsy

📖 Narcolepsy is an inherited or acquired REM sleep disorder (Table 16-1) that has been reported in many different breeds of dogs, a few mixed-breed dogs, and one cat. In Doberman pinschers and Labrador retrievers, this disorder is inherited as an autosomal dominant trait with incomplete penetrance and the initial clinical signs begin between 1 to 4 months of age. In other dogs, narcolepsy can be acquired late in life as the result of brain inflammation, injury, or neoplasia that may damage the brainstem areas responsible for normal sleep. Primary signs of narcolepsy include excessive daytime sleepiness, cataplexy, REM sleep at sleep onset, sleep paralysis, and hypnagogic hallucinations. Behavioral and polysomnography (PSG) studies indicate that dogs experience all signs of narcolepsy.

✓ Cataplexy is an acute loss of muscle tone and is the most common reason narcoleptic dogs are presented to veterinarians.

✓ Attacks of cataplexy are usually initiated by something exciting or pleasurable like food, play, greeting owners, or sex, not by negative or painful stimuli. The severity of signs varies from acute, episodic, brief periods of pelvic limb and neck collapse to acute onset of REM sleep with flaccid (areflexia) quadriplegia and twitching of eyelid and limb muscles. Affected animals may be awakened from severe attacks and appear normal between attacks but may sleep more during the day. The diagnosis is usually based on the characteristic clinical signs.

✓ Drugs that may minimize or abolish cataplexy include oral imiprimine (Tofranil, Novartis) 0.5–2 mg/kg every 8 to 12 hours in dogs or cats, clomipramine (Clomacalm, Pfizer) 1–3 mg/kg every 12 hours in dogs, fluoxetine (Prozac) 1 mg/kg every 24 hours in dogs and cats, buspirone (BuSpar) 2.5–10 mg in dogs or cats every 8 to 12 hours, or selegiline hydrochloride (Anipryl, Pfizer) 0.5–1.0 mg/kg once daily in the morning in dogs. Methylphenedate (Ritalin, Novartis) 0.25 mg/kg PO every 12 to 24 hours may be tried if excessive daytime sleepiness appears to be a problem. Response to treatment varies. Congenital narcolepsy in dogs stabilizes and does not worsen with age.

Rapid-Eye-Movement Behavior Disorder

✓ During normal REM sleep (Table 16-1), the major muscle groups are paralyzed so movement is minimal (Figure 16-1). If the inhibitory system originating in the brainstem becomes nonfunctional, significant motor activity can be released during REM sleep and result in REM behavior disorder. This disorder has been described in dogs and cats. Several golden retrievers have been affected since puppyhood. Other dogs and cats seem to develop the problem later in life.

✓ During REM sleep, movements may be so violent that the animal is propelled out of bed or across the floor. A few dogs become aggressive and will growl, bite blankets, or briefly attack but quickly awaken, and the aggression passes. However, as many animals sleep in the same bed or room as their owners, the disturbance may become difficult to bear. In addition, some animals may urinate during these episodes, which makes them even less tolerable.

Table 16-1
Basic Sleep Facts

- **Phase I:** The brain and muscles are relaxed.

- **Phase II:** The brain is very active, but the major muscles of the body are paralyzed so that only minor muscle twitching, paddling of the feet, and brief whimpering occur. Also known as rapid-eye-movement sleep because the eye muscles can be observed to twitch during this period.

- **Polysomnography (PSG):** Recording of the electroencephalogram, electromyogram, electro-oculogram, electrocardiogram, and respiratory parameters during sleep; used to objectively determine the phase of sleep.

✓ REM behavior disorders can be differentiated from nocturnal seizures by observation and PSG. With REM behavior disorder, animals appear normal when aroused. Abnormal events may not occur every time the animal is in REM sleep. Potassium bromide (KBr) 22–44 mg/kg PO every 12 hours has been the most effective treatment for controlling the signs in dogs. However, improvement may not occur for 1 to 2 months after KBr therapy is initiated. Oral gabapentin (Neurontin, Parke-Davis) 7.5–20 mg/kg in dogs or oral clonazepam (Klonopin, Roche) 0.01–0.1 mg/kg in dogs or cats given at bedtime may be tried but has been less successful. Gabapentin and clonazepam should be initiated at the lowest dose so daytime sedation does not occur. The dose can be slowly increased until REM behavior is reduced or absent or sedation occurs. In mild cases, many clients choose to confine the pet to a small crate at night to avoid injury to the pet or themselves or awakening of the household.

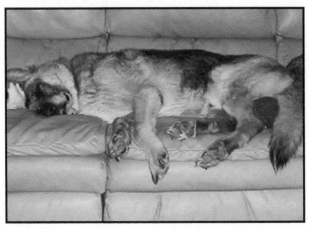

Figure 16-3 Although some twitching of distal limb muscles may be seen at times during REM sleep, violent movements often occur during REM behavior disorder.

NOTES

NOTES

NOTES